Atlas of
COMPLEX
ORTHODONTICS

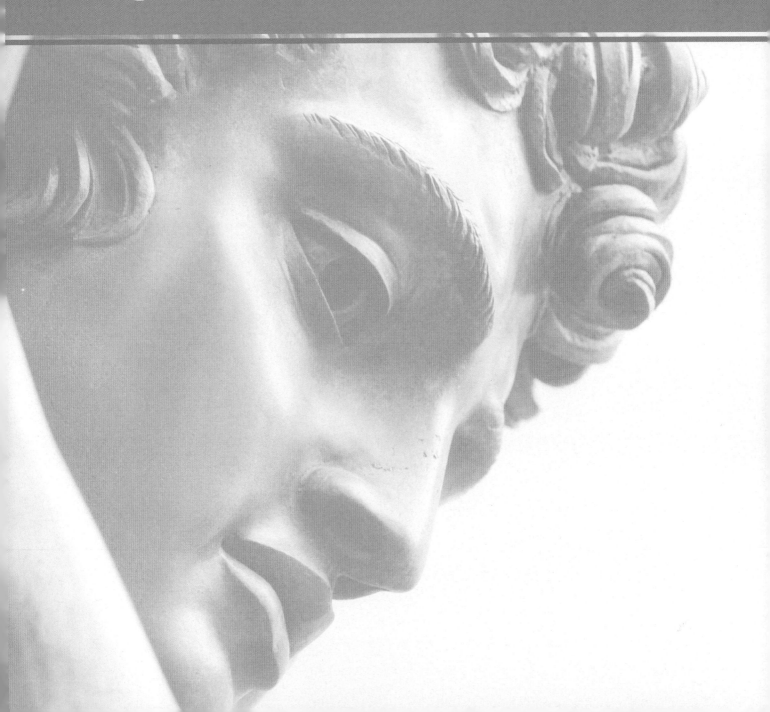

Atlas of
COMPLEX
ORTHODONTICS

Ravindra Nanda, BDS, MDS, PhD
Editor in Chief, Progress in Orthodontics
UConn Orthodontic Alumni Endowed Chair
Professor and Head
Department of Craniofacial Sciences
Chair, Division of Orthodontics
University of Connecticut School of Dental Medicine
Farmington, Connecticut

Flavio Andres Uribe, DDS, MDentSc
Charles Burstone Professor
Postgraduate Program Director
Division of Orthodontics
Department of Craniofacial Sciences
University of Connecticut School of Dental Medicine
Farmington, Connecticut

With significant contribution by
Sachin Agarwal, BDS, MDS, MDentSc (University of Connecticut, USA),
  Cert Orth (University of Connecticut, USA)
Senior Lecturer, Melbourne Dental School
University of Melbourne
Melbourne, Australia

ELSEVIER

ELSEVIER

3251 Riverport Lane
St. Louis, Missouri 63043

ATLAS OF COMPLEX ORTHODONTICS   ISBN: 978-0-323-08710-0

Library of Congress Cataloging-in-Publication Data
Names: Nanda, Ravindra, author. | Uribe, Flavio Andres, author. | Agarwal, Sachin, 1981- author.
Title: Atlas of complex orthodontics / Ravindra Nanda, Flavio Uribe ; with significant contribution by Sachin Agarwal.
Description: St. Louis, Missouri : Elsevier, [2017] | Includes index.
Identifiers: LCCN 2016002396 | ISBN 9780323087100 (hardcover : alk. paper)
Subjects: | MESH: Orthodontics, Corrective | Orthodontic Anchorage Procedures | Orthognathic Surgical Procedures | Malocclusion—surgery | Atlases | Case Reports
Classification: LCC RK521 | NLM WU 417 | DDC 617.6/43–dc23 LC record available at http://lccn.loc.gov/2016002396

Executive Content Strategist: Kathy Falk
Professional Content Development Manager: Jolynn Gower
Senior Content Development Specialist: Courtney Sprehe
Publishing Services Manager: Patricia Tannian
Senior Project Manager: Claire Kramer
Design Direction: Julia Dummitt

Printed in China

Last digit is the print number: 9   8   7   6   5   4   3   2   1

Working together
to grow libraries in
developing countries

www.elsevier.com • www.bookaid.org

To Catherine, for her love, support, and inspiration.
RN

I would like to dedicate this book to my wife, Patricia,
for her constant support and love since the day we met.
She has always been an inspiration and wonderful life partner.
FU

PREFACE

Contemporary orthodontics has evolved significantly in the last decade. New techniques and approaches are making their way into the practice of orthodontics, and this new technology has allowed the orthodontist to more effectively tackle complex cases. Despite this, the concepts of biomechanics remain the same and can be used in conjunction with some of these new tools, allowing for exciting and comprehensive treatment approaches that achieve predictable outcomes.

Today's orthodontists have to account for the biology of tooth movement and to understand the mechanics applied through a variety of devices; the use of surgery, with the application of virtual three-dimensional planning and surgery-first approach; the use of temporary anchorage devices; and the need for a full treatment plan that will satisfy the aesthetic and functional outcome for the patient.

Orthodontists are increasingly being confronted with more complicated cases. The case presentations that were once thought untreatable can now be addressed by the knowledgeable clinician; the science and research give the clinician many scenarios for a plausible outcome. Although clinicians can turn to the journal literature for such cases, what has really been needed in today's market is an atlas that presents a wide variety of advanced cases, along with the correct treatment planning. **The *Atlas of Complex Orthodontics* serves as a benchmark for both clinicians and residents who are looking to refine their skill set.**

KEY FEATURES

A **standardized presentation** for each case walks you through the pretreatment intraoral, extraoral, and smile analysis; the diagnosis and case summary (including the problem list and treatment plan); a brief discussion of the treatment options; the treatment sequence and biomechanical plan; and the final results.

More than 1500 clinical photographs, radiographs, and illustrations present each phase of treatment in stunning clarity, starting with the pretreatment workup, taking you through the treatment sequence, and ending with the final results of treatment.

Topics addressed include the following:

- The **management of patients with a deep bite**, which can have implications in the longevity of the dentition and can affect facial aesthetics. The management of this problem demands a careful diagnostic analysis, treatment plan, and selection of appropriate treatment therapy.
- The use of **temporary anchorage devices (TADs)**, which have been shown to be effective in correcting different types of malocclusion and also potentially reducing the time in orthodontic treatment. In addition, TADs allow the clinician to obtain the necessary anchorage, which increases the predictability of achieving the desired outcome in the treatment of complex malocclusions.
- **Surgery-First-Orthognathic-Approach (SFOA)**, a new paradigm in the combined orthodontic-orthognathic approach to jaw deformities. SFOA is an effective and time-saving procedure in the combined orthodontic-surgical approach to selected cases of mandibular prognathism. It achieves good facial aesthetics and occlusion without preoperative orthodontic treatment.
- A **multidisciplinary approach to treatment,** which draws appropriately from multiple disciplines to redefine problems outside of normal boundaries and reach solutions that are based on a new understanding of complex situations. The number of adult orthodontic patients continues to grow, and adult cases present unique challenges, such as missing teeth, root canals, and periodontal problems. Establishing a good multidisciplinary team is essential when dealing with these more complex cases.
- **Orthodontic finishing,** which is composed of individual perceptions and small detailing. Finishing distinguishes a true master of the profession from an average orthodontist. This step can be especially challenging because the minor changes performed are not generally as noticed by patients.

We would like to thank the following friends and residents who participated in the treatment of various patients depicted in this atlas: Sharifah Al Rushaid, Amir Assefnia, Avinash Bidra, Andrew Chapokas, Jing Chen, Aditya Chhibber, Jill Danaher, Amir Davoody, Mike Deluke, Thomas Dobie, Monica Dosanjh, Jonathan Feldman, Juan Fernando Restrepo, Pawandeep Gill, Michael Holbert, Nandakmar Janakiraman, Zachary Librizzi, Anna Manzotti, Rana Mehr, Christopher Olson, Ana Ortiz, Piero Palacios, Laura Posada, Greg Ross, Derek Sanders, David Shafer, Donald Sommerville, Junji Sugawara, Anthony Tang, Tom Taylor, Achint Utreja, Ashima Valiathan, Carlos Villegas, Neelesh Vinod Shah, and Allen Yaghoubzadeh.

CONTENTS

Atlas of
COMPLEX
ORTHODONTICS

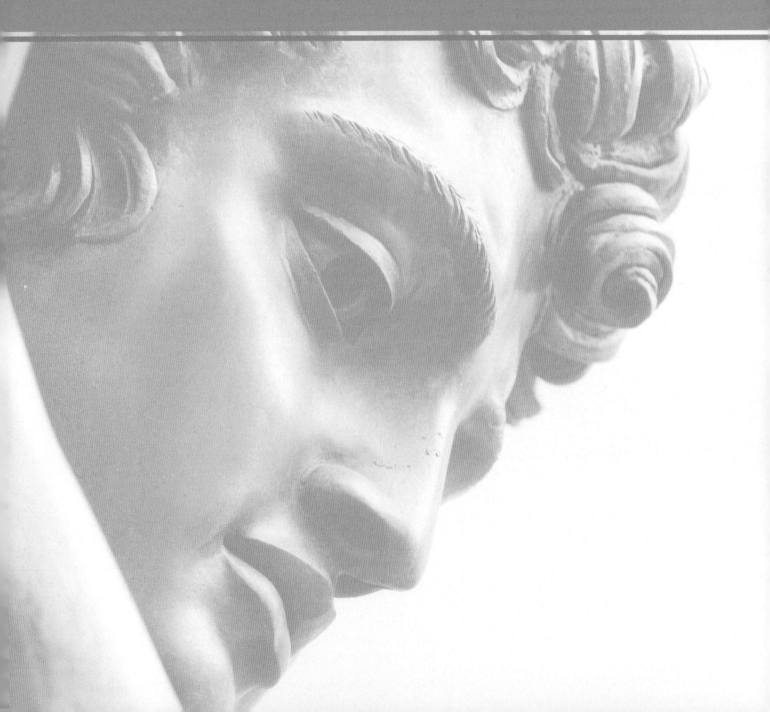

Section 1

Vertical Problems

CASE 1-1
Incisor Intrusion for the Excessive Gingival Display

A 13-year-old postpubertal female patient had a chief complaint of deep overbite and excess of gingival display on smiling. Medical and dental histories were noncontributory, and findings from a temporomandibular joint (TMJ) examination were normal with adequate range of jaw movements.

▪ PRETREATMENT

Extraoral Analysis (Fig. 1-1-1)

Facial Form	Mesoprosopic
Facial Symmetry	No gross asymmetries noticed
Chin Point	Coincidental with facial midline
Occlusal Plane	Normal
Facial Profile	Mild convexity due to a retrognathic mandible
Facial Height	Upper Facial Height/Lower Facial Height: Normal
	Lower Facial Height/Throat Depth: Normal
Lips	Competent, Upper: Normal; Lower: Protrusive
Nasolabial Angle	Normal
Mentolabial Sulcus	Normal

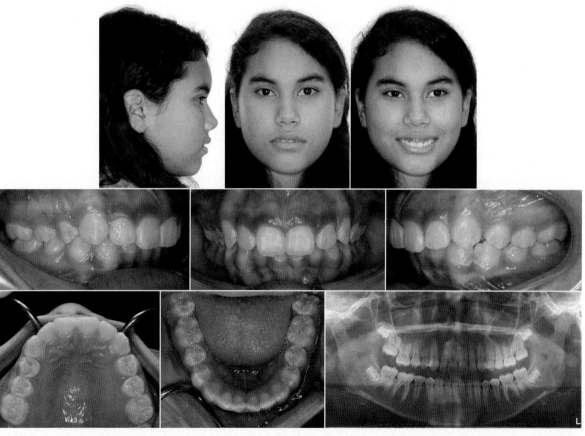

Figure 1-1-1   Pretreatment extraoral, intraoral photographs, and panoramic radiograph.

Smile Analysis (Fig. 1-1-2)

Smile Arc	Consonant, maxillary incisors impinging on lower lip
Incisor Display	Rest: 8 mm
	Smile: 4 mm of gingival display
Lateral Tooth Display	First premolar to first premolar
Buccal Corridor	Narrow
Gingival Tissue	Margins: Normal
	Papilla: Present
	Thin band of attached gingiva on labial aspect of the mandibular dentition
	Thin gingival biotype on labial aspect of the mandibular incisors
Dentition	Tooth size and proportion: Normal
	Tooth Shape: Normal
	Axial Inclination: Maxillary teeth inclined lingually
	Connector Space: Long connector between central incisors resulting in apically displaced papilla and small incisal embrasure
Incisal Embrasure	Slightly reduced between central incisors
Midlines	Upper dental midline coincidental with facial midline and lower dental midline 1 mm to the left

Intraoral Analysis (see Fig. 1-1-2)

Teeth Present	7654321/1234567
	7654321/1234567 (Unerupted 8s)
Molar Relation	Class I bilaterally
Canine Relation	Class I right, slight Class II left
Overjet	3 mm
Overbite	6 mm (100%)
Maxillary Arch	U shaped and symmetric
Mandibular Arch	U shaped with crowding of 1 mm and normal curve of Spee
Oral Hygiene	Fair

Functional Analysis

Swallowing	Normal adult pattern
Temporomandibular joint	Normal with adequate range of jaw movements

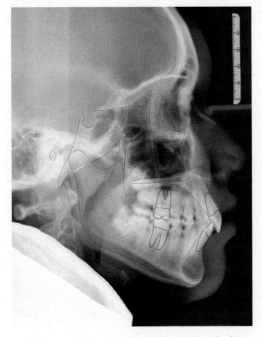

Parameter	Norm	Value
SNA (°)	82	82
SNB (°)	80	77
ANB (°)	2	5
FMA (°)	24	31
MP-SN (°)	32	40
U1-NA (mm/°)	4/22	4/11
L1-NA (mm/°)	4/25	7/31
IMPA (°)	95	95
U1-L1 (°)	130	131
OP-SN (°)	14	23
Upper Lip – E Plane (mm)	−4	−1.4
Lower Lip – E Plane (mm)	−2	3.6
Nasolabial Angle (°)	103	107
Soft Tissue Convexity (°)	135	130

Figure 1-1-2 Pretreatment lateral cephalogram with tracing and cephalometric analysis.

Diagnosis and Case Summary

A 13-year-old postpubertal female patient with convex soft tissue profile mainly due to a retrognathic mandible had a class I malocclusion, with increased gingival display on smiling and 100% deep bite due to supraerupted maxillary anterior teeth.

PROBLEM LIST			
Pathology/Others	Thin band of attached gingiva on labial aspect of the anterior mandibular dentition Thin biotype on labial of mandibular incisors		
Alignment	1 mm of crowding present in mandibular arch		
Dimension	**Skeletal**	**Dental**	**Soft Tissue**
Vertical	Increased FMA	OB: 6 mm Maxillary incisors supraerupted	Increased gingival display upon smiling and at rest. Gingival margins of maxillary central incisors slightly more incisal in relation to the lateral incisors
Anteroposterior	Convex profile due to slightly retrognathic mandible	Class II tendency of mandibular left canine	Protrusive lower lip
Transverse		Mandibular midline 1 mm to the left of facial	

FMA, Frankfurt-Mandibular plane angle; *OB*, overbite.

TREATMENT OBJECTIVES			
Pathology/Others	Monitor labial aspect of the mandibular incisors for gingival recession		
Alignment	Align mandibular arch to the relieve crowding.		
Dimension	**Skeletal**	**Dental**	**Soft Tissue**
Vertical		Intrude maxillary anterior teeth to correct overbite and reduce maxillary incisor display at rest and on smile	Reduce gingival display by intruding maxillary incisors. Refer for possible gingivectomy/crown lengthening
Anteroposterior		Correct Class II tendency on the left canines	Maintain
Transverse		Match lower midline to facial midline	

Treatment Options

The main objective in this patient is to reduce the overbite and gingival display due to the extruded maxillary incisors. Intrusion of the maxillary anterior teeth with a straight wire will result in intrusion of anterior teeth and extrusion of posterior teeth, which might result in an increased mandibular plane angle and limited intrusion of the anterior teeth, which is required for aesthetic objectives. Absolute intrusion with an intrusion arch results in a determinate force system leading to controlled intrusion of anterior teeth and minimum side effects on the posterior teeth.

TREATMENT SEQUENCE AND BIOMECHANICAL PLAN

Maxilla	Mandible
Band molars, bond maxillary arch, and segmental leveling with .016, .018, .016 × .022 inch NiTi arch wires.	
.017 × .025 inch CNA intrusion arch delivering 50 g of intrusive force to the anterior teeth.	
Continue intrusion of incisors.	Band molars, bond mandibular arch, and level with .016, .018, .016 × .022 inch NiTi arch wires.
Level with .017 × .025 inch NiTi.	Continue leveling with .017 × .025 inch NiTi arch wire.
Continue leveling with .019 × .025 inch NiTi.	Continue leveling with .019 × .025 inch NiTi arch wire.
.016 × .025 inch CNA wire with finishing bends.	.016 × .025 inch CNA arch wire with finishing bends.
Debond and deliver wrap around retainer.	Debond and fixed retainer.
6 months' recall appointment for retention check.	6 months' recall appointment for retention check.

CNA, Connecticut new archwire; NiTi, nickel-titanium.

■ TREATMENT SEQUENCE

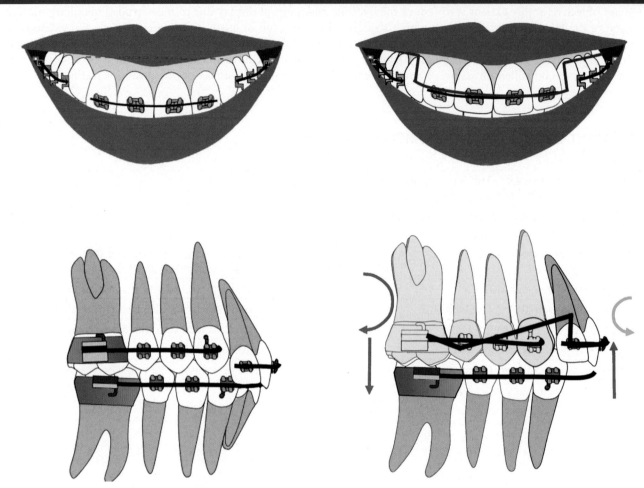

Figure 1-1-3 Intrusion arch results in clockwise rotation and extrusive force on the posterior segment and intrusive force that generates a counterclockwise moment resulting from this anterior segment. Intrusion of anterior teeth results in improvement of maxillary gingival display.

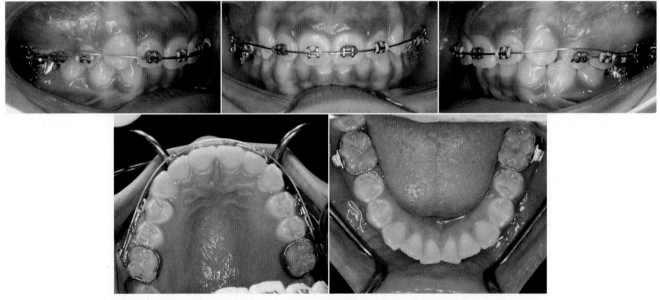

Figure 1-1-4 Intrusion arch tied to maxillary anterior teeth for absolute intrusion of the maxillary incisors. Note the stiff wire segments from maxillary molars to first premolars to counteract the side effects of the intrusion on the posterior dentition.

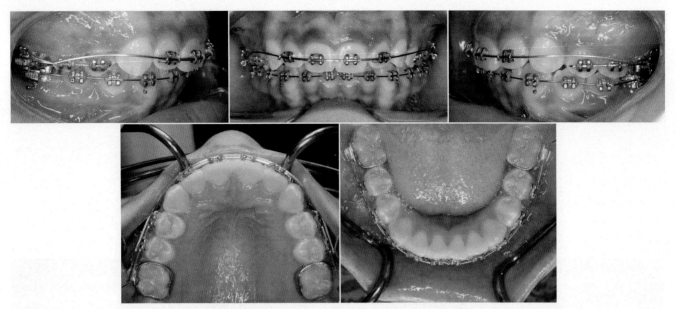

Figure 1-1-5 Connecticut new archwire (CNA) intrusion arch placed into the bracket slot. Intrusion arch exerts an intrusive force labial to the center of resistance.

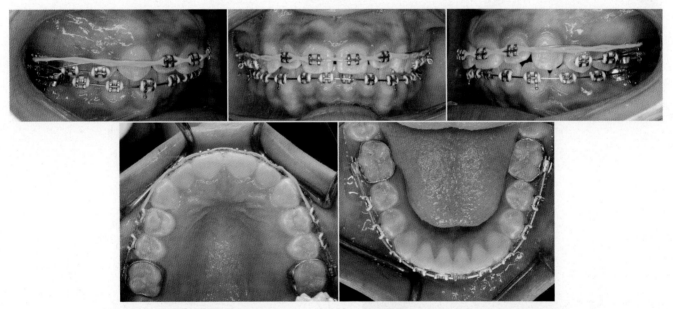

Figure 1-1-6 Intrusion of maxillary anterior teeth and leveling of mandibular arch. Note the correction of the overbite and leveling of the maxillary arch. Elastic chain exerts a distal force and prevents spaces from opening up. The result is an intrusive force passing along the incisors' center of resistance.

FINAL RESULTS

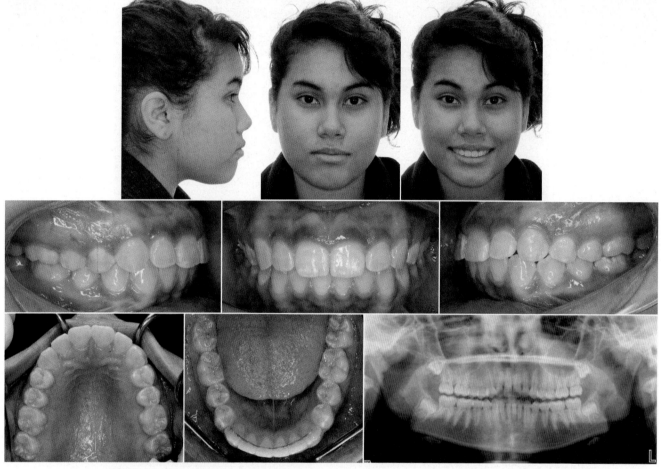

Figure 1-1-7   Posttreatment, extraoral and intraoral photographs and panoramic radiograph.

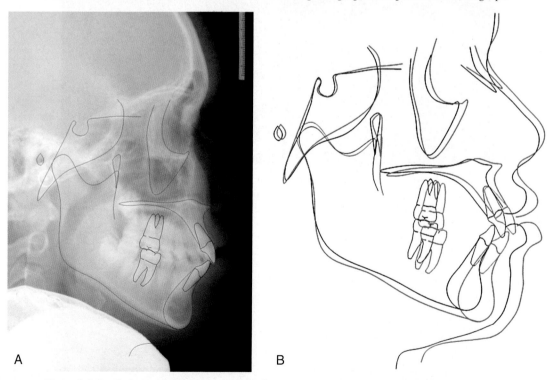

A   B

Figure 1-1-8   **A,** Posttreatment lateral cephalogram. **B,** Superimposition. *Black,* pretreatment; *red,* posttreatment.

How much intrusion is expected with an intrusion arch?
The amount of intrusion of the incisors in response to an intrusion arch depends on the location along the tooth where the vertical displacement is measured. Typically, around 2 mm of intrusion is expected with these mechanics when measured on the center of resistance. This could result in 4 mm of overbite correction if the incisal edge is also displaced labially with the intrusion. The change in the incisal edge would be similar to the change observed in the gingival margin. For the treatment of excessive gingival display, incisor intrusion with an intrusion arch can be combined with gingivectomy to maximize the correction if needed.

Intrusion Arch for Leveling the Mandibular Curve of Spee

A 12-year-old prepubertal male patient was referred by his general dentist regarding correction of his anterior deep bite. Medical and dental histories were noncontributory, and the findings of a temporomandibular joint (TMJ) examination were normal with adequate range of jaw movements.

▪ PRETREATMENT

Extraoral Analysis (Fig. 1-2-1)

Facial Form	Mesoprosopic
Facial Symmetry	No gross asymmetries noticed
Chin Point	Coincidental with facial midline
Occlusal Plane	Normal
Facial Profile	Convex due to retrognathic mandible
Facial Height	Upper Facial Height/Lower Facial Height: Normal
	Lower Facial Height/Throat Depth: Normal
Lips	Competent, Upper: Protrusive; Lower: Normal
Nasolabial Angle	Obtuse
Mentolabial Sulcus	Normal

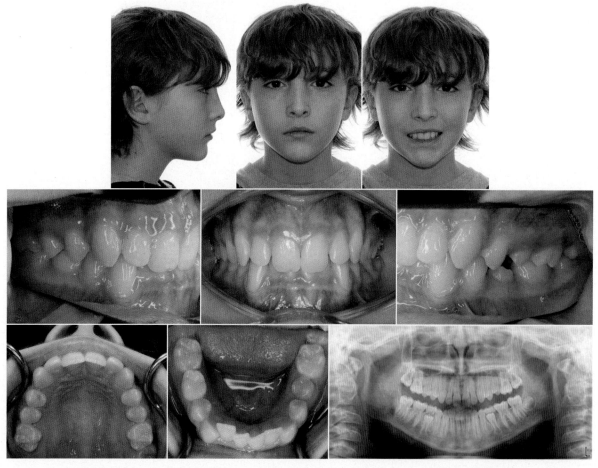

Figure 1-2-1　Pretreatment extraoral/intraoral photographs and panoramic radiograph.

Smile Analysis (Fig. 1-2-2)

Smile Arc	Consonant
Incisor Display	Rest: 3 mm
	Smile: 10 mm
Lateral Tooth Display	First premolar to first premolar
Buccal Corridor	Narrow
Gingival Tissue	Margins: Maxillary central incisors gingival margins are more incisal than adjacent teeth (discrepancy is also observed at the incisal level)
Papilla	Present
Dentition	Tooth size and proportion: Normal
Tooth Shape	Normal
Axial Inclination	Maxillary teeth inclined lingually
Connector Space and Contact Area	Normal
Incisal Embrasure	Normal
Midlines	Upper is coincidental, and lower midline is shifted to the right by 1 mm as compared with the facial midline

Intraoral Analysis (see Fig. 1-2-2)

Teeth Present	7654321/1234567 (Mandibular 8s developing, maxillary 8s missing)
	7654321/1234567
Molar Relation	Class I bilaterally
Canine Relation	Class I bilaterally
Overjet	3 mm
Overbite	8 mm
Maxillary Arch	U shaped symmetric with nor crowding or spacing
Mandibular Arch	U shaped with crowding and deep curve of Spee
Oral Hygiene	Fair

Functional Analysis

Swallowing	Normal adult pattern
Temporomandibular joint	Normal with normal range of jaw movements

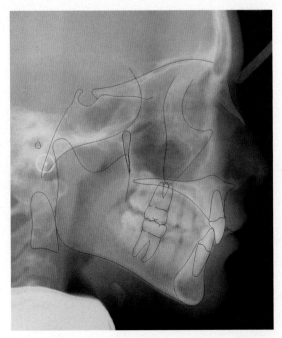

Parameter	Norm	Value
SNA (°)	82	84
SNB (°)	80	77
ANB (°)	2	5
FMA (°)	24	27
MP-SN (°)	32	32
U1-NA (mm/°)	4/22	−3/1.6
L1-NA (mm/°)	4/25	1/23
IMPA (°)	95	91
U1-L1 (°)	130	151
OP-SN (°)	14	20
Upper Lip – E Plane (mm)	−4	−2
Lower Lip – E Plane (mm)	−2	−1
Nasolabial Angle (°)	103	116

Figure 1-2-2   Pretreatment lateral cephalogram with tracing and cephalometric analysis.

Diagnosis and Case Summary

A 12-year-old prepubertal male patient presented with a convex skeletal and soft tissue profile mainly due to a retrognathic mandible and a dental Class I malocclusion. Maxillary incisors are retroclined and lingually placed. Mandibular arch is crowded, with a deep curve of Spee leading to an anterior deep bite. The interincisal angle is increased, the upper lip is retrusive, and the nasolabial angle is increased.

PROBLEM LIST			
Pathology/Others	Missing maxillary third molars		
Alignment	5 mm of crowding in mandibular arch		
Dimension	**Skeletal**	**Dental**	**Soft Tissue**
Anteroposterior	Skeletal Class II denture base	Retroclined maxillary incisors	Obtuse nasolabial angle Retrusive upper lip
Vertical		Overbite of 8 mm Deep curve of Spee	
Transverse		Mandibular midline shifted to right side by 1 mm	

TREATMENT OBJECTIVES			
Pathology/Others			
Alignment	Correct mandibular crowding by flaring the mandibular incisors.		
Dimension	**Skeletal**	**Dental**	**Soft Tissue**
Anteroposterior		Flare incisal edge by 1-2 mm and correct inclination of roots	
Vertical		Decrease overbite by leveling the curve of Spee	
Transverse		Improve mandibular midline to match facial midline	

Treatment Options

Correction of anterior deep bite could be carried out by either intruding the anterior teeth or extruding the posterior teeth.

In the present case, mandibular plane is normally inclined, so best strategy to correct the anterior deep bite is to intrude the anterior teeth. At smile, as well as at rest, there is no excessive exposure of maxillary incisors and there is deep mandibular curve of Spee, which means the reason of anterior deep bite is excessive curve of Spee.

Curve of Spee can be leveled either by intrusion of anterior teeth with help of an intrusion arch or by extrusion of posterior teeth with help of continuous arch wire having reverse curve of Spee swept in it. It was opted on this patient to level the mandibular curve of Spee by means of an intrusion arch.

TREATMENT SEQUENCE AND BIOMECHANICAL PLAN

Maxilla	Mandible
Band molars, bond maxillary arch, and start leveling with .016, .018, .016 × .022 inch NiTi arch wires.	Band molars, bond mandibular arch and segmental leveling with .016, .018, .016 × .022 inch NiTi arch wires.
Level with .017 × .025 inch NiTi arch wire.	Keep the segmental lateral incisor to lateral incisor wire, place .017 × .025 inch NiTi intrusion archwire, and apply 50 g of intrusive force to the anterior teeth.
Continue with .017 × .025 inch NiTi arch wire.	Continue intrusion of incisors.
Leveling with .019 × .025 inch NiTi arch wire.	Continue leveling with .019 × .025 inch NiTi arch wire.
.016 × .025 inch CNA with finishing bends.	.016 × .025 inch CNA with finishing bends.
Debond and wrap around retainer.	Debond and fixed retainer.
Six-month recall appointment for retention check.	Six-month recall appointment for retention check.

CNA, Connecticut new arch wire; NiTi, nickel titanium.

■ TREATMENT SEQUENCE

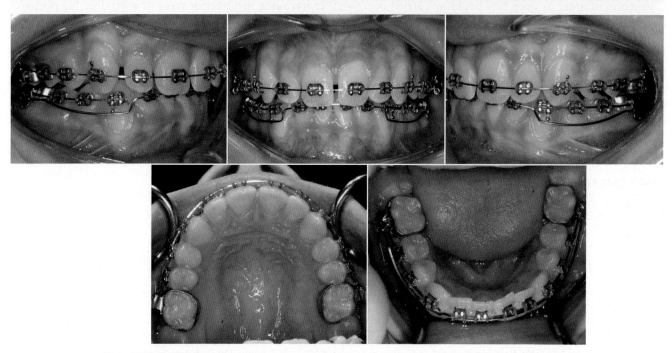

Figure 1-2-3 Intrusion arch wire in mandibular arch applying 50 g of intrusive force on mandibular anterior teeth.

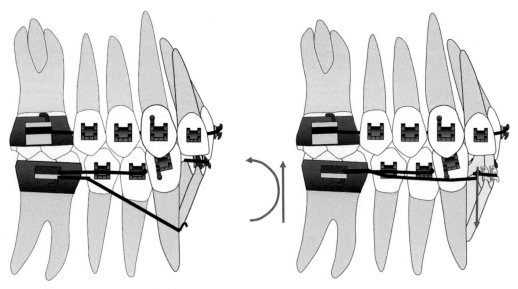

Figure 1-2-4 After significant intrusion of mandibular anterior teeth and bite opening, continuous wire is placed in mandibular arch for final alignment.

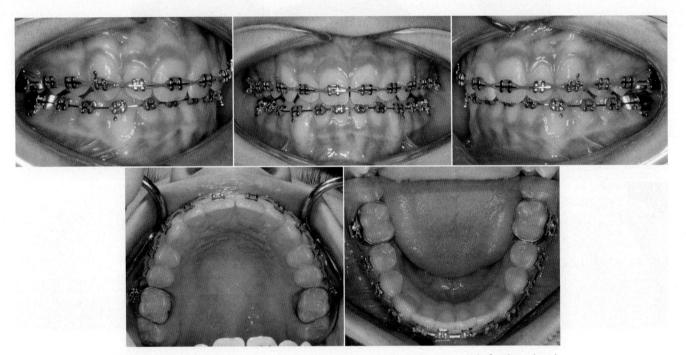

Figure 1-2-5   Continuous 16 × 22 inch Connecticut new arch wires with finishing bends at the final stages of treatment.

■ FINAL RESULTS

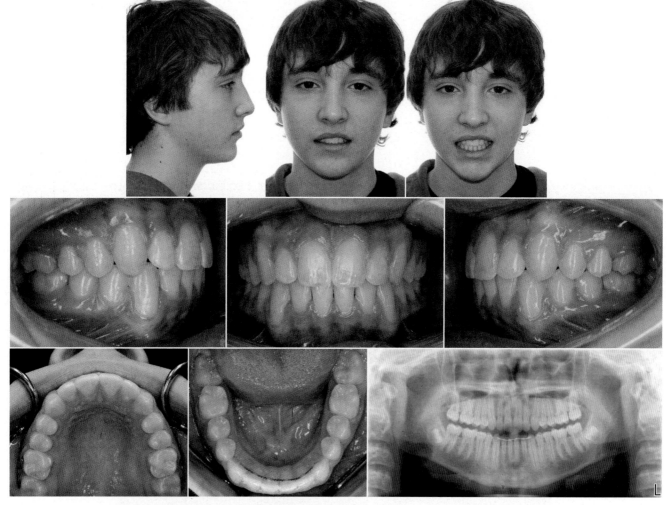

Figure 1-2-6   Posttreatment extraoral/intraoral photographs and panoramic radiograph.

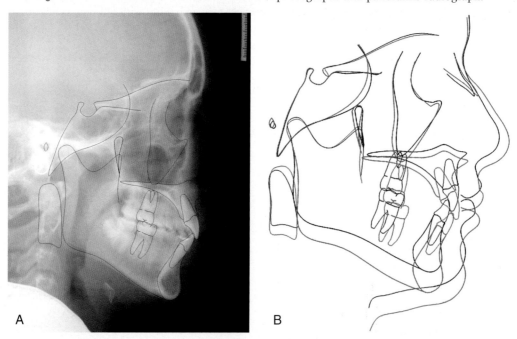

A   B

Figure 1-2-7   **A,** Posttreatment lateral cephalogram; **B,** Superimposition. *Black,* pretreatment; *red,* posttreatment.

What is the advantage of leveling the curve of Spee with an intrusion arch as compared with the continuous straight wire?

The curve of Spee can be leveled either by an intrusion arch, which results in pure intrusion of the anterior teeth, or with the help of a continuous arch wire with an incorporated reverse curve of Spee, which results in relative intrusion of the anterior teeth (some amount of posterior extrusion). The choice depends on the treatment objectives related to the correction of the deep bite. If pure intrusion of the anterior teeth is desired, an intrusion arch has shown to be the most effective appliance for this objective. Reverse curve of Spee arch wires, on the other hand, are effective in leveling of the arch but through extrusion of the posterior teeth. Therefore, although reduction of the overbite is reduced with both appliances, the mechanism of action varies and therefore the specific objectives drive the specific use.

In this patient, maximum intrusion of the lower incisors was desired due to the magnitude of overbite and the specific objective of minimal intrusion of the maxillary incisors. Thus the majority of the overbite correction is required from intrusion of the mandibular incisors.

Increase of the Vertical Dimension with Implants and Midline Correction with a Miniplate in a Patient with Multiple Missing Teeth*

A 39-year-old male patient with multiple missing teeth was referred for an interdisciplinary approach by the prosthodontist. The patient's chief complaint was to replace the missing teeth and achieve an aesthetic smile. Medical and dental histories were noncontributory, and findings from the temporomandibular (TMJ) examination were normal with adequate range of jaw movements.

■ PRETREATMENT

Extraoral Analysis (Fig. 1-3-1)

Facial Form	Leptoprosopic
Facial Symmetry	No gross asymmetries noticed
Chin Point	Coincidental with facial midline
Occlusal Plane	Normal
Facial Profile	Convex due to retrognathic mandible
Facial Height	Upper Facial Height/Lower Facial Height: Normal
	Lower Facial Height/Throat Depth: Normal
Lips	Competent, Upper: Normal; Lower: Retrusive
Nasolabial Angle	Obtuse
Mentolabial Sulcus	Normal

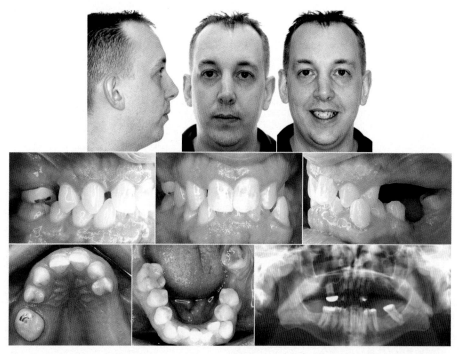

Figure 1-3-1 Pretreatment extraoral/intraoral photographs and panoramic radiograph.

*Portions of Case 1-3 from Uribe F, Janakiraman N, Nanda R. Interdisciplinary approach for increasing the vertical dimension of occlusion in an adult patient with several missing teeth. *Am J Orthod Dentofacial Orthop*. 2013;143:867-876.

Smile Analysis (Fig. 1-3-2)

Smile Arc	Flat
Incisor Display	Rest: 0 mm
	Smile: 9 mm
Lateral Tooth Display	First premolar to first premolar
Buccal Corridor	Large; accentuated by missing teeth in maxillary left quadrant
Gingival Tissue	Gingival Margins: Canine margins are low (more incisal)
	Slight discrepancy in gingival heights between maxillary central incisors
Dentition	Tooth size and proportion: maxillary canines are small mesiodistally
Tooth Shape	Normal, except for maxillary canines that are conical
Axial Inclination	Mandibular incisors are inclined lingually
Connector Space and Contact Area	No contact between maxillary central incisor and canines
Incisal Embrasure	Normal
Midlines	Upper shifted to the right by 1 mm and lower dental midline shifted to the left side by 4 mm with respect to the facial midline

Intraoral Analysis (see Fig. 1-3-2)

Teeth Present	6431/134
	654321/123457
Molar Relation	Class II right side; left side N/A
Canine Relation	Class II left side; Class I on right side
Overjet	2 mm
Overbite	5 mm
Maxillary Arch	U shaped with spacing
Mandibular Arch	U shaped with crowding
Oral Hygiene	Fair
Other	Brown discolorations on facial middle third of central incisors
	Broken porcelain of full coverage crown of right maxillary first molar
	Adequate buccolingual width of edentulous ridges with slightly reduced height

Functional Analysis

Swallowing	Normal
Temporomandibular joint	With adequate range of jaw movements

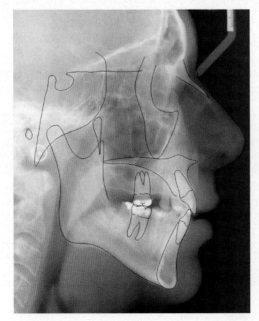

Parameter	Norm	Value
SNA (°)	82	82
SNB (°)	80	78
ANB (°)	2	4
FMA (°)	24	31
MP-SN (°)	32	35
U1-NA (mm/°)	4/22	3/21
L1-NA (mm/°)	4/25	6/18
IMPA (°)	95	84
U1-L1 (°)	130	136
OP-SN (°)	14	16
Upper Lip – E Plane (mm)	−4	−4.2
Lower Lip – E Plane (mm)	−2	−.8
Nasolabial Angle (°)	103	113
Soft Tissue Convexity (°)	135	126

Figure 1-3-2 Pretreatment lateral cephalogram with tracing and cephalometric analysis.

Diagnosis and Case Summary

A 39-year-old adult male patient had a convex skeletal and soft tissue profile due to retrusive mandible. Intraorally, there are multiple teeth missing, a Class II molar on the right side, a Class I canine on the right side, a Class II on the left side, and spacing due to missing maxillary lateral incisors in the maxillary arch and crowding in the mandibular arch. The maxillary midline is shifted to the right side by 1 mm, and the mandibular midline is shifted to the left side by 4 mm. A retrusive lower lip and an obtuse nasolabial angle are evident. A deep overbite is also present.

PROBLEM LIST			
Pathology/Other	Missing maxillary right second and third molar, second premolar and lateral incisor		
	Missing maxillary left lateral incisor an all teeth distal to the left first premolar		
	Missing mandibular left first molar, right second molar, and both third molars		
	Fractured occlusal porcelain of maxillary right first molar crown		
	Large restorations present with respect to mandibular right first molar and left second molar		
	Brown discoloration on middle facial third of central incisors		
	Overerupted mandibular left second molar		
Alignment	Maxillary spacing		
	Moderate lower crowding		
Vertical	Slight convexity due to retrognathic mandible	No interocclusal space between maxillary posterior edentulous ridge and mandibular left second molar	Asymmetric smile of the upper lip (left side lower)
		Deep overbite	
Anteroposterior		Class II canine relation on the left side	Obtuse nasolabial angle
		Class II molar relation on the right side	
Transverse		Mandibular left canine is in crossbite	
		Mandibular midline shifted to the left by 4 mm as compared with the facial midline	
		Cross bite tendency on right first molars	
		Maxillary midline 1 mm to the right of facial	

TREATMENT OBJECTIVES			
Pathology/ Other	Perform canine substitution for missing maxillary lateral incisors		
	Restore missing right maxillary second premolar, left second premolar, and first molar and mandibular left first molar with implants		
	Extract mandibular left second molar		
	Replace maxillary right first molar crown		
	Extract mandibular left second molar		
Alignment	Close maxillary spaces due to missing lateral incisors by protracting maxillary canines mesially		
	Distalize the right mandibular segment by 4 mm to alleviate crowding		
Dimension	**Skeletal**	**Dental**	**Soft Tissue**
Vertical		Provisional crowns on the right maxillary first molar, left maxillary first premolar and first molar endosseous dental implants to support an increase in the vertical dimension of occlusion by 2 mm.	
		Correct deep bite by increasing vertical dimension of occlusion by 2 mm	
Anteroposterior		Distalization of the maxillary right first molar by 3 mm to maintain the Class II molar relation and 3-mm protraction of maxillary right first premolar, canine into Class II canine relation	
		Open up space for maxillary right second premolar implant	
		Distalize mandibular right buccal segment by 4 mm to relieve anterior crowding	
Transverse		Bring mandibular left canine into the arch and correct the crossbite	
		Distalize the right mandibular segment to shift the midline to right side	

Treatment Options

One option could be opening of the space for the missing lateral incisors for implant-supported crowns instead of canine substitution. This approach, though, would necessitate use of the skeletal anchorage units in both quadrants of the maxillary arch to retract the canines with maximum anchorage.

Extraction of a mandibular incisor could have been another option, but it would still require 2 mm of distalization of the mandibular right buccal segment to achieve an adequate alignment. With this option, it is likely that a remnant overjet would be present at the end of treatment.

The third option was to mesialize the maxillary canines and substitute these in place of the missing laterals. Distalization of the right buccal segment in the mandibular arch was to be accomplished with skeletal anchorage placed in the external oblique ridge. On the left side of the mandible, the second molar was to be extracted because of its significant supraeruption, and a prosthetic implant placed in the first molar site. A prosthetic implant-supported bridge on the left posterior maxillary quadrant in conjunction with a porcelain fused to metal crown on the right would help in opening the vertical dimension of occlusion.

Finally, left mandibular second molar intrusion and protraction into the first molar extraction space was an option. Intrusion of the molar by 4 mm and 6 mm of protraction into long-standing edentulous space would be difficult and time consuming; thus extraction of the second molar with a prosthodontic implant for the missing first molar was considered.

The multidisciplinary team, together with the patient, decided to pursue the third option.

TREATMENT SEQUENCE AND BIOMECHANICAL PLAN

Maxilla	Mandible
Temporary crown on right first molar to open the bite.	
Place implants for maxillary left second premolar and first molar to obtain a bilateral occlusion at new vertical dimension of occlusion. Place abutments and temporary bridge over endosseous implants.	Bond mandibular arch, bypass left canine and align with .016, .018, .016, × .022 inch Niti arch wires.
Bond maxillary arch and align with .016, .018, .016, × .022 inch Niti arch wires.	Place .017 × .022 inch SS arch wire and a TAD 5-mm distal to right first molar and start distalization of the right segment.
Place .017 × .022 inch SS arch wire and push coil between right first molar and first premolar to open space for right second premolar implant.	Align left lateral incisor and canine and shift midline to right side by 4 mm.
Place implant for maxillary right second premolar.	Extract left second molar and place implant for mandibular left first molar.
Debond and wrap around retainer.	Debond and bonded 3-3 lingual retainer.
Restoration with crowns over the implants and veneers from canine to canine (lateral incisor shape). Place permanent crown on right first molar.	Restoration of left first molar with a crown.
6-month recall appointment for retention check.	6-month recall appointment for retention check.

■ TREATMENT SEQUENCE

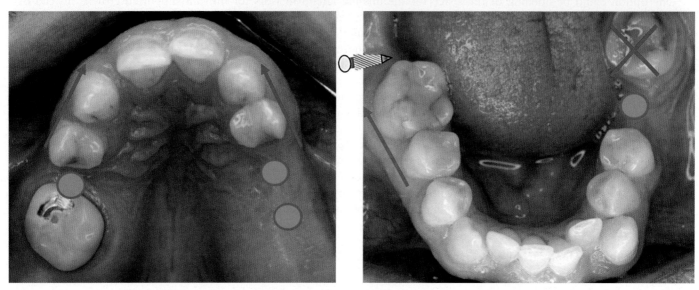

Figure 1-3-3   Proposed orthodontic movements. In the maxillary arch, mesialize maxillary canines and substitute in place of missing laterals and replacement of missing teeth with prosthetic implants. In the mandibular arch distalization of the right side with the help of skeletal anchorage, replacing left first molar with prosthetic implant and extraction of left second molar.

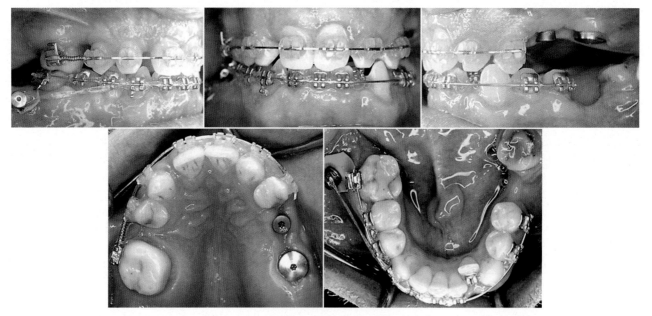

Figure 1-3-4   Push-coil between maxillary right first molar and first premolar to open up space for a right maxillary second premolar implant. In the mandibular arch, distalization of right segment occurs with the help of skeletal anchorage (miniplate).

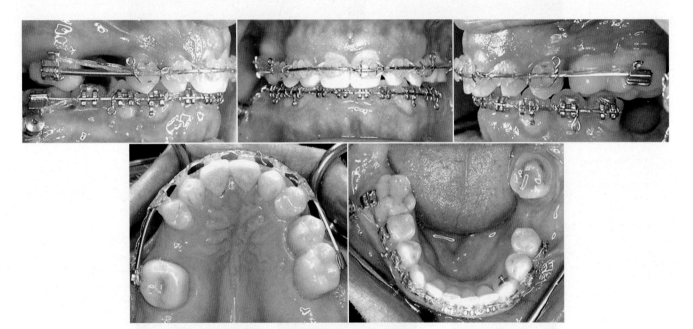

Figure 1-3-5 Maxillary canine substitution in place of the missing lateral incisors. Completed alignment of the mandibular teeth with significant improvement of the mandibular midline.

FINAL RESULTS

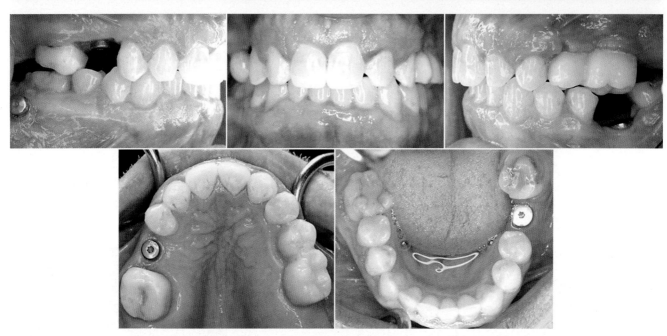

Figure 1-3-6   Posttreatment intraoral photographs.

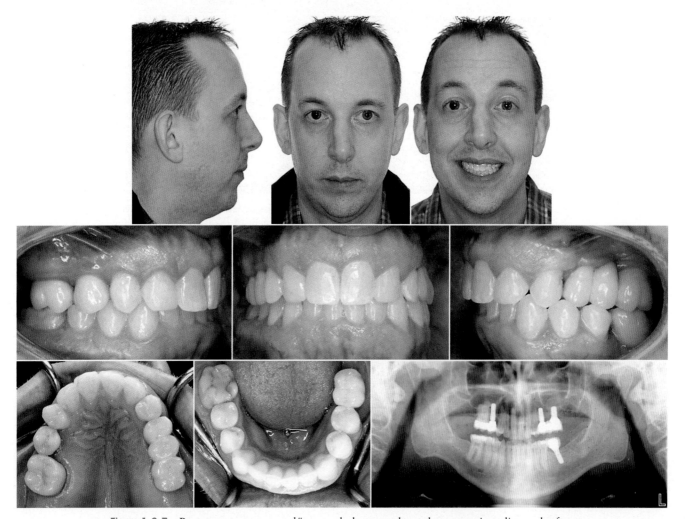

Figure 1-3-7   Posttreatment extraoral/intraoral photographs and panoramic radiograph after placement of all restorations.

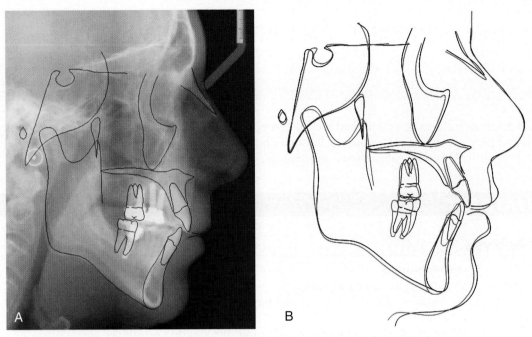

Figure 1-3-8   **A,** Posttreatment lateral cephalogram; **B,** Superimposition. *Black,* retreatment; *red,* posttreatment.

Why was the vertical dimension of occlusion increased in this patient?
The patient had a deep overbite and significant loss of teeth in the posterior buccal segments. For the overbite to be reduced, it was necessary to increase the vertical dimension of occlusion because there was no anchorage to intrude the anterior teeth in the mandible. This was accomplished by placing maxillary endosseous implants on the left side early in treatment to support the occlusion together with a new crown on the maxillary right first molar.

Deep Bite Correction with Anterior Bite Stops

A 14-year-old postpubertal female patient had a chief complaint of irregular teeth in the anterior region of her upper jaw. Medical and dental histories were noncontributory, and findings from a temporomandibular joint (TMJ) examination were normal, with normal range of jaw movements.

■ PRETREATMENT

Extraoral Analysis (Fig. 1-4-1)

Facial Form	Mesoprosopic
Facial Symmetry	No gross asymmetries noticed
Chin Point	Coincidental with the facial midline
Occlusal Plane	Normal
Facial Profile	Convex due to prognathic maxilla and retrognathic mandible
Facial Height	Upper Facial Height/Lower Facial Height: Short lower facial height
	Lower Facial Height/Throat Depth: Short lower facial height
Lips	Competent, Upper: Normal; Lower: Normal
Nasolabial Angle	Obtuse
Mentolabial Sulcus	Normal

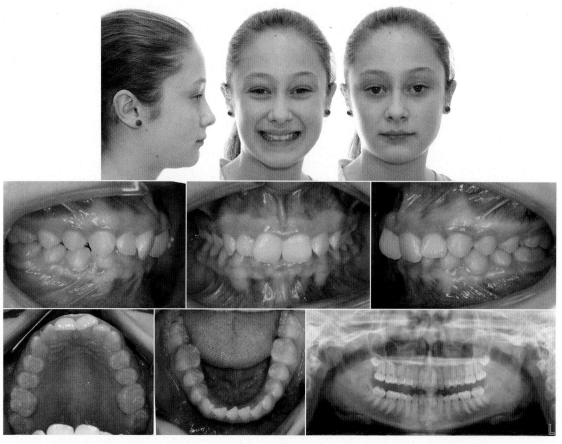

Figure 1-4-1   Pretreatment extraoral/intraoral photographs and panoramic radiograph.

Smile Analysis (Fig. 1-4-2)

Smile Arc	Consonant
Incisor Display	Rest: 4 mm
	Smile: 9 mm
Lateral Tooth Display	First premolar to first premolar
Buccal Corridor	Wide
Gingival Tissue	Gingival Margins: Canine margins are at same level as lateral incisors
Papilla	Present but at a low (gingival) level between central incisors
Dentition	Tooth size and proportion: slightly short length of maxillary incisors
Tooth Shape	Normal
Axial Inclination	Maxillary and mandibular incisors are inclined lingually
Connector Space and Contact Area	Contact area between central incisors displaced gingivally due to low contact as result of converging roots and diverging crowns
Incisal Embrasure	Open (between maxillary central incisors) due to diverging crowns
Midlines	Maxillary and mandibular midlines are coincidental with the facial midline

Intraoral Analysis (see Fig. 1-4-2)

Teeth Present	7654321/1234567 (Developing maxillary third molars and late development of mandibular right third molar, crypt observed. No evidence of mandibular left third molar.)
	7654321/1234567
Molar Relation	Class I on left side and Class II End on right side
Canine Relation	Class I on left side and Class II End on right side
Overjet	2 mm
Overbite	6 mm
Maxillary Arch	Shaped symmetric with crowding of 4 mm
Mandibular Arch	U shaped with crowding of 6 mm and deep curve of Spee
Oral Hygiene	Fair

Functional Analysis

Swallowing	Normal adult pattern
Temporomandibular joint	Normal with normal range of jaw movements

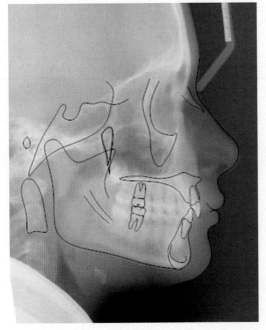

Parameter	Norm	Value
SNA (°)	82	83
SNB (°)	80	78
ANB (°)	2	5
FMA (°)	24	16
MP-SN (°)	32	28
U1-NA (mm/°)	4/22	−1/5
L1-NA (mm/°)	4/25	−2/16
IMPA (°)	95	90
U1-L1 (°)	130	154
OP-SN (°)	14	18
Upper Lip – E Plane (mm)	−4	−1
Lower Lip – E Plane (mm)	−2	−1
Nasolabial Angle (°)	103	113
Soft Tissue Convexity (°)	135	130

Figure 1-4-2 Pretreatment lateral cephalogram with tracing and cephalometric analysis.

Diagnosis and Case Summary

This 14-year-old postpubertal female patient has a convex soft tissue profile mainly due to a slightly prognathic maxilla and a retrognathic mandible. A dental Class II division I subdivision right malocclusion with reduced mandibular plane angle indicating a hypodivergent growth pattern. Crowding of 4 mm is present in the maxillary arch, and crowding of 6 mm is present in the mandibular arch. A 100% deep bite due to supraerupted and retroclined maxillary incisors and deep curve of Spee is evident.

PROBLEM LIST			
Pathology/Other	Delayed formation of mandibular third molars		
Alignment	4 mm of crowding in maxillary arch and 6 mm of crowding in mandibular arch		
Dimension	**Skeletal**	**Dental**	**Soft Tissue**
Vertical	Hypodivergent growth pattern	100% overbite Deep curve of Spee Supererupted incisors	Low papilla between central incisors Reduced length of maxillary incisors
Anteroposterior	Skeletal Class II due to prognathic maxilla	Class II end on relationship on right side Obtuse interincisal angle	Obtuse nasolabial angle
Transverse			

TREATMENT OBJECTIVES			
Pathology/Other	Monitor formation of mandibular third molars		
Alignment	Flare maxillary and mandibular anterior teeth to align maxillary and mandibular arch to relieve crowding		
Dimension	**Skeletal**	**Dental**	**Soft Tissue**
Vertical	Increase mandibular plane angle and lower facial height	Decrease overbite by extruding posterior teeth Level curve of Spee by extruding posterior teeth	Monitor papillary height changes between central incisors Monitor gingival levels on maxillary incisors
Anteroposterior		Mesialize mandibular right buccal segment into Class I molar and canine relation Improve interincisal angle by flaring maxillary and mandibular incisors	Improve nasolabial angle
Transverse			

Treatment Options

Correction of the deep overbite can be performed by either intrusion of the incisors or extrusion of the posterior teeth. Because the patient is hypodivergent, correction of the deep bite by the extrusion of posterior teeth will not only correct the deep bite but also improve the mandibular inclination. For extrusion of the posterior teeth, it is necessary to disocclude the dentition, which could be accomplished by placing bonded anterior occlusal stop on the maxillary anterior teeth. After disocclusion of posterior teeth, vertical settling elastics can erupt posterior teeth into the interocclusal space.

A second option for extrusion of the posterior teeth is to use an intrusion arch. The intrusion arch exerts intrusion force on the anterior segment and extrusion force on the posterior segment of the arch. However, anterior intrusion is predominant with this approach.

In this patient a combination of both options described was selected. Anterior bite stops bonded to the lingual surface of the maxillary incisors allow for eruption of the posterior teeth. The intrusion arch would help with the extrusion of the maxillary molars and tip back of the first molars, especially in the right Class II subdivision side. A heavy base arch wire premolar to premolar would counteract any intrusion tendency in the maxillary anterior teeth.

TREATMENT SEQUENCE AND BIOMECHANICAL PLAN

Maxilla	Mandible
Band molars, bond maxillary arch, level the arch with .016, .016 × .022, .019 × .025 inch NiTi arch wires. Bond anterior bite stops on lingual of central incisors to disocclude posterior teeth by 3 mm and favor extrusion of posterior teeth.	Band molars, bond maxillary arch, level the arch with .016, .016 × .022, .019 × .025 inch NiTi arch wires.
Place .017 × .025 inch SS base arch wire from first premolar to first premolar, place .016 × .022 inch NiTi intrusion arch wire into the auxilliary slot of first molars, tie it onto the anterior teeth, and reinforce tip back with Class II elastics.	Continue leveling with .019 × .025 inch CNA arch wire, Class II elastics for the correction of the buccal segment, and extrusion of mandibular posterior teeth.
Settle the occlusion and debond, wrap around retainer.	Debond and fixed retainer.
6-month recall appointment for retention check.	6-month recall appointment for retention check.

CNA, Connecticut new arch wire; *NiTi,* nickel titanium; *SS,* stainless steel.

■ TREATMENT SEQUENCE

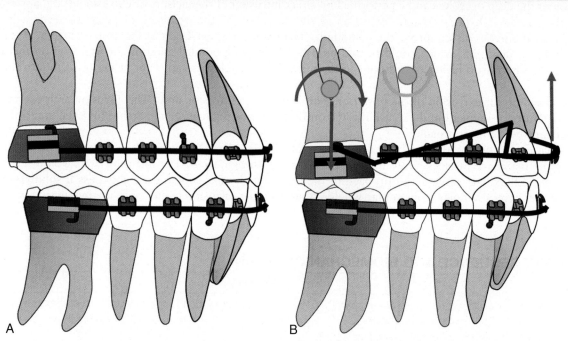

Figure 1-4-3 **A,** Posterior teeth are disoccluded by placing an anterior bite stop on the lingual surface of maxillary anterior teeth. **B,** Intrusion arch from the maxillary first molars results in extrusive force and clockwise moment the maxillary molars and intrusive force and counterclockwise moment due to force on the anterior second premolar to second premolar segment. Extrusive force results in extrusion of maxillary first molars into the posterior interocclusal space. Sequentially, all the remaining teeth are extruded into the interocclusal space, resulting in improvement of the anterior deep bite and normalization of the mandibular plane angle.

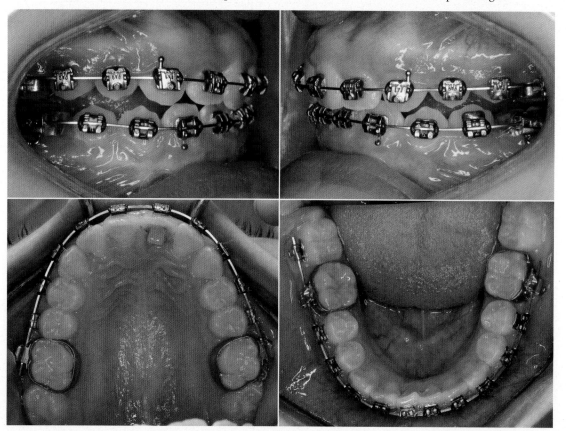

Figure 1-4-4 Disocclusion of the posterior teeth by placing an anterior bite stop on the lingual surface of the maxillary anterior teeth.

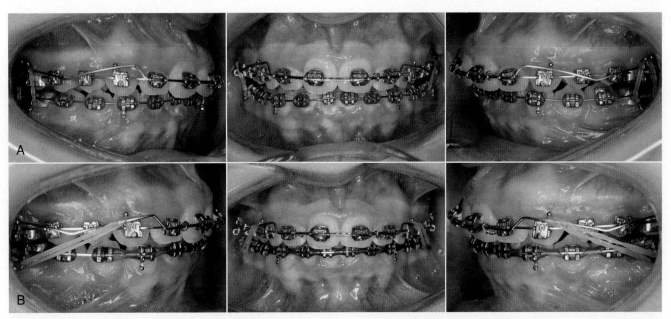

Figure 1-4-5 **A,** Base arch wire placed in the maxillary arch from first premolar to first premolar with NiTi intrusion arch wire placed into the axillary slot of first molars and tied on to the anterior teeth resulting in minimal intrusion of maxillary anterior teeth tip back of the maxillary molar for Class II correction and extrusion of the posterior teeth. **B,** Class II elastics helps to correct buccal occlusion and extrude mandibular posterior teeth.

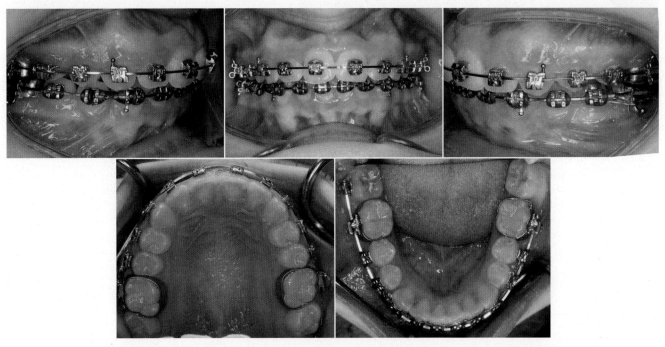

Figure 1-4-6   Finishing stage and settling of occlusion after Class II correction.

FINAL RESULTS

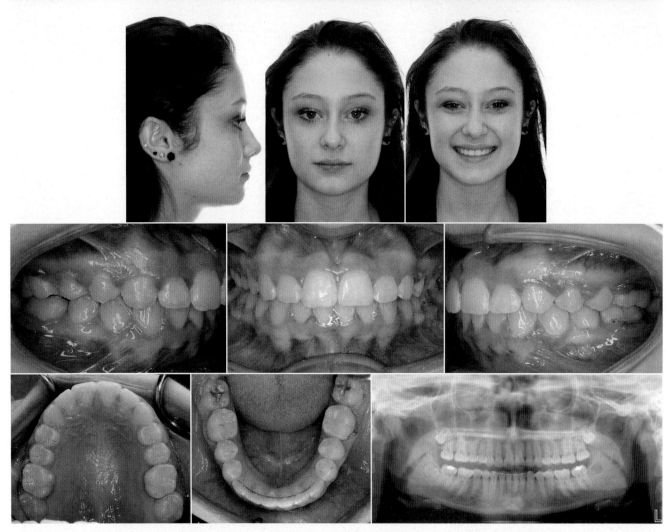

Figure 1-4-7 Posttreatment extraoral/intraoral photographs and panoramic radiograph. Note that gingival levels are higher in the maxillary central incisors, favorably increasing the length of the clinical crown. Maxillary lateral incisors and canines would require gingivectomy/crown lengthening to maximize smile aesthetics. The height of the interproximal papilla between central incisors has normalized with treatment.

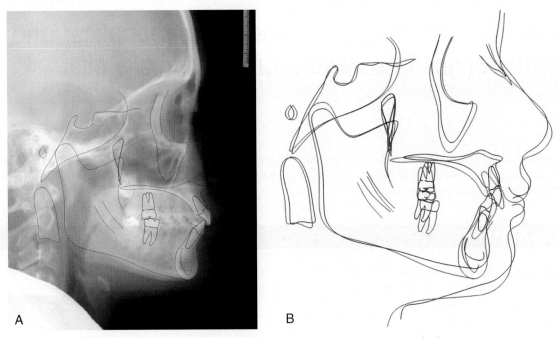

Figure 1-4-8 **A,** Posttreatment lateral cephalogram; **B,** Superimposition. *Black,* pretreatment; *red,* posttreatment.

Why were anterior bite stops used to open the bite in this patient?
This patient had a significant deep bite with a brachiofacial pattern. In addition, a slightly reduced incisor display at smile was evident. In order to correct her deep overbite, the options were limited to mandibular intrusion or extrusion of the posterior teeth. A combination of the two options was necessary to be able to correct the severity of the deep bite. Vertical elastics on the molars were used to erupt these teeth into a new vertical dimension of occlusion.

Combined Orthognathic Surgery, Orthodontics, and Prosthodontics in a Severe Brachiofacial Pattern

A 56-year-old male patient was referred by his prosthodontist for correction of an anterior deep bite. Medical and dental histories were noncontributory, and findings from the temporomandibular joint (TMJ) examination were normal with adequate range of jaw movements.

■ PRETREATMENT

Extraoral Analysis (Fig. 1-5-1)

Facial Form	Euryprosopic
Facial Symmetry	No gross asymmetry noticed
Chin Point	Coincidental with facial midline
Occlusal Plane	Normal
Facial Profile	Convex due to retrognathic mandible. Prominent chin button
Facial Height	Upper Facial Height/Lower Facial Height: Increased
	Lower Facial Height/Throat Depth: Decreased, Increased cervicomental angle
Lips	Competent, Upper: Protrusive; Lower: Retrusive
Nasolabial Angle	Normal
Mentolabial Sulcus	Deep

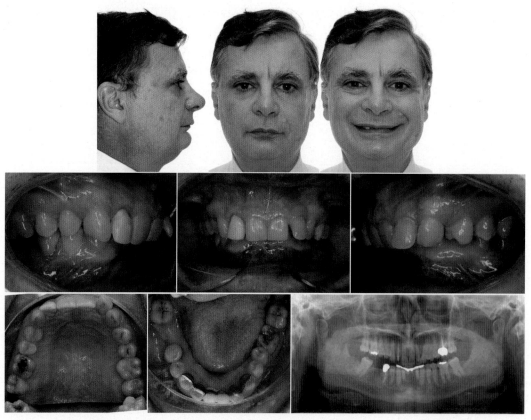

Figure 1-5-1   Pretreatment extraoral/intraoral photographs and panoramic radiograph.

Smile Analysis (Fig. 1-5-2)

Smile Arc	Flat
Incisor Display	Rest: −2 mm
	Smile: 5 mm
Lateral Tooth Display	First premolars
Buccal Corridor	Slightly wide
Gingival Tissue	Gingival Margins: Maxillary lateral incisor margins are higher.
Papilla	Present between maxillary central incisors
Dentition	Tooth size and proportion: normal
Tooth Shape	Normal
Axial Inclination	Maxillary teeth inclined lingually
Connector Space and Contact Area	No contact between left lateral incisor and central incisor
Incisal Embrasure	Minimal
Midlines	Upper and lower midlines are coincidental with facial midline
Occlusal Plane	Flat and maxillary and mandibular occlusal planes converge anteriorly

Intraoral Analysis (see Fig. 1-5-2)

Teeth Present	7654321/1234567
	754321/1234567 (Mandibular central incisors are replaced by Maryland bridge)
Molar Relation	Class I left side and undetermined right side
Canine Relation	Class II bilaterally
Overjet	5 mm
Overbite	8 mm
Maxillary Arch	U shaped, symmetric
Mandibular Arch	U shaped, symmetric and deep curve of Spee
Oral Hygiene	Fair
Other	Root canal therapy and full coverage restorations on maxillary left first molar, mandibular right second premolar, and maxillary right lateral incisor

Functional Analysis

Swallowing	Normal adult pattern
Temporomandibular joint	Normal with normal range of jaw movements

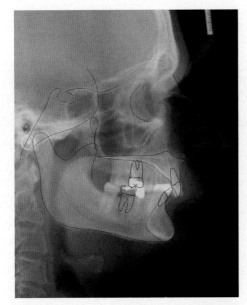

Parameter	Norm	Value
SNA (°)	82	83
SNB (°)	80	75
ANB (°)	2	8
FMA (°)	24	13
MP-SN (°)	32	20
U1-NA (mm/°)	4/22	−1/10
L1-NA (mm/°)	4/25	4/30
IMPA (°)	95	113
U1-L1 (°)	130	132
OP-SN (°)	14	7
Upper Lip – E Plane (mm)	−4	0
Lower Lip – E Plane (mm)	−2	−4
Nasolabial Angle (°)	103	108

Figure 1-5-2 Pretreatment lateral cephalogram with tracing and cephalometric analysis.

Diagnosis and Case Summary

A 56-year-old male patient with multiple missing mandibular teeth presented with a convex skeletal and soft tissue profile mainly due to a retrognathic mandible. He had an accentuated brachiofacial pattern with short lower facial height and reduced mandibular plane angle dental Class II division 2 malocclusion with retroclined maxillary central incisors. The upper lip is protrusive, whereas the lower lip is retrusive.

PROBLEM LIST

Pathology/Others	Missing mandibular central incisors and right first molar
	Maryland bridge bonded to mandibular lateral incisors and canines
	Root canal treatment of maxillary right lateral incisor and left first molar and mandibular right second premolar
	Unaesthetic provisional crown on maxillary right lateral incisor
	Metal tattoo present with respect to mandibular anterior labial gingiva

Alignment

Dimension	Skeletal	Dental	Soft Tissue
Anteroposterior	Convex profile due to retrognathic mandible	Class II canine relationship bilaterally and molar on the left side	Protrusive upper lip and retrusive lower lip
	Thick chin button	Overjet of 5 mm	Deep mentolabial sulcus
		Retroclined maxillary incisors	Thick soft tissue chin
		Labially inclined prosthesis replacing mandibular incisors	
		Deep curve of Spee	
Vertical	Reduced mandibular plane angle	Overbite of 8 mm	Insufficient incisal show upon smiling
	Reduced upper facial height	Flat occlusal plane	No incisor display at rest (−2 mm in relation to upper lip)
			Redundant lips
Transverse		Buccal cross bite with respect to maxillary left first premolar	Increased cervicomental angle

TREATMENT OBJECTIVES

Pathology/ Others	Replace missing teeth with prosthetic implants
	Evaluate root canal treatment of maxillary right lateral incisor, left first molar and mandibular second premolar
	Replace unaesthetic crown on maxillary right lateral incisor
	Remove Maryland bridge present in mandibular anterior region

Alignment

Dimension	Skeletal	Dental	Soft Tissue
Anteroposterior	Surgical correction of skeletal to advance the mandible	Correct dental Class II relationship and overjet by mandibular advancement	Improve lower lip retrusion and mentolabial sulcus with wedge genioplasty
		Flare maxillary anterior teeth to improve the inclination	
		Level curve of Spee postsurgically by extrusion of posterior teeth	
Vertical	LeFort I osteotomy with maxillary down grafting to increase lower anterior facial height and improve mandibular plane angle	Improve the overbite by leveling the curve of Spee by extrusion of posterior teeth postsurgically	Improve incisal show by LeFort I osteotomy and maxillary down grafting
			Increase lower facial height with an additional wedge genioplasty
Transverse		Improve buccal crossbite with respect to maxillary left first premolar	Improve cervicomental angle with mandibular advancement

Treatment Options

In the present case, for the skeletal vertical dimension to be increased, a LeFort I osteotomy and down fracture of maxillary arch are required. For the skeletal Class II relationship to be corrected, mandibular advancement is necessary. A wedge genioplasty is also beneficial to increase total facial height.

For the mandible anteriorly to be advanced, the overbite needs to be addressed. In this patient the maxillary and mandibular occlusal planes converge anteriorly, which requires a clockwise rotation of the mandibular occlusal plane. This can be obtained by correcting the overbite anteriorly surgically and leaving interocclusal space in the posterior region for extrusion of the mandibular buccal segments with orthodontic tooth movement. Extrusion of the posterior teeth postsurgically in a deep bite patient leads to an increase in lower anterior facial height and improvement in mandibular plane angle.

TREATMENT SEQUENCE AND BIOMECHANICAL PLAN

Maxilla	Mandible
Band molars and bond maxillary arch.	Band molars and bond mandibular arch.
Level using .016, .018, .016 × .022, .019 × .025 inch NiTi arch wires.	Level using .016, .018, .016 × .022, .019 × .025 inch NiTi arch wires.
Place .019 × .025 inch SS surgical wire.	Place .019 × .025 inch SS surgical wire.
Orthognathic surgery: LeFort I osteotomy with down fracture of the maxilla with graft.	Orthognathic surgery: BSSO advancement to attain ideal overjet and overbite.
Postsurgically: Cut the occlusal stent distal to maxillary lateral incisors, and keep the remaining of stent tied to the maxillary anterior teeth.	Postsurgically: Cut the mandibular arch wire distal to canines and start vertical elastics to extrude the mandibular posterior segments.
Continue leveling using .019 × .025 inch CNA.	.016 × .022 inch CNA with step between anterior and posterior teeth.
.016 × .022 inch CNA with finishing bends.	.016 × .022 inch CNA with step between anterior and posterior teeth. Place finishing bends on .016 × .022 inch CNA.
Debond and wrap around retainer.	Debond and deliver Hawley retainer.
New restoration of maxillary right lateral incisor.	Replace missing teeth with prosthetic implants.
6-month recall appointment for retention check.	6-month recall appointment for retention check.

BSSO, Bilateral sagittal split osteotomy; *CNA,* connecticut new arch wire; *SS,* stainless steel.

■ TREATMENT SEQUENCE

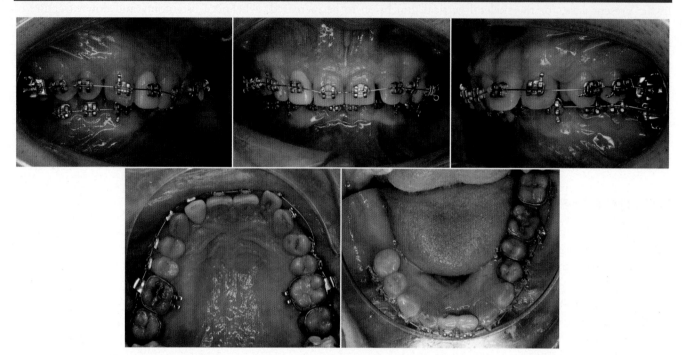

Figure 1-5-3   Presurgical leveling. Note: Mandibular right second molar had to be extracted because of a vertical root fracture.

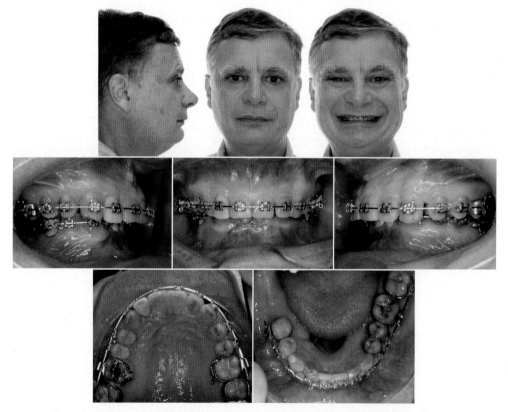

Figure 1-5-4   Presurgical leveling with .019 × .025-inch stainless steel arch wire.

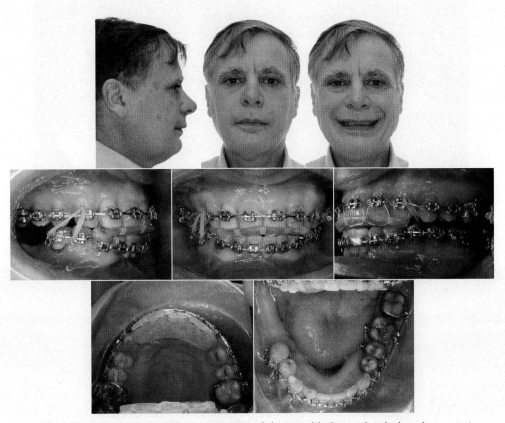

Figure 1-5-5 Postsurgical clockwise rotation of the mandibular occlusal plane by extrusion of mandibular posterior teeth.

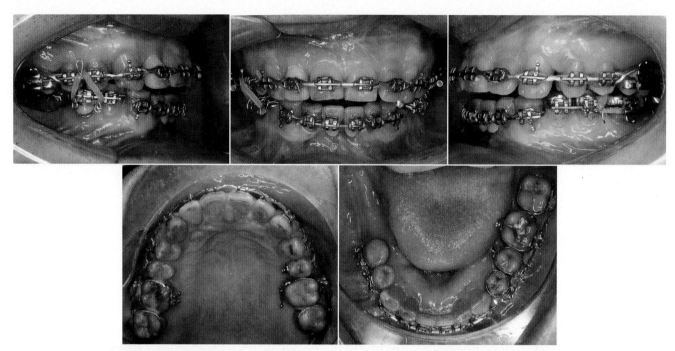

Figure 1-5-6 Continued postsurgical clockwise rotation of the mandibular occlusal plane by extrusion of the mandibular posterior.

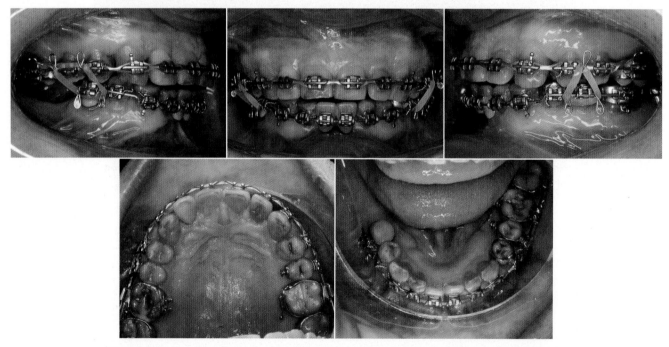

Figure 1-5-7 Continued postsurgical clockwise rotation of the mandibular occlusal plane by extrusion of the mandibular posterior.

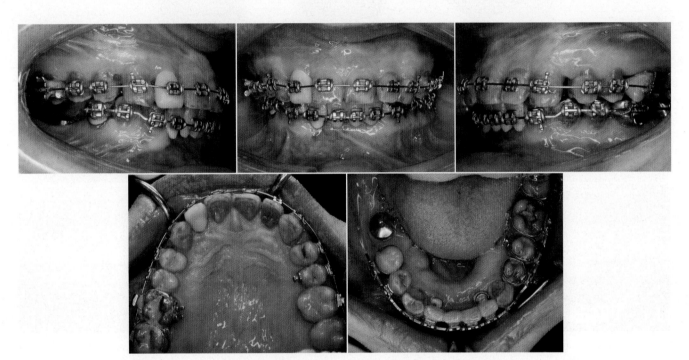

Figure 1-5-8   Postsurgical settling of occlusion. The step between mandibular anterior and posterior teeth is maintained. Dental implant placed in lower right mandibular first molar region. Note: In the anterior incisor region, it was decided by the prosthodontist to extract the lateral incisors and place two dental implants in these sites to support two central incisor pontics.

FINAL RESULTS

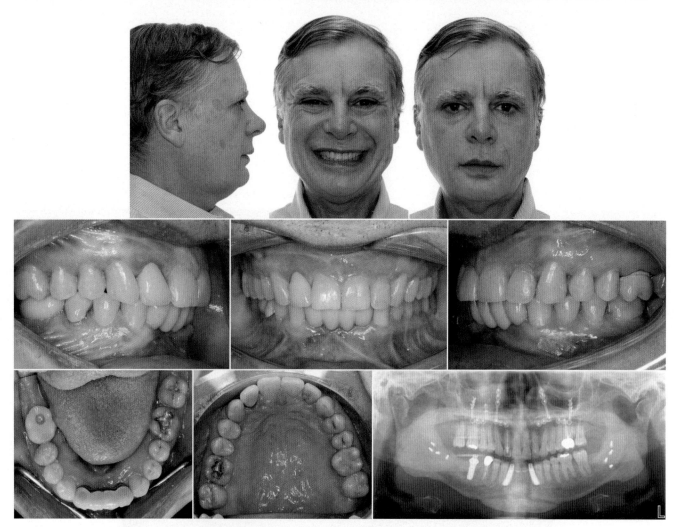

Figure 1-5-9 Posttreatment extraoral/intraoral photographs and panoramic radiograph. Restorative work completed, including crowns on mandibular right first molar implant, crowns on mandibular incisor segment supported by dental implants on lateral incisors, and crown on maxillary right central incisor.

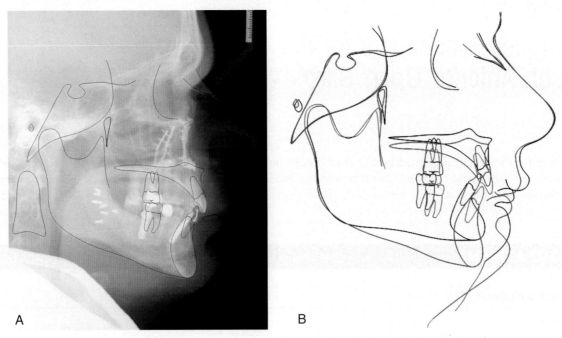

A

B

Figure 1-5-10   **A,** Posttreatment lateral cephalogram. **B,** Superimposition. *Black,* pretreatment; *red,* posttreatment.

Why was orthognathic surgery done in this patient?
This patient presented with a severe brachiofacial pattern and anterior deep bite. Aesthetically, a deep mentolabial fold with minimal incisal display at rest and smile was evident. For the severity of the short face syndrome to be addressed, this patient had to be corrected with orthognathic surgery, maximizing the downfracturing of the maxilla, clockwise rotation of the mandible, and wedge genioplasty. All these movements contributed to a maximal aesthetic and occlusal change. Without orthognathic surgery, the occlusal correction would had been limited with negligible impact on the facial and smile aesthetics.

Why was a stent left after surgery?
The stent was left to serve as a guide for the vertical dimension on the anterior teeth. Specifically, the surgical stent was left as a reference as to where the posterior teeth needed to be extruded into occlusion because the patient had moderate wear on the mandibular incisors. The stent was cut distal to the maxillary canines to allow the eruption of the posterior teeth, which was accomplished with Class II elastics to favor primarily an occlusal plane change in the mandible.

CASE 2-1
Targeted Mechanics for the Correction of an Anterior Open Bite*

A 28-year-old male patient presented with a chief complaint that he wants to fix his open bite. The patient's medical history was only significant for a mild form of asthma. He had regular dental checkups, with recent root canal treatment performed for maxillary left first molar. Findings from a temporomandibular joint (TMJ) examination were normal with adequate range of jaw movements.

▪ PRETREATMENT

Extraoral Analysis (Fig. 2-1-1)

Facial Form	Mesoprosopic
Facial Symmetry	No gross asymmetries noticed
Chin Point	Coincidental with facial midline
Occlusal Plane	Normal
Facial Profile	Straight
Facial Height	Upper Facial Height/Lower Facial Height: Reduced
	Lower Facial Height/Throat Depth: Normal
Lips	Competent, Upper: Protrusive; Lower: Protrusive
Nasolabial Angle	Acute
Mentolabial Sulcus	Normal

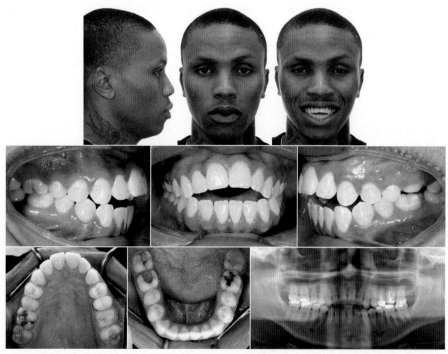

Figure 2-1-1   Pretreatment extraoral/intraoral photographs and panoramic radiograph.

---

*Portions of Case 2-1 from Librizzi ZT, Janakiraman N, Rangiani A, Nanda R, Uribe FA. Targeted Mechanics for Limited Posterior Treatment with Mini-Implant Anchorage. *J Clin Orthod.* 2015;49:777-783.

Smile Analysis (Fig. 2-1-2)

Smile Arc	Reverse
Incisor Display	Rest: 0 mm
	Smile: 8 mm
Lateral Tooth Display	First molar to first molar
Buccal Corridor	Narrow
Gingival Tissue	Margins: Maxillary central and lateral incisor margins are high compared with canines
Papilla	Present
	Slight recession in the gingival margin of the mandibular left central incisor
Dentition	Tooth size and proportion: Normal. Crown preparation for provisional full coverage restoration on maxillary left first molar (provisional crown missing).
	Full coverage crown on maxillary left second premolar
	Root canal therapy on maxillary left second premolar and first molar
Tooth Shape	Normal
Axial Inclination	Maxillary teeth inclined labially
Connector Space and Contact Area	Normal
Incisal Embrasure	Normal
Midlines	Upper and lower midline are coincidental with facial midline

Intraoral Analysis (see Fig. 2-1-2)

Teeth Present	7654321/1234567
	7654321/1234567
Molar Relation	Class I bilaterally
Canine Relation	Class II end on bilaterally
Overjet	4 mm
Overbite	6 mm
Maxillary Arch	U shaped, symmetric with 2 mm of spacing
Mandibular Arch	U shaped, symmetric with 2 mm of spacing and normal curve of Spee
Oral Hygiene	Good

Functional Analysis

Swallowing	Anterior tongue posture for seal during swallowing
Temporomandibular joint	Normal with normal range of jaw movements
Habits	History of thumb sucking habit, stopped approximately 1 year ago

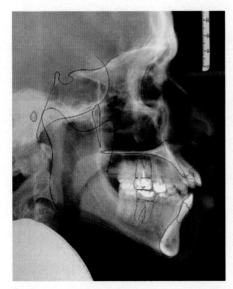

Parameter	Norm	Value
SNA (°)	85	86
SNB (°)	81	83
ANB (°)	4	3
FMA (°)	28	24
MP-SN (°)	38	32
U1-NA (mm/°)	7/22	11/34
L1-NA (mm/°)	9/33	9/34
IMPA (°)	98	93
U1-L1 (°)	119	113
OP-SN (°)	16	8
Upper Lip – E Plane (mm)	0	3
Lower Lip – E Plane (mm)	4	7
Nasolabial Angle (°)	90	86

Figure 2-1-2   Pretreatment lateral cephalogram with tracing and cephalometric analysis.

Diagnosis and Case Summary

A 28-year-old male patient had an orthognathic soft and hard tissue profile with dental Class I molar and Class II end on canine relationship. He exhibited an anterior open bite of 6 mm due to undererupted and proclined upper incisors and lower incisors and spacing of 2 mm present in the upper and lower arch. The patient has a history of thumb sucking, which he stopped 1 year before consultation.

PROBLEM LIST			
Pathology/Others	Mildly restored dentition, root canal treatment on maxillary left first molar with preparation for crown and absent provisional Root canal treatment with full coverage crown on maxillary left second premolar All the third molars have been removed		
Alignment	2 mm spacing upper, I-2 mm lower		
Dimension	**Skeletal**	**Dental**	**Soft Tissue**
Vertical	Decreased ramus height Reduced UFH:LFH	6-mm anterior open bite Reverse smile arch 1 posterior and 2 anterior occlusal planes Undererupted maxillary and mandibular incisors	
Anteroposterior		4 mm of overjet Proclined upper incisors Class II end on canine relationship bilaterally Acute interincisal angle	Upper and lower lips protrusive relative to E-plane
Transverse		Constriction of maxillary intercanine width	

LFH, lower facial height; *UFH,* upper facial height.

TREATMENT OBJECTIVES			
Pathology/Others	Place post and core and fabricate permanent full-coverage restoration on maxillary left first molar Monitor for caries development		
Alignment	Close up maxillary and mandibular spacing		
Dimension	**Skeletal**	**Dental**	**Soft Tissue**
Vertical		Extrude maxillary and mandibular anterior teeth to close anterior open bite, improve smile arc, and level occlusal plane	
Anteroposterior		Retract maxillary and mandibular anterior teeth to correct the overjet and proclination of maxillary and mandibular anterior teeth	Improve upper and lower lip protrusion
Transverse		Improve constriction of maxillary intercanine width	

Treatment Options

In the present case, anterior and posterior teeth have different occlusal planes that require correction by means of segmental mechanics. Moreover, the long-standing thumb sucking habit has resulted in undereruption of the maxillary anterior teeth. Extrusion of anterior teeth can be accomplished with an extrusion arch with buccal seating and anterior box elastics. In this option, compliance with elastic wear is needed from the patient.

A second option could also use an extrusion arch to close the anterior open bite and temporary anchorage devices (TADs) to stabilize the first molars, counteracting the mesial moment generated by the extrusive force. Furthermore, TAD stabilization of the first molar obviates the need to bond the entire buccal segment and the use of the vertical elastics on the buccal segments necessary to counteract the counterclockwise moment on the posterior teeth.

Extraction of first premolars could reduce lip protrusion; however, the patient was satisfied with his lip position and declined this option.

TREATMENT SEQUENCE AND BIOMECHANICAL PLAN

Maxilla	Mandible
Place temporary crown for maxillary left first molar.	
Separators and bond 3-3.	Separators and bond 3-3.
Fit bands and pick up impression for tongue crib.	Band first molars. Segmental leveling of incisors.
Segmental leveling of incisors up to .016 × .022 inch SS arch wire.	Segmental leveling of incisors up to .016 × .022 inch SS arch wire.
Cement tongue crib, place TADs between second premolar and first molar, stabilize first molar with TADs using .019 × .025 inch SS arch wire. Place .017 × .025 inch NiTi extrusion arch wire.	Place TADs between second premolar and first molar, stabilize first molar with TADs with .019 × .025 inch SS wire. Place .017 × .025 inch NiTi extrusion arch wire.
Finishing with seating elastics.	Finishing with seating elastics.
Debond and 4-4 fixed retainer.	Debond and 3-3 fixed retainer.
Final restoration of maxillary left first molar. 6-month recall appointment for retention check.	6-month recall appointment for retention check.

NiTi, nickel-titanium alloy; *SS,* stainless steel; *TAD,* temporary anchorage devices.

▪TREATMENT SEQUENCE

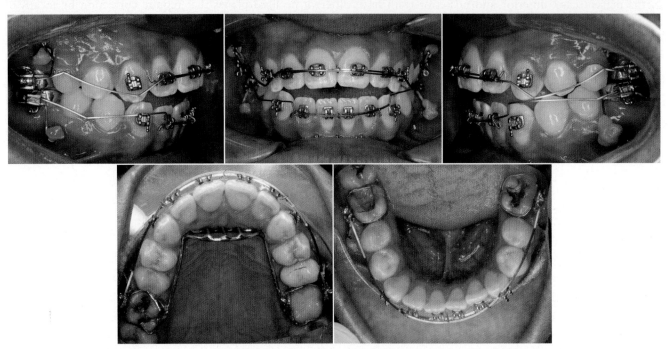

Figure 2-1-3 Intraoral photographs showing extrusion arch from first molar to anterior teeth for closure of the anterior open bite. First molar stabilized with temporary anchorage devices. Tongue crib in the maxillary arch to control the thumb-sucking habit.

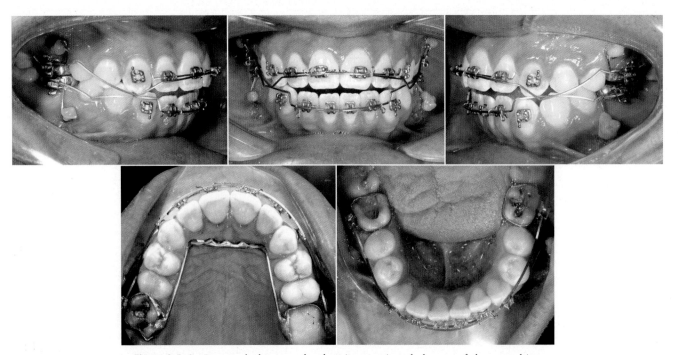

Figure 2-1-4 Intraoral photographs showing continued closure of the open bite.

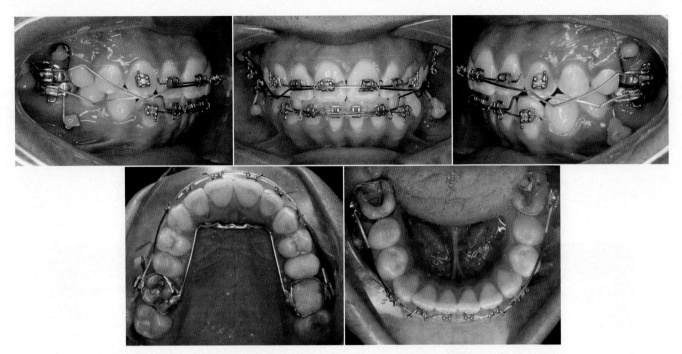

Figure 2-1-5   Intraoral photographs showing closure of the open bite.

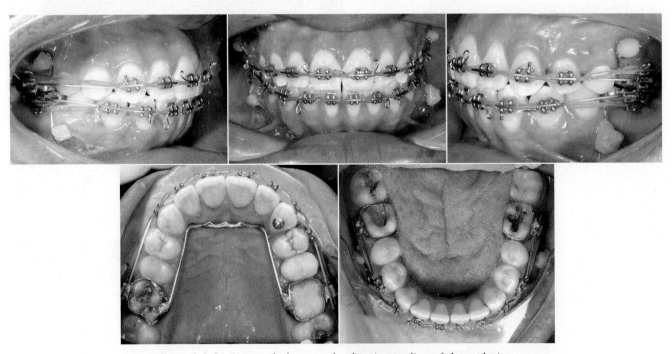

Figure 2-1-6   Intraoral photographs showing settling of the occlusion.

FINAL RESULTS

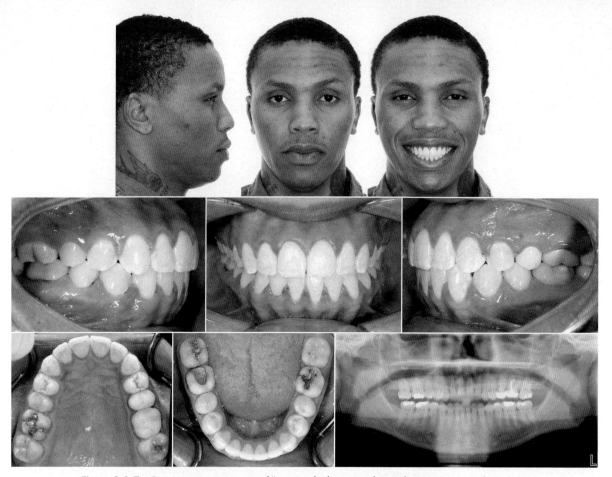

Figure 2-1-7   Posttreatment extraoral/intraoral photographs and panoramic radiograph.

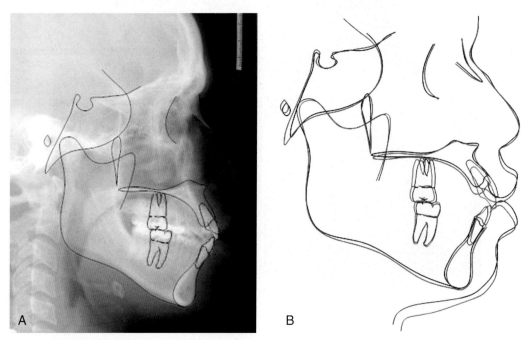

Figure 2-1-8   **A,** Posttreatment lateral cephalogram. **B,** Superimposition. *Black,* pretreatment; *red,* posttreatment.

Why were miniscrews used in this patient for anterior open bite closure?
The primary reason for a miniscrew in each quadrant was to counteract the counterclockwise moment on the maxillary molars and clockwise moment in the mandibular molars inherent to the mechanics applied. Specifically, the extrusive force in the incisors (which is desired) results in a side effect on the posterior end (molars), which in this patient was counteracted by indirect anchorage provided by the miniscrews. Because the buccal segment was in perfect occlusion, the premolars were bonded only at the end of treatment during the refinement of the occlusion. This targeted approach dramatically reduced the treatment time for this patient to 10 months.

Anterior Open Bite Correction by Mini-Implant–Assisted Posterior Intrusion

A 16-year-old postpubertal male patient presented with a chief complaint that his upper and lower front teeth did not come together. The patient had history previous orthodontic treatment performed with maxillary premolar extractions. His medical history was noncontributory, and findings from a temporomandibular joint (TMJ) examination were normal with adequate range of jaw movements.

■ PRETREATMENT

Extraoral Analysis (Fig. 2-2-1)

Facial Form	Leptoprosopic
Facial Symmetry	No gross asymmetries noticed
Chin Point	Coincidental with facial midline
Occlusal Plane	Normal
Facial Profile	Convex due to a retrognathic mandible
Facial Height	Upper Facial Height/Lower Facial Height: Reduced
	Lower Facial Height/Throat Depth: Increased
Lips	Incompetent, Upper: Normal; Lower: Protrusive
Nasolabial Angle	Obtuse
Mentolabial Sulcus	Normal

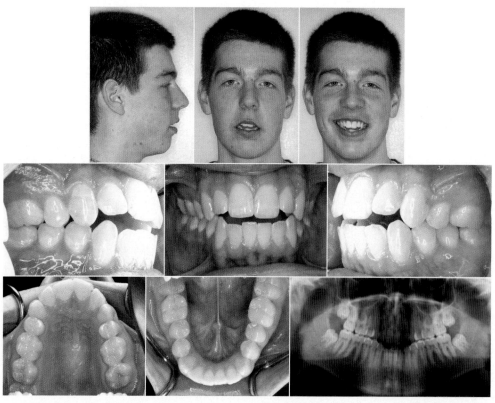

Figure 2-2-1 Pretreatment extraoral/intraoral photographs and panoramic radiograph.

Smile Analysis (Fig. 2-2-2)

Smile Arc	Reverse
Incisor Display	Rest: 4 mm
	Smile: 10 mm
Lateral Tooth Display	First molar to first molar
Buccal Corridor	Narrow
Gingival Tissue	Margins: Incisor gingival margins are high. Thin labial gingival tissue on mandibular first premolars and anterior teeth
Papilla	Present
Dentition	Tooth size and proportion: Normal
Tooth Shape	Normal
Axial Inclination	Maxillary incisors are inclined normally
Connector Space and Contact Area	Normal
Incisal Embrasure	Normal
Midlines	Upper midline is coincidental, and lower dental midline is shifted to the left by 1 mm as compared with the facial midline

Intraoral Analysis (see Fig. 2-2-2)

Teeth Present	8765321/123567
	7654321/1234567 (Unerupted maxillary left 8 and mandibular 8s)
Molar Relation	Class II bilaterally
Canine Relation	Class I bilaterally
Overjet	3 mm
Overbite	−3 mm
Maxillary Arch	U shaped, symmetric with accentuated curve of Spee
Mandibular Arch	U shaped, symmetric, with reverse curve of Spee
Oral Hygiene	Fair

Functional Analysis

Swallowing	Normal adult pattern
Temporomandibular joint	Normal with normal range of jaw movements

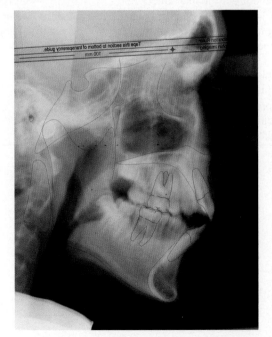

Parameter	Norm	Value
SNA (°)	82	80
SNB (°)	80	74
ANB (°)	2	6
FMA (°)	24	29
MP-SN (°)	32	36
U1-NA (mm/°)	4/22	4/21
L1-NA (mm/°)	4/25	11/36
IMPA (°)	95	106
U1-L1 (°)	130	115
OP-SN (°)	14	18
Upper Lip – E Plane (mm)	−4	−3
Lower Lip – E Plane (mm)	−2	0
Nasolabial Angle (°)	103	115
Wits Appraisal (mm)	−1	5

Figure 2-2-2   Pretreatment lateral cephalogram with tracing and cephalometric analysis.

Diagnosis and Case Summary

A 16-year-old postpubertal male patient presented with convex skeletal and soft tissue profile mainly due to a retrognathic mandible. He had a Class I malocclusion with an anterior open bite (resulting in two maxillary occlusal planes [i.e., incisal and posterior]); increased mandibular plane angle; increased lower anterior facial height; and flared and anteriorly placed mandibular incisors leading to reduced interincisal angle. His upper lip is normal, lower lip is protrusive, and nasolabial angle is increased. An increased interlabial gap is present.

PROBLEM LIST			
Pathology/Others			
Alignment	Mild mandibular crowding		
Dimension	**Skeletal**	**Dental**	**Soft Tissue**
Anteroposterior	Convex skeletal profile due to retrognathic mandible Wits appraisal = 5 mm	Flared and anteriorly placed mandibular incisors Reduced interincisal angle	Protrusive lower lip Obtuse nasolabial angle
Vertical	Increased lower anterior facial height Increased mandibular plane angle	Overbite = –3 mm Incisal planes for the maxilla and mandible diverge from single posterior occlusal plane	Increased interlabial gap
Transverse		Mandibular midline 1 mm to the left of facial midline	

TREATMENT OBJECTIVES			
Pathology/Others			
Alignment			
Dimension	**Skeletal**	**Dental**	**Soft Tissue**
Anteroposterior	Reduce skeletal convexity with autorotation of the mandible in counterclockwise direction	Improve overjet by autorotation of the mandible counterclockwise Distalize mandibular anterior teeth to correct the inclination	
Vertical	Reduce lower anterior facial height and mandibular plane angle by intruding the posterior teeth	Achieve a single occlusal plane by intruding posterior teeth and maintaining the vertical position of the anterior teeth Achieve positive overbite by intrusion of the posterior teeth	Reduce interlabial gap with mandibular autorotation
Transverse		Improve mandibular midline by differentially distalizing the dental arch more on the right side	

Treatment Options

The anterior open bite can be corrected by either extruding the anterior teeth or intruding the posterior teeth and allowing the mandible to autorotate counterclockwise and close the anterior open bite.

In the present case, the amount of maxillary incisor show at rest and on smiling is ideal. This precludes any extrusion of maxillary incisors to prevent excessive gingival show at smile.

Maxillary teeth have two occlusal planes (i.e., incisal and posterior). For the maxillary occlusal plane to be leveled, the maxillary posterior teeth must be selectively intruded, which will prevent incisors from extruding and will cause the mandible to autorotate in a counterclockwise direction, normalize the mandibular plane angle, reduce the lower anterior facial height, and result in correction of the anterior open bite.

TREATMENT SEQUENCE AND BIOMECHANICAL PLAN

Maxilla	Mandible
Band molars, place transpalatal arch made out of .032 inch SS round wire and bond maxillary arch.	Band molars, place lingual arch made out of .032 inch SS round wire and bond mandibular arch.
Segmental alignment with .016, .018, .016 × .022, .019 × .025 inch NiTi arch wires.	Segmental alignment with .016, .018, .016 × .022, .019 × .025 inch NiTi arch wires.
.019 × .025 inch SS segmental stabilizing arch wire.	.019 × .025 inch SS segmental stabilizing arch wire.
Refer the patient to oral surgeon for placement of bone plates between first and second molars.	Refer the patient to oral surgeon for placement of bone plates between first and second molars.
Initiate intrusion of maxillary posterior teeth by placing 100 g of intrusive by connecting first molars to the bone plate with the help of an elastomeric thread.	Stabilize mandibular arch by connecting mandibular molars to the bone plate with help of .014 inch ligature wire.
Continue maxillary posterior intrusion with cantilever arms extended from the miniplates made of .036 inch SS to achieve parallel intrusion.	Distalize mandibular right side with help of elastomeric thread to improve the midline.
.016 × .022 inch continuous CNA arch wire with finishing bends.	.016 × .022 inch continuous CNA arch wire with finishing bends.
Debond and wrap around retainer.	Debond and deliver Hawley retainer.
6-month recall appointment for retention check.	6-month recall appointment for retention check.

CNA, Connecticut new arch wire; *NiTi,* nickel titanium; *SS,* stainless steel.

■ TREATMENT SEQUENCE

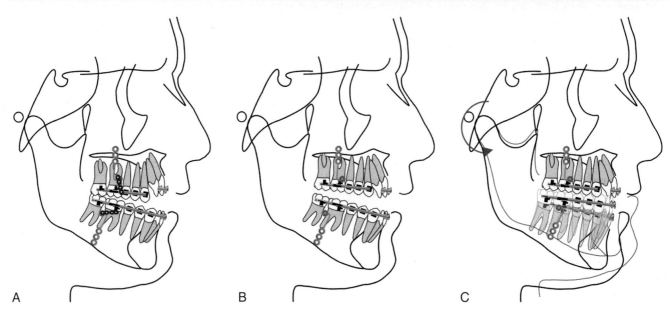

Figure 2-2-3 Biomechanical plan. **A,** Intrusion of maxillary posterior teeth by connecting the maxillary molars with bone plates with help of elastomeric thread. **B,** Intrusions of maxillary posterior teeth level the maxillary anterior and posterior occlusal planes and create interocclusal space for autorotation of mandible. **C,** Autorotation of mandible in counterclockwise direction corrects the anterior open bite and normalizes the anterior facial height of the face.

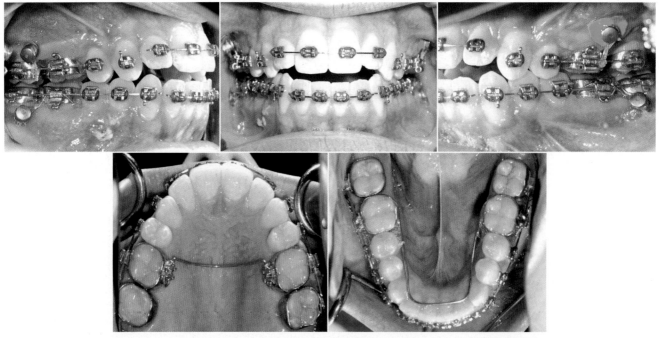

Figure 2-2-4 Intrusion of maxillary posterior teeth by connecting the maxillary molars with bone plates with help of elastomeric thread. Green piece of rubber dam was placed on maxillary left plate to keep the tissue from growing over the attachment head.

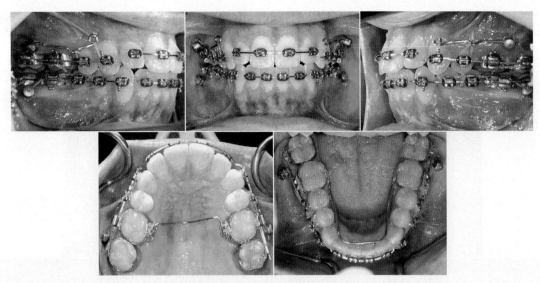

Figure 2-2-5   Cantilever arms from bone plates extended anteriorly to transfer intrusive force to maxillary canines and second premolars for parallel intrusion of the buccal segments.

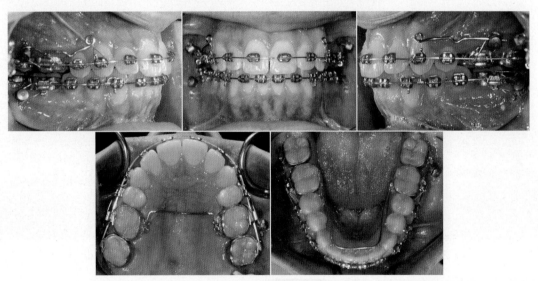

Figure 2-2-6   Maxillary occlusal plane leveled and stabilized by connecting maxillary arch with bone plates with .012 inch stainless steel ligature.

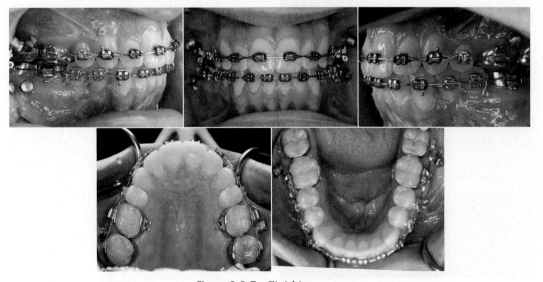

Figure 2-2-7   Finishing stage.

■ FINAL RESULTS

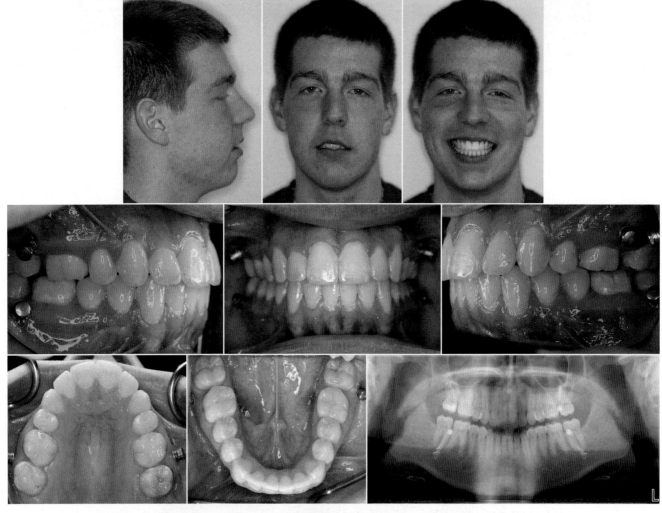

Figure 2-2-8   Posttreatment extraoral/intraoral photographs and panoramic radiograph.

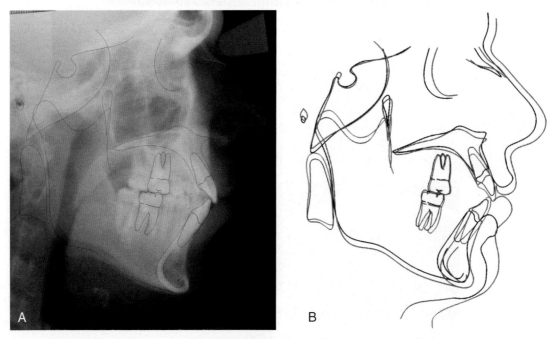

Figure 2-2-9   **A,** Posttreatment lateral cephalogram. **B,** Superimposition. *Black,* Pretreatment; *red,* posttreatment.

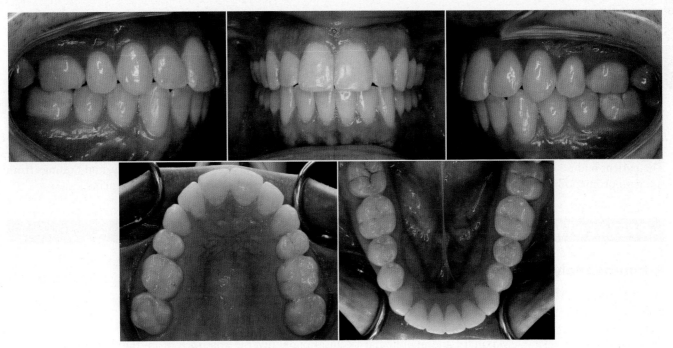

Figure 2-2-10   Three-year postretention intraoral photographs.

What is the advantage of attachment heads on the miniplates?
Patients with an anterior open bite who have a single posterior occlusal plane and two anterior diverging occlusal planes require parallel intrusion of the posterior segments. This is often a difficult task because forces are applied directly from a miniplate, which is usually located between the first and second molars. When an intrusive force is delivered from this area, it has either a retraction component if tied to the premolar or canines or a tipping effect (distal tip) on the posterior segment to intrude if tied directly to the first or second molar. The reason for this is that it is difficult to coincide with the center of resistance of this segment. To counteract any tipping of this segment, a rigid wire from the attachment head is extended. From this wire, different force vectors can be applied for a translatory effect on the posterior teeth to intrude.

CASE 2-3
Miniplate-Supported Posterior Intrusion with Posterior Acrylic Plate for Open Bite Correction

A 22-year-old postpubertal female patient's chief complaint was that her upper and lower front teeth did not contact. The patient had no history of previous orthodontic treatment. Medical history was noncontributory, and findings from the temporomandibular joint (TMJ) examination were normal with adequate range of jaw movements.

▪ PRETREATMENT

Extraoral Analysis (Fig. 2-3-1)

Facial Form	Leptoprosopic
Facial Symmetry	No gross asymmetries noticed
Chin Point	Coincidental with facial midline
Occlusal Plane	Maxillary and mandibular occlusal plane diverge anteriorly from the first premolar
Facial Profile	Convex due to retrognathic mandible
Facial Height	Upper Facial Height/Lower Facial Height: Reduced
	Lower Facial Height/Throat Depth: Increased
Lips	Incompetent, Upper: Protrusive; Lower: Protrusive
Nasolabial Angle	Acute
Mentolabial Sulcus	Shallow

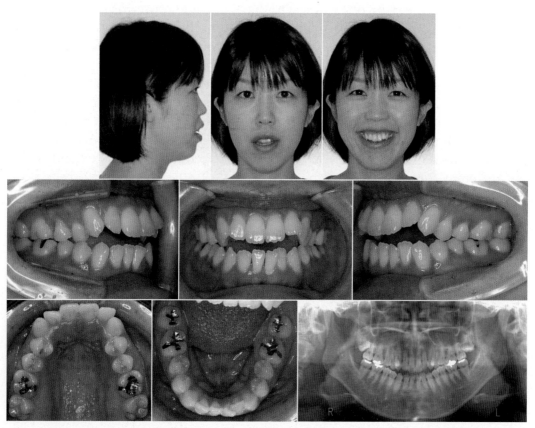

Figure 2-3-1   Pretreatment extraoral/intraoral photographs and panoramic radiograph.

Smile Analysis (Fig. 2-3-2)

Smile Arc	Reverse
Incisor Display	Rest: 5 mm
	Smile: 14 mm (100% with 4 mm of gingival display)
Lateral Tooth Display	First molar to first molar
Buccal Corridor	Narrow
Gingival Tissue	Margins: Maxillary lateral incisors have more apical displacement of the gingival margins compared with central and canines
	Mild recession in maxillary buccal segments
Papilla	Present on maxilla. Small black triangles on mandibular anteriors
Dentition	Tooth size and proportion: Normal
	Tooth shape: Normal
Axial Inclination	Maxillary incisors are inclined normally. Mandibular incisors are flared and inclined to the left side
Connector Space and Contact Area	Normal
Incisal Embrasure	Normal
Midlines	Upper midline is coincidental, and lower dental midline is shifted to the left by 1 mm as compared to the facial midline

Intraoral Analysis (see Fig. 2-3-2)

Teeth Present	7654321/1235467 (Unerupted maxillary 8s with significant mesial angulation)
	7654321/1234567
Molar Relation	Class I bilaterally
Canine Relation	Class II ends on bilaterally
Overjet	3 mm
Overbite	−3 mm
Maxillary Arch	U shaped, symmetric, 4 mm of crowding. Occlusal plane diverges anteriorly from the first premolar
Mandibular Arch	U shaped, symmetric, 3 mm of crowding and with reverse curve of Spee
Oral Hygiene	Fair

Functional Analysis

Swallowing	Normal adult pattern
Temporomandibular joint	Normal with normal range of jaw movements

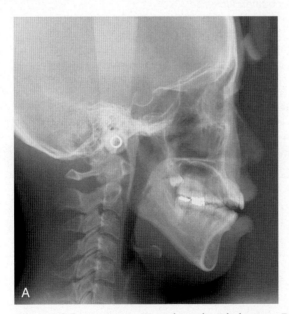
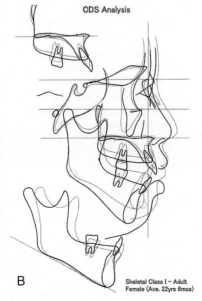

Figure 2-3-2 **A,** Pretreatment lateral cephalogram. **B,** Cephalometric tracing superimposed on the composite tracing of the average for Japanese norms.

Diagnosis and Case Summary

A 22-year-old postpubertal female patient presented with a convex skeletal soft tissue profile mainly due to a retrognathic mandible. She had a dental Class I malocclusion with an anterior open bite (resulting in two maxillary occlusal planes, i.e., incisal and posterior), increased mandibular plane angle, increased lower anterior facial height, and flared and anteriorly placed mandibular incisors leading to a reduced interincisal angle. Posterior maxillary and mandibular dentoalveolar heights are excessive. Upper and lower lips are protrusive, and the nasolabial angle is acute.

PROBLEM LIST

Pathology/Others	Slight recession in labial aspect of maxillary teeth in the buccal segment Significant mesial angulation of maxillary third molars		
Alignment	4 mm of crowding in maxillary arch and 3 mm of crowding in mandibular arch		
Dimension	**Skeletal**	**Dental**	**Soft Tissue**
Anteroposterior	Skeletal Class II	Overjet = 3 mm End on Class II canine relation, bilaterally Flared and labially placed mandibular incisors Reduced interincisal angle	Protrusive upper and lower lips Acute nasolabial angle
Vertical	Increased lower anterior facial height Increased mandibular plane angle	Overbite = −3 Maxillary occlusal plane has a step, incisal and posterior Increased maxillary and mandibular posterior dentoalveolar heights	Large interlabial gap
Transverse		Lower dental midline is shifted to the left by 1 mm, as compared with the facial midline	

TREATMENT OBJECTIVES

Pathology/Others	Monitor recession in labial aspect of maxillary buccal segments Extract maxillary third molars		
Alignment	Distalize maxillary posterior teeth to create space for alignment of the dental arch		
Dimension	**Skeletal**	**Dental**	**Soft Tissue**
Anteroposterior	Reduce the skeletal convexity by autorotation of mandible in counterclockwise direction	Improve overjet by autorotation of mandible counterclockwise Distalize maxillary and mandibular posterior teeth to create space to improve incisor inclination	
Vertical	Improve increased lower anterior facial height and increased mandibular plane angle by intruding the posterior teeth and counterclockwise rotation of mandible	Improve anterior overbite and step in occlusal plane by selectively intruding maxillary posterior teeth and autorotation of mandible in counterclockwise direction Reduce vertical dentoalveolar heights of buccal segments with miniplate supported intrusion	Reduce interlabial gap through mandibular autorotation
Transverse		Improve mandibular midline by distalizing mandibular dental arch on the right side	

Treatment Options

An anterior open bite can be corrected either by extruding the anterior teeth or by intruding the posterior teeth and allowing the mandible to autorotate counterclockwise and close the anterior open bite.

In the present case, the amount of maxillary incisor show at rest, as well as at smiling, is ideal. This means that any extrusion of maxillary incisors will result in excessive incisors/gum show at rest.

Maxillary teeth have two sets of occlusal planes (i.e., incisal and posterior). For leveling the maxillary occlusal plane, maxillary posterior teeth have to be selectively intruded, which will prevent incisors from extruding and cause the mandible to autorotate in a counterclockwise direction, normalize the mandibular plane angle, reduce the lower anterior facial height, and will result in correction of the anterior open bite.

The second option in the present case could have been a LeFort I osteotomy with posterior impaction along with mandibular advancement and optional genioplasty. Although the surgical option could have normalized the skeletal harmony of the face, the pretreatment skeletal discrepancy was not severe enough to justify orthognathic surgery. Results of posterior intrusion and orthognathic surgery were expected to be comparable.

TREATMENT SEQUENCE AND BIOMECHANICAL PLAN

Maxilla	Mandible
Bond posterior teeth, segmental alignment with .016, .018 inch NiTi arch wires.	Bond posterior teeth, segmental alignment with .016, .018 inch NiTi arch wires.
Place SAS bone plates bilaterally next to first molars. Cement posterior acrylic plate (occlusal acrylic coverage with right and left side connected with .040 inch SS round wire). Deliver 100 g of intrusive force by connecting the posterior acrylic plate with miniplates of the SAS system through NiTi closed coil springs.	Place SAS bone plates bilaterally next to the first molars. Continue alignment with .016 × .022, .019 × .025 inch NiTi arch wires.
Place .019 × .025 inch SS arch wire, passively bent. Place .032 × 032 CNA palatal arch to maintain transverse dimension. Continue intrusive force. Start 50 g of distalizing force by connecting the arch wire hook with the SAS system with elastomeric thread.	Continue alignment with .019 × .025 inch NiTi arch wire.
Bond anterior teeth and start alignment with .017 × .025 inch NiTi arch wire. Continue distalization force.	Continue alignment with .019 × .025 inch SS arch wire. Distalization of the mandibular buccal segment to create space to relieve anterior crowding.
.016 × .022 inch CNA with finishing bends.	.016 × .022 inch CNA with finishing bends.
Debond and wrap around retainer.	Debond and deliver Hawley retainer.
6-month recall appointment for retention check.	6-month recall appointment for retention check.

CNA, Connecticut new arch wire; *NiTi,* nickel titanium; *SAS,* skeletal anchorage system; *SS,* stainless steel.

■ TREATMENT SEQUENCE

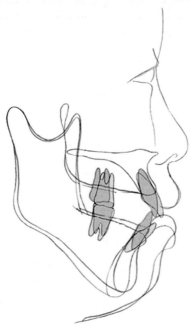

Figure 2-3-3   Visualized treatment objective. *Blue*, pretreatment; *red*, goal.

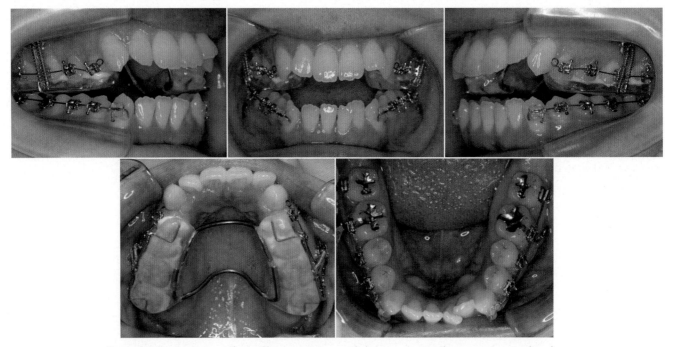

Figure 2-3-4   Intrusion of maxillary posterior teeth by connecting the posterior acrylic plate *to* the bone miniplates through nickel titanium coil springs.

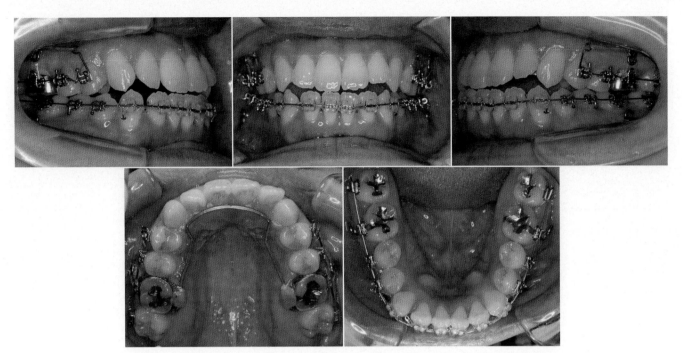

Figure 2-3-5 Distalization of maxillary posterior teeth by connecting arch wire hooks to the skeletal anchorage system through an elastomeric chain. Palatal arch connecting maxillary first molars to control the transverse dimension.

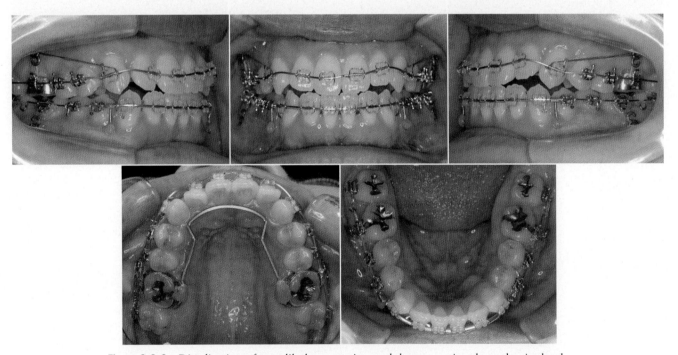

Figure 2-3-6 Distalization of mandibular posterior teeth by connecting the arch wire hooks to the skeletal anchorage system through an elastomeric chain.

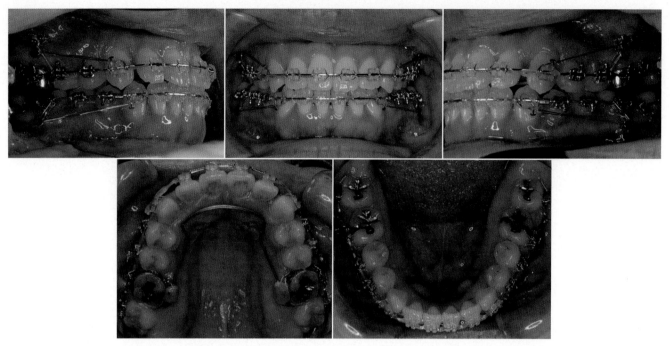

Figure 2-3-7 Finishing stage and settling of the occlusion.

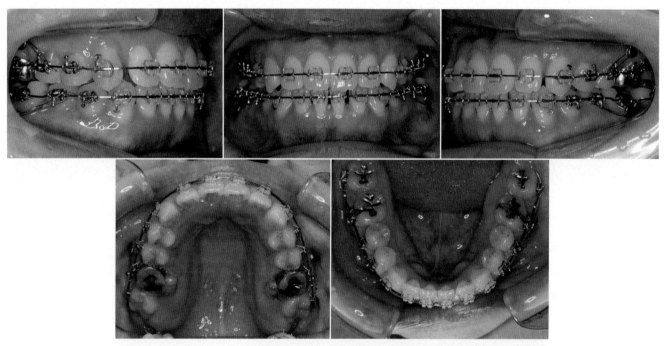

Figure 2-3-8 Finishing stage and settling of the occlusion.

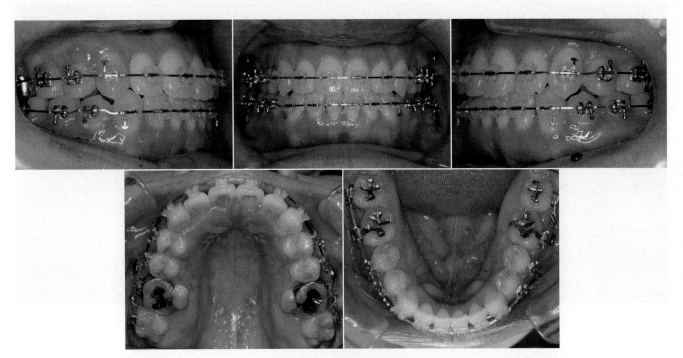

Figure 2-3-9 Finishing stage.

■ FINAL RESULTS

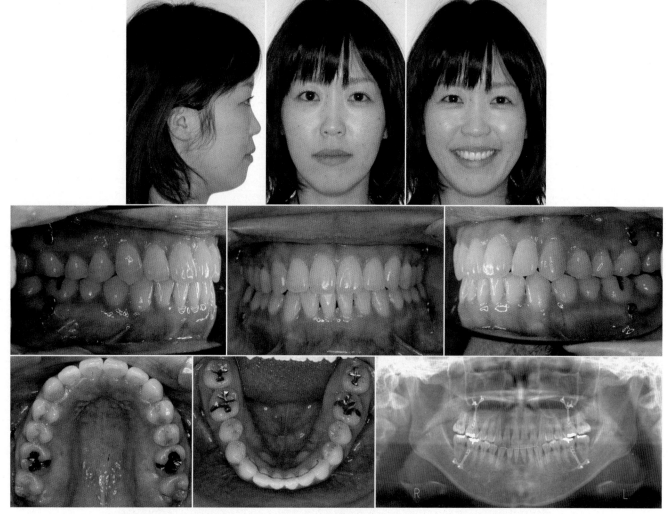

Figure 2-3-10 Posttreatment extraoral/intraoral photographs and panoramic radiograph.

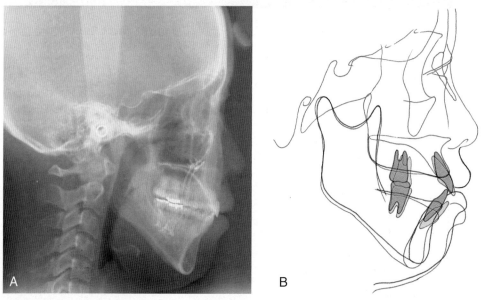

Figure 2-3-11 **A,** Posttreatment lateral cephalogram. **B,** Superimposition. *Blue,* pretreatment; *red,* posttreatment.

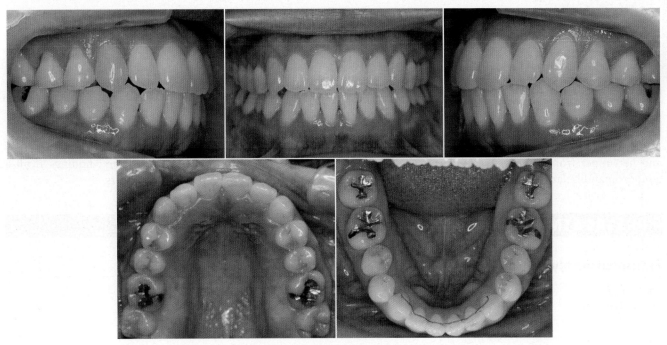

Figure 2-3-12   One-year posttreatment intraoral photographs.

?

Why do we need a posterior acrylic plate during the intrusion?

The acrylic plate has four specific functions during posterior intrusion of the buccal segments. First, it incorporates the posterior segments as a single rigid unit to be intruded. Second, the labial tipping of the posterior teeth (side effect from the moment of the applied intrusive force) is minimized by connecting both buccal segments. Third, the occlusal coverage of the posterior teeth may aid in preventing the extrusion of the mandibular segments and may also aid in the intrusion of the maxillary teeth by transferring the occlusal forces from the musculature. Finally, the transpalatal arches displace the tongue inferiorly, and as a result of normal function of the tongue, an intrusive load is transferred indirectly to the buccal segments.

Correction of a Class III Malocclusion with Vertical Excess with the Surgery-First Approach

A 22-year-old postpubertal female patient's chief complaint was that her lower teeth were in front of the upper teeth and her upper front teeth were crowded. Medical and dental histories were noncontributory, and findings from a temporomandibular joint (TMJ) examination were normal with adequate range of jaw movements.

■ PRETREATMENT

Extraoral Analysis (Fig. 2-4-1)

Facial Form	Leptoprosopic
Facial Symmetry	No gross asymmetries noticed
Chin Point	On with the facial midline
Occlusal Plane	Normal
Facial Profile	Concave due to prognathic mandible
Facial Height	Upper Facial Height/Lower Facial Height: Reduced
	Lower Facial Height/Throat Depth: Increased
Lips	Incompetent, Upper: Protrusive; Lower: Protrusive
Nasolabial Angle	Normal
Mentolabial Sulcus	Shallow
Malar Prominences	Deficient

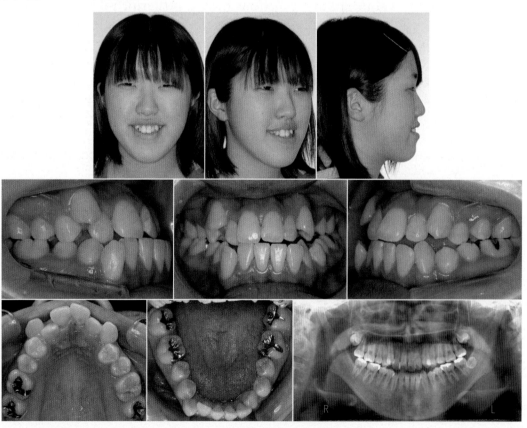

Figure 2-4-1   Pretreatment extraoral/intraoral photographs and panoramic radiograph.

Smile Analysis (Fig. 2-4-2)

Smile Arc	Consonant
Incisor Display	Rest: 7 mm
	Smile: 12 mm
Lateral Tooth Display	Second premolar to second premolar
Buccal Corridor	Normal
Gingival Tissue	Margins: Maxillary canine margins are high
Papilla	Present
Dentition	Tooth size and proportion: Normal
Tooth Shape	Normal
Axial Inclination	Maxillary teeth inclined labially
Connector Space and Contact Area	Normal
Incisal Embrasure	Normal
Midlines	Upper midline shifted to right side by 3 mm as compared with the facial midline

Intraoral Analysis (see Fig. 2-4-2)

Teeth Present	7654321/1234567 (Unerupted 8s, missing mandibular right third molar)
	7654321/1234567
Molar Relation	Class III bilaterally
Canine Relation	Class III bilaterally
Overjet	0 mm
Overbite	0 mm
Maxillary Arch	U shaped, asymmetric, anterior crossbite and 10 mm of crowding
Mandibular Arch	U shaped with crowding of 5 mm and normal curve of Spee
Oral Hygiene	Fair

Functional Analysis

Swallowing	Normal adult pattern
Temporomandibular joint	Normal with adequate range of jaw movements

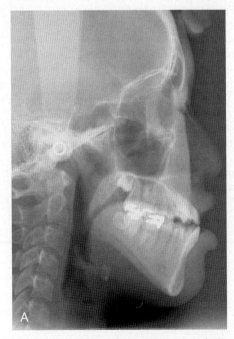 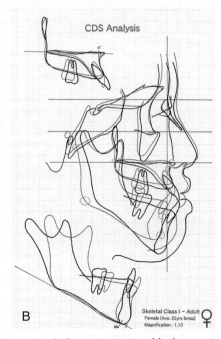

Figure 2-4-2   **A,** Pretreatment lateral cephalogram. **B,** Cephalometric tracing (*black*) superimposed on the composite tracing (*red*) of the average for Japanese norm according to the age.

Diagnosis and Case Summary

A 22-year-old female patient had a concave soft hard and soft tissue profile mainly due to mandibular prognathism. She had a dental Class III relationship with an edge-to-edge anterior bite and labially inclined maxillary incisors. The maxillary midline had shifted to the right side, and crowding was present in both arches.

PROBLEM LIST			
Pathology/Others	Missing tooth bud of mandibular right 8		
Alignment	10 mm of crowding present in maxillary arch Ectopic eruption of maxillary canines 5 mm of crowding present in mandibular arch		
Dimension	**Skeletal**	**Dental**	**Soft Tissue**
Anteroposterior	Convex profile due to mandibular prognathism	Overjet: 0 mm Molar relationship: Class III bilaterally Canine relation: Class III bilaterally Flared maxillary incisors Maxillary lateral incisors in crossbite	Concave soft tissue profile Protrusive lower upper lip
Transverse		Maxillary left first premolar in crossbite Maxillary midline shifted to the right side by 3 mm	
Vertical	Increased lower anterior facial height Increased mandibular plane angle	Overbite: 0 mm Increased incisor display at rest and smile	Incompetent lips

TREATMENT OBJECTIVES			
Pathology/Others	Extract all impacted 8s		
Alignment	Relieve mandibular crowding by distalization of the posterior teeth and create space in the anterior region of the arch for alignment of the anterior teeth		
Dimension	**Skeletal**	**Dental**	**Soft Tissue**
Anteroposterior	Maintain the maxilla Set back the mandible Anteriorly sliding genioplasty	Distalize the maxillary posterior teeth by 6 mm and mandibular posterior teeth by 3 mm to create space in the anterior region for alignment and correction of the molar relation in Class I relationship (postsurgical molar occlusion will be end-on Class II) Correct the maxillary incisor inclination by retracting the anterior teeth into the space created by distalization of posterior teeth Improve the anterior overjet	Correct the concave soft tissue profile and protrusive lower lip by surgical correction of the skeletal discrepancy
Transverse	Maintain	Correct the crossbite of the maxillary left first premolar Shift the maxillary midline to the left by 3 mm by more distalization of posterior teeth on left side	Maintain
Vertical	Genioplasty for correction of increased anterior facial height	Improve anterior overbite	Maintain

Treatment Options

Orthognathic surgery is indicated for the correction of skeletal facial concavity, paranasal deficiency, and Class III malocclusion. Two surgical approaches were available. The first one is the conventional orthognathic surgery approach in which, first, the teeth are aligned and leveled into an ideal relationship with their respective basal arches, and then surgical correction is performed. This treatment approach usually takes approximately 2 to 3 years to complete.

The second alternative could be the "Surgery First Approach" in which there is no presurgical orthodontic phase. The patient is banded and bonded a few weeks before the surgery, and the dental correction is done after the surgical procedure. Some of the advantages of this approach are reduced total treatment time, elimination of the unesthetic period of decompensation of the dental arches, and addressing the patient's chief complaint early in treatment.

Alignment and correction of the crowding in the maxillary and mandibular arch can be performed with the help of extraction, as well as distalization of the posterior segment. Both extraction and distalization option can be combined with conventional surgery, as well as a surgery-first approach. The patient was treated with a surgery-first nonextraction (miniplate-supported distalization) approach.

TREATMENT SEQUENCE AND BIOMECHANICAL PLAN

Maxilla	Mandible
Bond all maxillary teeth and take impression and face bow transfer for surgical stent fabrication.	Bond all mandibular teeth.
Place .017 × .025 inch SS arch wire with surgical hooks soldered on maxillary arch the day before surgery. Place .032 × .032 inch SS TPA to bonded lingual brackets on the first molars.	Place .017 × .025 inch SS arch wire with surgical hooks soldered on mandibular arch the day before surgery.
Orthognathic surgery. Place SAS (skeletal anchorage system) bone plates.	Orthognathic surgery. Place SAS (skeletal anchorage system) bone plates.
Four weeks after surgery, remove the stent and check for appliance breakages, remove the surgical wires, replace all the debonded brackets, place .016 × .022 inch NiTi arch wires and ligate securely. Wear intermaxillary elastics to seat the occlusion.	Four weeks after surgery, remove the stent and check for appliance breakages, remove the surgical wires, replace all the debonded brackets, place .016 × .022 inch NiTi arch wires and ligate securely. Wear intermaxillary elastics to seat the occlusion.
Continue leveling with .017 × .025 inch NiTi arch wire. Distalize the posterior teeth with the help of elastomeric chain from SAS plates.	Continue leveling with .017 × .025 inch NiTi arch wire. Distalize the posterior teeth with the help of an elastomeric chain from SAS plates.
Continue leveling with .019 × .025 inch NiTi arch wire.	Continue leveling with .019 × .025 inch NiTi arch wire.
.016 × .022 inch CNA with finishing bends.	.016 × .022 inch CNA with finishing bends.
Debond and wrap around retainer. Remove SAS plates.	Debond and wrap around retainer. Remove SAS plates.
6-month recall appointment for retention check.	6-month recall appointment for retention check.

CNA, Connecticut new arch wire; NiTi, nickel titanium; SS, stainless steel; TPA, transpalatal arch.

■TREATMENT SEQUENCE

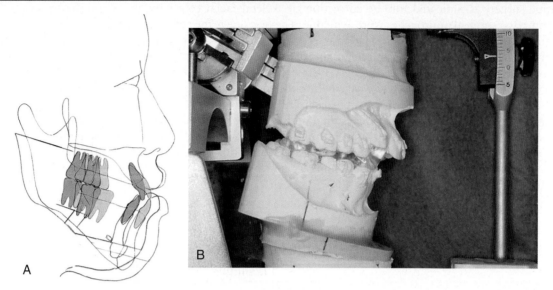

Figure 2-4-3 **A,** Visualized treatment objective. *Blue,* pretreatment; *red,* goal. **B,** Model surgery showing the amount of skeletal movement.

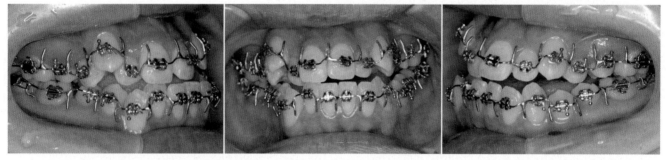

Figure 2-4-4 Passive .017 × .025 inch stainless steel surgical arch wire with soldered surgical hooks placed the day before surgery.

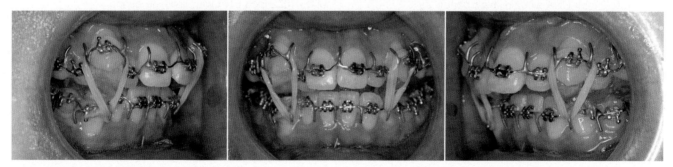

Figure 2-4-5 Two weeks after the surgery. Stent in place with buccal seating elastics.

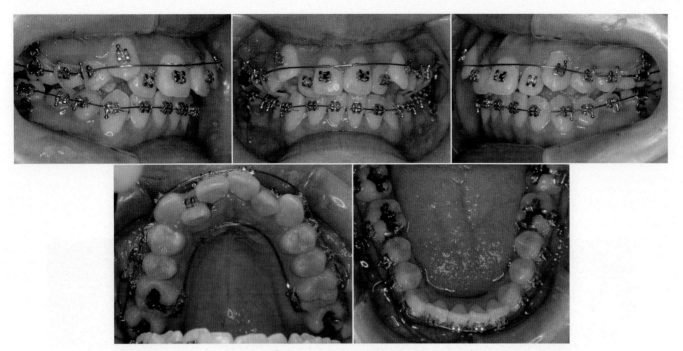

Figure 2-4-6 One month after the surgery. Distalization of the posterior teeth with the help of an elastomeric chain from the skeletal anchorage system plates to the premolars and molars. A .032 × .032 inch Connecticut new arch wire lingual arch in the maxillary arch was used to control the transverse dimension.

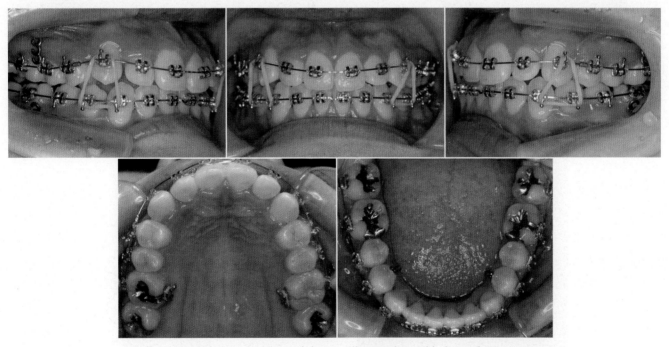

Figure 2-4-7 Leveling of the maxillary and mandibular arches.

■FINAL RESULTS

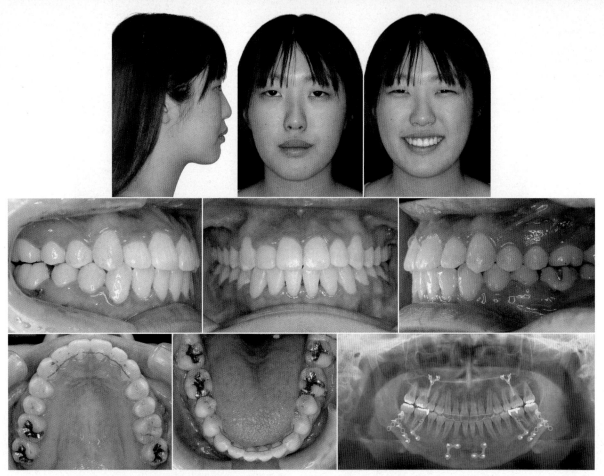

Figure 2-4-8   Posttreatment extraoral/intraoral photographs and panoramic radiograph.

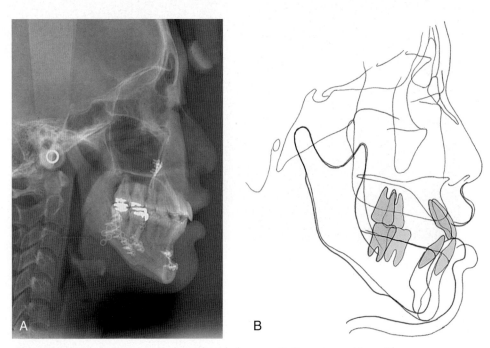

Figure 2-4-9   **A,** Posttreatment lateral cephalogram; **B,** Superimposition. *Blue,* pretreatment; *red,* posttreatment.

Why is the patient overcorrected to a Class II immediately after surgery?
The reason for this is that because of the crowding in the maxilla, the buccal segments including the canine are to be distalized after surgery. The skeleton is normalized after surgery, and it is the orthodontist who will bring occlusion to the proper relationship using the miniplates for distalization of the maxillary teeth. The overcorrection with surgery in a Class III patient is also necessary as slight relapses of the surgical movements are observed during the postsurgical orthodontics phase.

CASE 3-1
Biomechanical Treatment of an Asymmetric Open Bite

A 24-year-old female patient was referred by her general dentist for assessment of anterior open bite. Medical and dental histories were noncontributory, and findings from the temporomandibular joint (TMJ) examination were normal with normal range of jaw movements.

■ PRETREATMENT

Extraoral Analysis (Fig. 3-1-1)

Facial Form	Mesoprosopic
Facial Symmetry	No gross asymmetries noticed
Chin Point	Coincidental with facial midline
Occlusal Plane	Maxillary incisor plane canted
Facial Profile	Convex due to prognathic maxilla
Facial Height	Upper Facial Height/Lower Facial Height: Reduced
	Lower Facial Height/Throat Depth: Increased
Lips	Competent, Upper: Protrusive; Lower: Protrusive
Nasolabial Angle	Normal
Mentolabial Sulcus	Deep
Other	Increased cervicomental angle

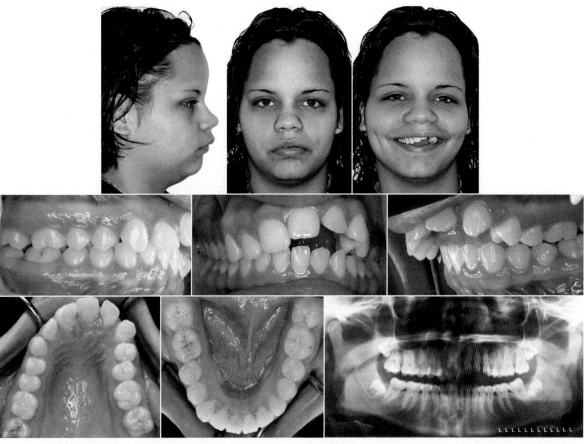

Figure 3-1-1   Pretreatment extraoral/intraoral photographs and panoramic radiograph.

Smile Analysis (Fig. 3-1-2)

Smile Arc	Reverse
Incisor Display	Rest: 0 mm
	Smile: 6 mm (asymmetric)
Lateral Tooth Display	Maxillary molar to molar
Buccal Corridor	Medium
Gingival Tissue	Margins: Irregular
	Papilla: Present in all teeth
Dentition	Tooth size and proportion: Normal
	Tooth shape: Normal
	Axial inclination: Maxillary teeth inclined labially
	Connector space and contact area: Open contacts in maxillary anterior region
Incisal Embrasure	Open
Midlines	Upper and lower dental midlines are coincidental with facial midline

Intraoral Analysis (see Fig. 3-1-2)

Teeth Present	7654321/1234567 Unerupted third molars
	7654321/1234567
Molar Relation	Class II bilaterally
Canine Relation	Class II bilaterally
Overjet	8 mm
Overbite	−5 mm
Maxillary Arch	Asymmetric with spacing and normal curve of Spee
Mandibular Arch	U shaped with adequate arch length and normal curve of Spee
Oral Hygiene	Fair

Functional Analysis

Swallowing	Tongue thrust present
Temporomandibular joint	Normal with adequate range of jaw movements

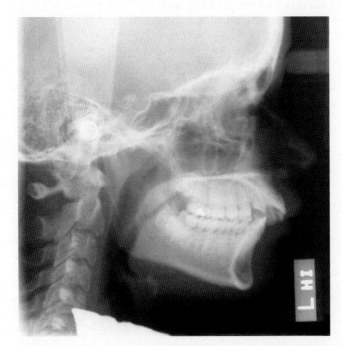

Parameter	Norm	Value
SNA (°)	82	92
SNB (°)	80	81
ANB (°)	2	11
FMA (°)	24	16.5
MP-SN (°)	32	20
U1-NA (mm/°)	4/22	5/28
L1-NA (mm/°)	4/25	7/24
IMPA (°)	95	101
U1-L1 (°)	130	118
OP-SN (°)	14	−0.5
Upper Lip – E Plane (mm)	−4	3
Lower Lip – E Plane (mm)	−2	0
Nasolabial Angle (°)	103	102
Soft Tissue Convexity (°)	135	128

Figure 3-1-2   Pretreatment lateral cephalogram and cephalometric analysis.

Diagnosis and Case Summary

A 24-year-old female patient with skeletal and dental Class II malocclusion with convex soft tissue profile mainly due to prognathic maxilla. The mandibular plane angle is reduced, occlusal plane is flat, and an asymmetric anterior open bite is present, resulting in a reverse smile arc.

PROBLEM LIST			
Pathology/Other	Tongue thrust habit		
Alignment	4-mm spacing present in maxillary arch		
Dimension	**Skeletal**	**Dental**	**Soft Tissue**
Anteroposterior	Class II denture base due to prognathic maxilla	Full cusp Class II molar and canine relation OJ: 8 mm Proclined maxillary incisors Acute interincisal angle	Protrusive upper lip
Vertical	Excessive lower facial height	Anterior open bite: 5 mm Cant of maxillary incisor plane Reduced incisor display on the left anterior segment of the maxilla	
Transverse		Asymmetric maxillary arch form	

OJ, overjet.

TREATMENT OBJECTIVES			
Pathology/Other	Correction of tongue thrust habit		
Alignment	Align and close spaces in maxillary arch		
Dimension	**Skeletal**	**Dental**	**Soft Tissue**
Anteroposterior		Maintain Class II molar relation Retract maxillary incisors to decrease overjet, correct proclination of incisors and acute interincisal angle	Retraction of maxillary incisors to correct protrusion of upper lip
Vertical		Extrusion of left maxillary lateral incisor and canine to correct asymmetric anterior open bite Intrusion of maxillary right lateral incisor and canine to correct the incisal plane cant	
Transverse		Expansion of maxillary arch to coordinate it to mandibular arch form	

Treatment Options

The use of a tongue crib allows control of the tongue thrusting habit, resulting in some spontaneous closure of the open bite. Correction of the overjet and improvement of the soft tissue profile can be obtained by either extraction of maxillary first premolars or distalization of the entire maxillary arch with help of TADs (temporary anchorage devices).

Although both the procedures are expected to achieve the same aesthetic results, distalization of the maxillary arch can lead to longer duration of treatment. With the extraction option, anchorage can be obtained by means of an intrusion arch while the canines and anterior teeth are retracted.

Cant of the maxillary anterior incisal plane can be corrected with help of cantilever mechanics. After considering advantages and disadvantages of both treatment options, the patient chose to undergo extraction of the maxillary first premolars and use of the nickel titanium (NiTi) intrusion arch for controlling anchorage during maxillary anterior retraction.

TREATMENT SEQUENCE AND BIOMECHANICAL PLAN

Maxilla	Mandible
Tongue crib for 3 months and reassess open bite (Fig. 3-1-3).	
Extraction of first premolars.	
Band molars and bond second premolar to second premolar.	Band molars and bond mandibular arch.
Sectional leveling of maxillary right lateral incisor and canine with .016-inch NiTi arch wire.	Level with .016-inch NiTi arch wire.
Continue sectional leveling with .016 × .022 inch NiTi arch wire.	Continue leveling with .016 × .022 inch NiTi arch wire.
.017 × .022 inch CNA base arch wire bypassing maxillary right lateral incisor and canine.	Continue leveling with .017 × .025 inch NiTi arch wire.
Intrusion of maxillary right lateral incisor and canine with help of a .016 × .022 inch CNA cantilever from the auxiliary tube of the right first molar (Fig. 3-1-4).	Continue leveling with .017 × .025 inch NiTi arch wire.
Stainless steel .017 × .025 inch main arch wire with .016 × .022 inch NiTi intrusion arch wire placed in the auxiliary arch wire slot for anchorage control. Individual maxillary canine retraction with elastomeric chain (Fig. 3-1-5).	Continue leveling using .019 × .025 inch NiTi arch wire.
CNA .017 × .025 inch mushroom loop arch wire to close the extraction spaces (Fig. 3-1-6).	Continue leveling with .019 × .025 inch NiTi.
.017 × .025 inch CNA with finishing bends.	.017 × .025 inch CNA arch wire with finishing bends.
Debond and wrap around retainer.	Debond and fixed retainer.
6-month recall appointment for retention check.	6-month recall appointment for retention check.

CNA, Connecticut new arch wire; *NiTi,* nickel titanium.

■TREATMENT SEQUENCE

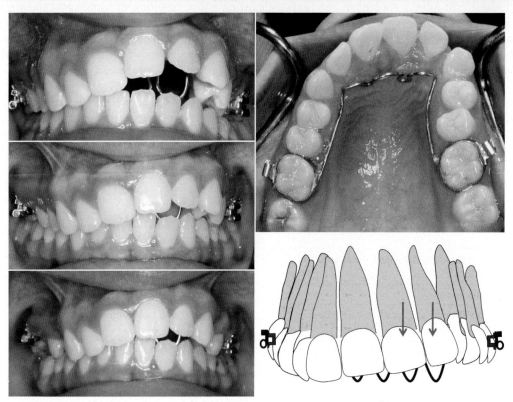

Figure 3-1-3 Crib to prevent anterior displacement of the tongue and allow maxillary anterior teeth to erupt, thus partially correcting the maxillary anterior open bite and anterior incisal plane cant.

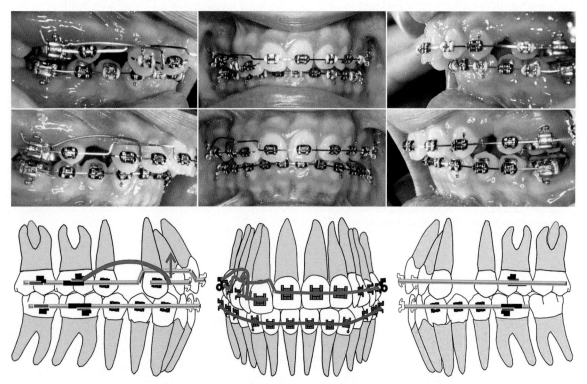

Figure 3-1-4 Cantilever from the auxiliary tube of the molar is used to segmentally intrude the maxillary right canine and lateral incisor and to further correct the cant of the maxillary anterior teeth.

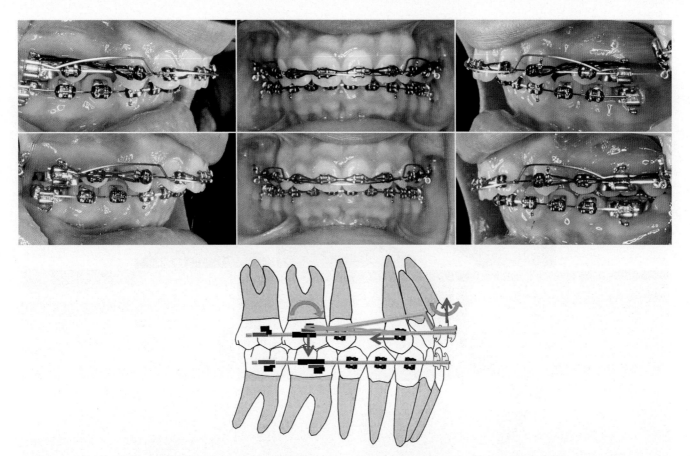

Figure 3-1-5   The intrusion arch produces a clockwise moment, which helps in reinforcing anchorage during the canine retraction stage.

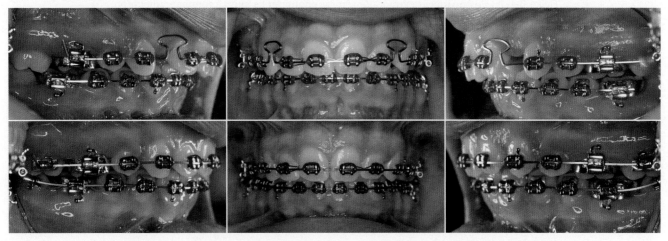

Figure 3-1-6   Retraction of maxillary anterior teeth using mushroom loop arch wire.

■ FINAL RESULTS

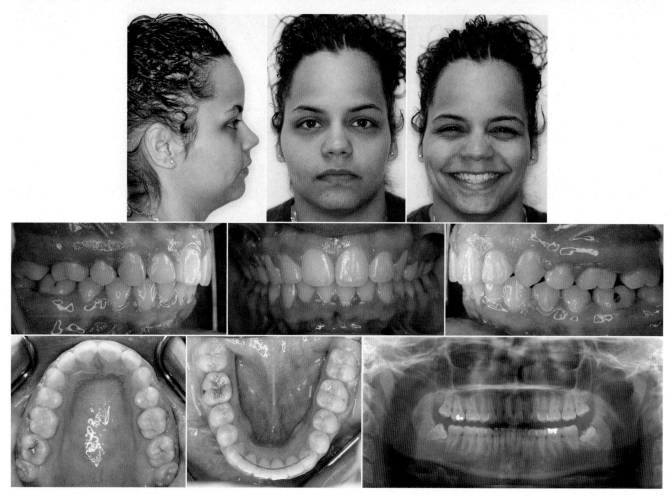

Figure 3-1-7   Posttreatment extraoral/intraoral photographs and panoramic radiograph.

Why is a tongue crib indicated?
In the presence of a tongue-thrusting habit, the tongue tends to protrude between the anterior teeth to attain oral seal during swallowing. The tongue crib helps to keep away the tongue from the teeth, allowing vertical eruption of teeth.

Why extraction of first the premolar instead of distalization of the maxillary arch?
For Class I molar relationship in a nonextraction approach to be attained, 5-mm distalization of entire the maxillary arch was required. Such a large movement of so many teeth is best performed in a two-step approach. First, distalization of the posterior teeth is performed. In the second step, retraction of anterior the teeth is addressed. Both of these steps are expected to take 6 to 8 months each, increasing total treatment time. Furthermore, to achieve the objective of maintaining the anteroposterior inclination of the lower incisors, distalization would need to be TAD supported.

Why were lower incisors not retracted?
Lower incisors were well aligned before the start of treatment, in spite of increased incisor mandibular plane angle (IMPA); hence we can expect them to remain stable later in life since no further flaring occurred during treatment.

CASE 4-1
Orthognathic Surgery for Significant Vertical Excess, Facial Convexity, and Large Interlabial Gap

A 17-year-old postpubertal male patient's chief complaint was "my lips don't come together." Medical and dental histories were noncontributory, and findings from a temporomandibular joint (TMJ) examination were normal with adequate range of jaw movements.

■ PRETREATMENT

Extraoral Analysis (Fig. 4-1-1)

Facial Form	Leptoprosopic
Facial Symmetry	No gross asymmetries noticed
Chin Point	Coincidental with the facial midline
Occlusal Plane	Steep
Facial Profile	Convex due to retrognathic mandible
Facial Height	Upper Facial Height/Lower Facial Height: Reduced
	Lower Facial Height/Throat Depth: Increased
Lips	Incompetent, Upper: Protrusive; Lower: Protrusive. Mental strain on closure
Nasolabial Angle	Obtuse
Mentolabial Sulcus	Deep

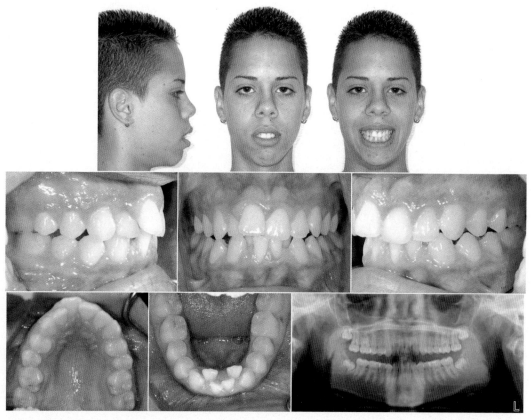

Figure 4-1-1 Pretreatment extraoral/intraoral photographs and panoramic radiograph.

Smile Analysis (Fig. 4-1-2)

Smile Arch	Flat
Incisor Display	Rest: 9 mm
	Smile: 12 mm
Lateral Tooth Display	Second premolar to second premolar
Buccal Corridor	Normal
Gingival Tissue	Gingival margins: Normal architecture
	Papilla: Present
	Reduced attached gingiva with slight recession on labial of mandibular central incisors
Dentition	Tooth size and proportion: Normal
	Tooth shape: Normal
	Axial inclination: Maxillary and mandibular teeth inclined labially
	Connector space and contact area: Normal
Incisal Embrasure	Not observed between maxillary central incisors as these teeth overlap
Midlines	Lower midline shifted to the left side by 2 mm as compared with facial midline

Intraoral Analysis (see Fig. 4-1-2)

Teeth Present	7654321/1234567
	7654321/1234567 Unerupted 8s
Molar Relation	Class III on the right
Canine Relation	Class I bilaterally
Overjet	5 mm
Overbite	3 mm
Maxillary Arch	U shaped, asymmetric with 5 mm of crowding
Mandibular Arch	U shaped, crowding of 10 mm and normal curve of Spee
Oral Hygiene	Fair

Functional Analysis

Swallowing	Normal adult pattern
Temporomandibular joint	Normal with adequate range of jaw movements

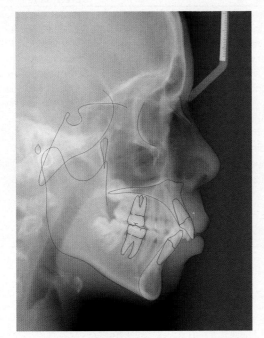

Parameter	Norm	Value
SNA (°)	82	78
SNB (°)	80	71
ANB (°)	2	7
FMA (°)	24	28
MP-SN (°)	32	40
U1-NA (mm/°)	4/22	6/24
L1-NA (mm/°)	4/25	9/30
IMPA (°)	95	95
U1-L1 (°)	130	118
OP-SN (°)	14	21
Upper Lip – E Plane (mm)	−4	4
Lower Lip – E Plane (mm)	−2	6
Nasolabial Angle (°)	103	107
Wits appraisal (mm)	−1	5

Figure 4-1-2 Pretreatment lateral cephalogram with tracing and cephalometric analysis.

Diagnosis and Case Summary

A 17-year-old male patient had convex skeletal and soft tissue profile mainly due to a retrognathic mandible. He had a Class I malocclusion with high mandibular plane angle, labially positioned and flared maxillary and mandibular incisors, reduced interincisal angle, and protrusive lips with a large interlabial gap.

PROBLEM LIST			
Pathology/Others	Reduced attached gingiva with slight recession on labial of mandibular central incisors		
Alignment	5 mm of crowding present in maxillary arch and 10 mm of crowding in mandibular arch		
Dimension	**Skeletal**	**Dental**	**Soft Tissue**
Anteroposterior	Convex profile with retrognathic mandible	OJ: 5 mm Class III molar relationship on the right Upper and lower incisors are labially placed Upper and lower incisors are proclined Acute interincisal angle	Convex soft tissue profile Protrusive upper and lower lip
Transverse		Mandibular midline shifted to the left side by 2 mm Crossbite tendency on molar/premolar region	
Vertical	High mandibular plane angle Long lower facial height Excessive maxillary vertical height	Excessive incisor display at rest and smile Steep occlusal plane	Large interlabial gap Mentalis strain upon lip closure

OJ, overjet.

TREATMENT OBJECTIVES			
Pathology/Others	Monitor labial gingiva of mandibular incisors		
Alignment	Relieve the mandibular crowding by extraction of first premolars in all the quadrants		
Dimension	**Skeletal**	**Dental**	**Soft Tissue**
Anteroposterior	Correct the skeletal convexity by mandibular autorotation and anterior sliding genioplasty	Reduce overjet and improve the inclination of maxillary and mandibular incisor, improve interincisal angle by retraction of the anterior teeth into extraction space	Correct the convex soft tissue profile by surgical correction of the skeletal discrepancy Correction of protrusive upper and lower lips by retracting anterior teeth
Transverse		Shift the mandibular midline by 2 mm to the right Coordinate arches in premolar area	
Vertical	Improve mandibular plane angle by reducing the vertical height of the maxilla and autorotation of the mandible Anterior sliding genioplasty to reduce the lower facial height	Improve incisal display at rest and smile by maxillary impaction	Reduce interlabial gap and mentalis strain

Treatment Options

Correction of the vertical maxillary excess, retrognathic profile, and significant intralabial gap would necessitate orthognathic surgery to address the aesthetics in the dentofacial deformity. Vertical maxillary impaction would reduce the upper facial height and reduce the amount of incisor show at rest. For the skeletal convexity to be corrected, mandibular autorotation as a result of maxillary impaction along with genioplasty (if necessary to improve chin projection).

Extraction of premolars would be necessary to create space in the dental arches to relieve the maxillary and mandibular crowding, correct the incisal inclination, and reduce the amount of lip protrusion.

TREATMENT SEQUENCE AND BIOMECHANICAL PLAN

Maxilla	Mandible
Extract first premolars.	Extract first premolars.
Band molars, bond maxillary arch, level with .016 inch NiTi arch wire.	Band molars and bond mandibular arch. Level with .016 inch NiTi arch wire.
Continue leveling with .016 × .022 inch NiTi arch wire.	Continue leveling using .016 × .022 inch NiTi arch wire, push coil between central and lateral incisor.
Continue leveling with .017 × .025 inch NiTi arch wire.	Continue leveling with .017 × .025 inch NiTi arch wire.
Continue leveling with .019 × .025 inch NiTi arch wire.	Continue leveling with .019 × .025 inch NiTi arch wire.
Place .019 × .025 inch SS arch wire, retract anterior teeth, and close extraction spaces with elastomeric chain.	Place .019 × .025 inch SS arch wire, retract anterior teeth with help of elastomeric chain.
Place .019 × .025 inch SS arch wire with surgical hooks. Iowa spaces distal to lateral incisors to ensure proper occlusion after surgery.	Place .019 × .025 SS arch wire with surgical hooks.
Orthognathic surgery, maxillary impaction.	Orthognathic surgery: genioplasty.
.016 × .022 inch CNA with finishing bends.	.016 × .022 inch CNA with finishing bends.
Debond and wrap around retainer.	Debond and fixed retainer.
6-month recall appointment for retention check.	6-month recall appointment for retention check.

CNA, Connecticut new arch wire; *NiTi,* nickel titanium; *SS,* stainless steel.

■ TREATMENT SEQUENCE

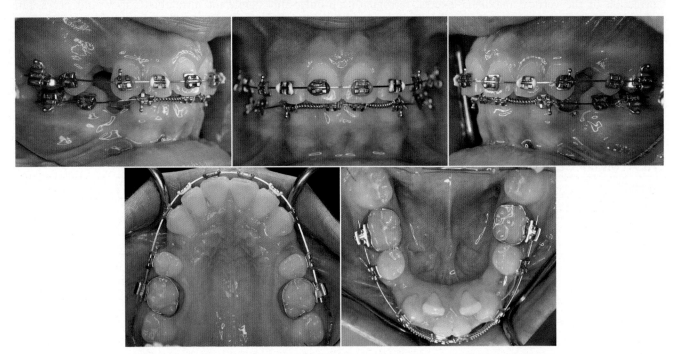

Figure 4-1-3   Initial alignment in both arches after extraction of first premolars.

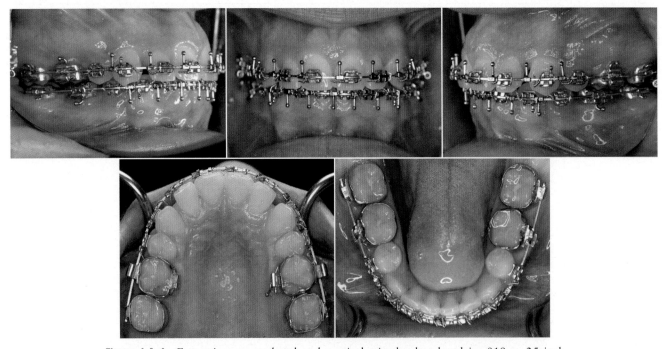

Figure 4-1-4   Extraction space closed and surgical wire hooks placed in .019 × .25 inch stainless steel wire. Iowa spaces present distal to maxillary lateral incisors before surgery.

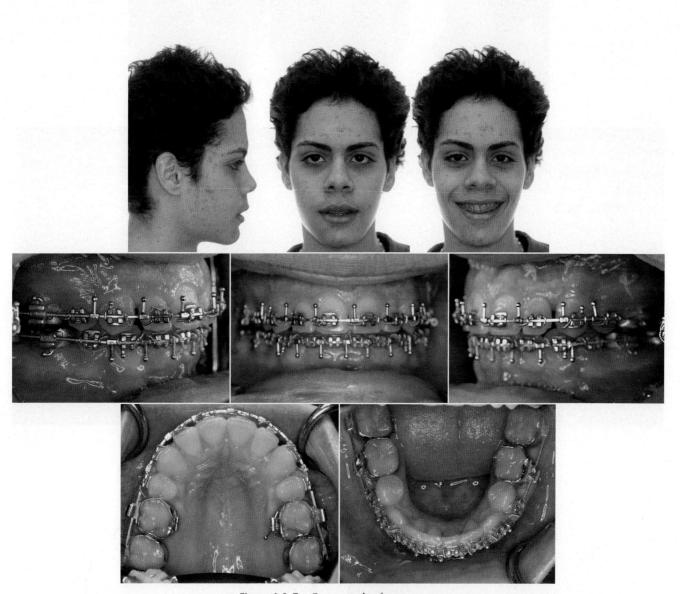

Figure 4-1-5   One month after surgery.

◼ FINAL RESULTS

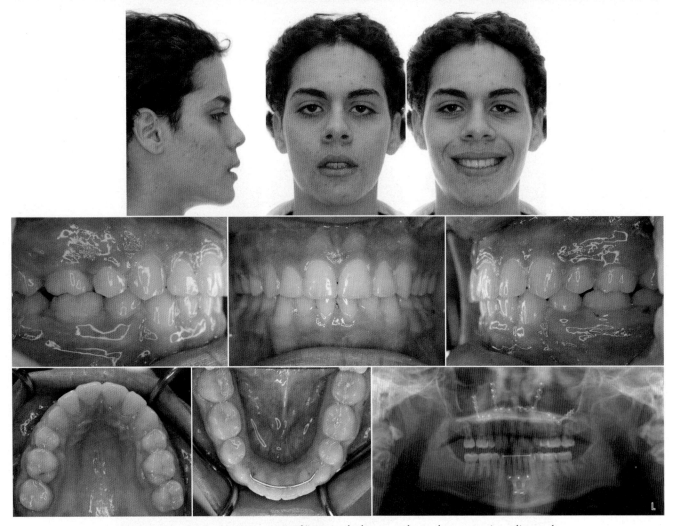

Figure 4-1-6   Posttreatment extraoral/intraoral photographs and panoramic radiograph.

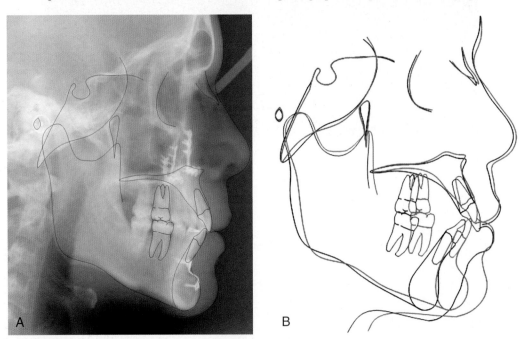

Figure 4-1-7   **A,** Posttreatment lateral cephalogram. **B,** Superimposition. *Black,* pretreatment; *red,* posttreatment.

What options are available to reduce an excessive interlabial gap?
Orthognathic surgery is perhaps the best approach to reduce an excessive interlabial gap, especially in patients with vertical maxillary excess and retrognathic mandible. In these patients maxillary impaction and the resulting autorotation improve significantly lip competence and aesthetics. Often an anterior sliding genioplasty contributes to further reduce the profile convexity and anterior facial height.

Although retraction of the incisors after extraction of premolars may improve in itself the interlabial gap, usually the impact of the correction is far less evident than the change observed with orthognathic surgery.

Section 2

Anteroposterior Problems

CASE 5-1
Intrusion and Retraction of the Anterior Maxillary Teeth by Means of a Three-Piece Intrusion Assembly

A 14-year-old female patient's chief complaint was crowding in the front region of the mandible. Medical and dental histories were noncontributory, and findings from the temporomandibular joint (TMJ) examination were normal with adequate range of jaw movements.

■ PRETREATMENT

Extraoral Analysis (Fig. 5-1-1)

Facial Form	Mesoprosopic
Facial Symmetry	No gross asymmetries noted
Chin Point	Coincidental with facial midline
Occlusal Plane	Normal
Facial Profile	Convex due to retrognathic mandible
Facial Height	Upper Facial Height/Lower Facial Height: Reduced
	Lower Facial Height/Throat Depth: Normal
Lips	Competent, Upper: Protrusive; Lower: Protrusive
Nasolabial Angle	Normal
Mentolabial Sulcus	Shallow

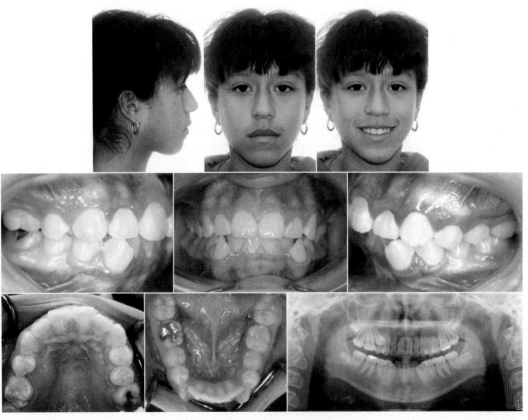

Figure 5-1-1   Pretreatment extraoral/intraoral photographs and panoramic radiograph.

Smile Analysis (Fig. 5-1-2)

Smile Arc	Consonant
Incisor Display	Rest: 1 mm
	Smile: 10 mm
Lateral Tooth Display	Maxillary: First premolar to first premolar
Buccal Corridor	Minimal
Gingival Tissue	Margins: Maxillary left central and lateral have slight more incisal position
	Papilla: Present in all teeth
Dentition	Tooth size and proportion: Normal
	Tooth shape: Normal
	Axial Inclination: Normal
Connector Space and Contact Area	Closed contacts
Incisal Embrasure	Normal
Midlines	Upper dental midline is coincidental with facial midline. Lower dental midline is 1 mm left of the facial midline

Intraoral Analysis (see Fig. 5-1-2)

Teeth Present	764321/1234567
	7654321/1234567 Unerupted third molars and impacted right maxillary second premolar
Molar Relation	Class II end on right side and Class I on left side
Canine Relation	Class II end on right side and Class I on left side
Overjet	4 mm
Overbite	3 mm
Maxillary Arch	Asymmetric crowding with impacted right second premolar
Mandibular Arch	U shaped with blocked-out canines and normal curve of Spee
Oral Hygiene	Fair

Functional Analysis

Swallowing	Adult
Temporomandibular joint	Normal with adequate range of jaw movements

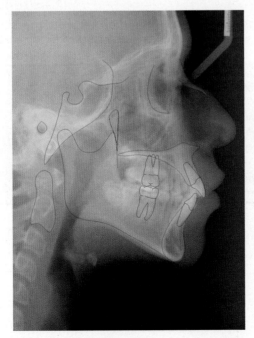

Parameter	Norm	Value
SNA (°)	82	77
SNB (°)	80	71
ANB (°)	2	6
FMA (°)	24	28
MP-SN (°)	32	45
U1-NA (mm/°)	4/22	4/22
L1-NA (mm/°)	4/25	8/31
IMPA (°)	95	94
U1-L1 (°)	130	120
OP-SN (°)	14	30
Upper Lip – E Plane (mm)	−4	1.9
Lower Lip – E Plane (mm)	−2	0.6
Nasolabial Angle (°)	103	90
Soft Tissue Convexity (°)	135	124

Figure 5-1-2   Pretreatment lateral cephalogram with tracing and cephalometric analysis.

Diagnosis and Case Summary

A 14-year-old female patient came with a convex hard and soft tissue profile mainly due to retrognathic mandible and a dental Class II subdivision malocclusion. Increased mandibular plane angle and severe crowding were present in the maxillary and mandibular arch.

PROBLEM LIST			
Pathology/Others	Deep lingual fossa maxillary incisors Brown discoloration cusp tip right maxillary canine and distobuccal cusp of right maxillary first molar		
Alignment	Maxilla: Crowding of 8 mm Mandible: Crowding of 14 mm Impacted maxillary second premolar		
Dimension	**Skeletal**	**Dental**	**Soft Tissue**
Anteroposterior	Class II denture base due to retrognathic mandible	Class II End molar and canine on right side OJ: 4 mm Proclined mandibular incisors Acute interincisal angle End to end relationship of mandibular canines with maxillary lateral incisors	Protrusive upper and lower lips
Vertical	Increased lower anterior facial height		
Transverse		Labially placed mandibular canines Lower midline 1 mm to the left of facial midline	

OJ, overjet.

TREATMENT OBJECTIVES			
Pathology/Others	Reinforce oral hygiene Inform patient regarding brown discolorations Evaluate prominent marginal ridges on maxillary incisors to achieve proper buccal occlusion (contour if necessary)		
Alignment	Correction of maxillary and mandibular crowding with extractions of premolars (all first premolars except in the maxillary right quadrant where the second premolar is to be extracted)		
Dimension	**Skeletal**	**Dental**	**Soft Tissue**
Anteroposterior	Maintain	Correction of Class II end on molar relation on right side Slight retraction of maxillary anterior teeth to reduce overjet Maintain mandibular incisor inclination Eliminate edge to edge relationship between mandibular canines and maxillary lateral incisors	Maintain
Vertical			
Transverse		Align mandibular canines into the arch Correct lower dental midline with space closure	

Treatment Options

Correction of maxillary and mandibular crowding and slight improvement of the overjet and soft tissue profile make this a high-anchorage case and necessitate 4 premolar extraction. On the maxillary right side, either first or second premolar extraction can be done as both are expected to result in a similar outcome. Space remaining after correction of crowding needs to be closed by retraction of all the anterior teeth for correction of overjet. Anchorage on the right side would be critical. In the mandibular arch, all the extraction space is necessary to accommodate the labially placed canines.

TREATMENT SEQUENCE AND BIOMECHANICAL PLAN

Maxilla	Mandible
Extraction of right second premolar (impacted) and left first premolar.	Extraction of first premolars.
Band molars and bond maxillary arch.	Band molars and bond mandibular arch.
Leveling of maxillary arch with .016, .018, .016, × .022 inch NiTi arch wires (Fig. 5-1-3).	Leveling of maxillary arch with .016, .018 inch NiTi arch wires (Fig. 5-1-3).
Continue leveling with .017 × .025 inch NiTi arch wire.	Continue leveling with .017 × .025 inch NiTi arch wire, place elastomeric chain for closing of remanent spaces.
Stainless steel .017 × .025 inch section arch wire from lateral to lateral, .017 × .025 inch CNA cantilever arch wire from auxiliary slot of the molar tube with 40 g of intrusion force. Elastomeric chain with retraction force of 40 g attached from molar tube hook to the anterior sectional wire (Fig. 5-1-5).	
Finishing with CNA .016 × .022 inch arch wire (Fig. 5-1-8).	Finishing with CNA .016 × .022 inch arch wire (Fig. 5-1-8).
Debond and wrap around retainer.	Debond and fixed retainer.
6-month recall appointment for retention check.	6-month recall appointment for retention check.

CNA, Connecticut new arch wire; NiTi, nickel titanium.

■ TREATMENT SEQUENCE

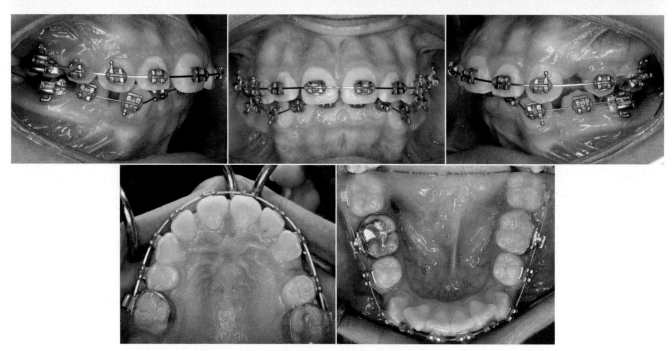

Figure 5-1-3 Initial alignment after extraction of all first premolars (except in the upper right quadrant where the impacted second premolar was extracted).

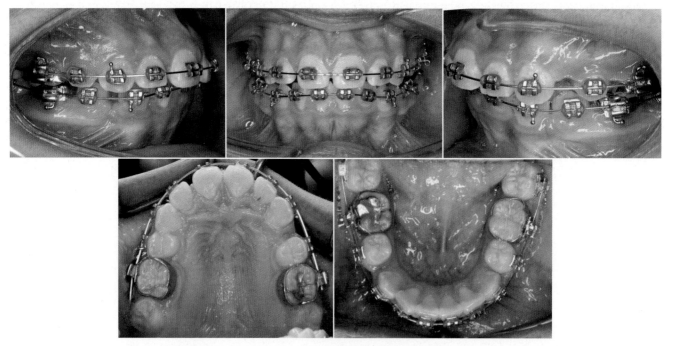

Figure 5-1-4 Correction of labially placed mandibular canines.

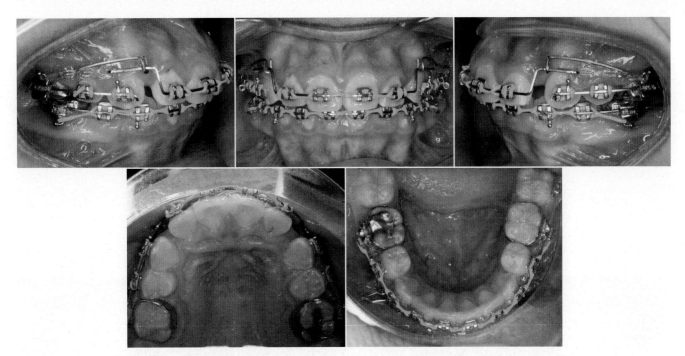

Figure 5-1-5 Three-piece intrusion retraction mechanics. Closure of mandibular extraction spaces with help of elastomeric chain.

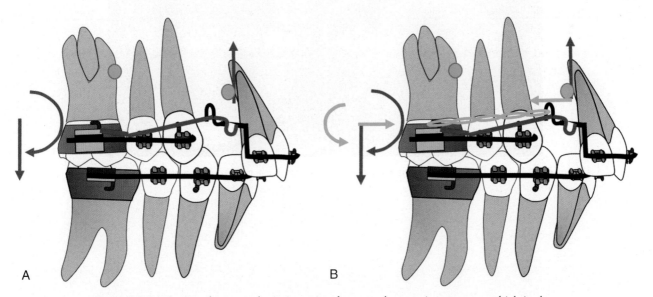

A   B

Figure 5-1-6 **A,** Cantilever results in intrusion force on the anterior segment, which is close to the resistance of the anterior segment, clockwise moment, and extrusion force on the posterior segment. **B,** Retractive force creates a resultant force acting through the center of resistance, parallel to the long axes of the anterior teeth, and a counterclockwise moment on the posterior teeth (*green*). The resultant clockwise moment on the posterior segment reinforces the posterior anchorage.

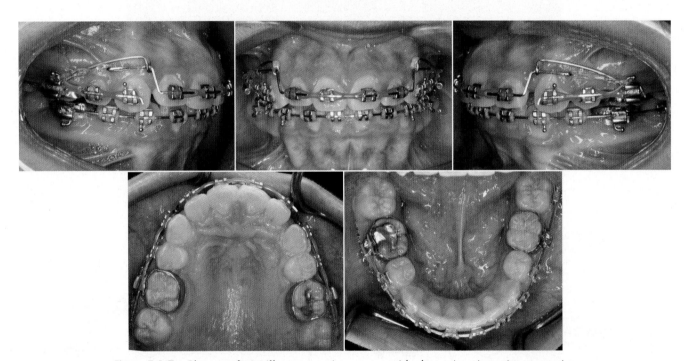

Figure 5-1-7 Closure of maxillary extraction spaces with three-piece intrusion retraction mechanics.

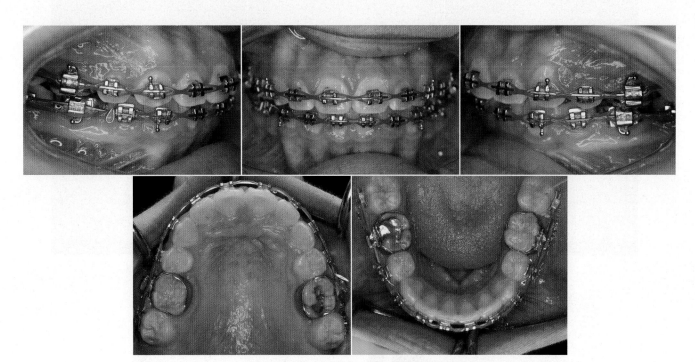

Figure 5-1-8   Final finishing and detailing.

■ FINAL RESULTS

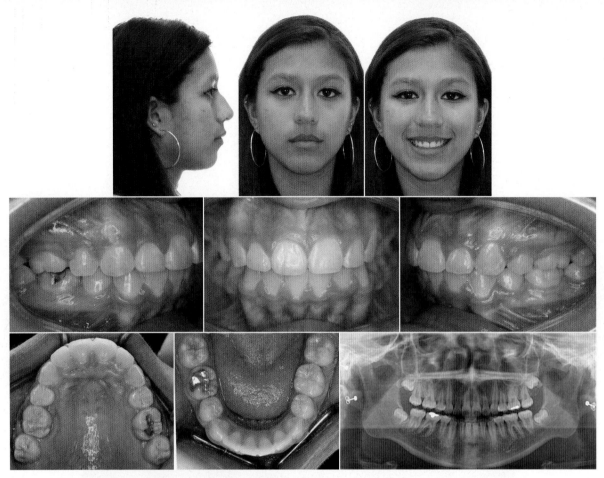

Figure 5-1-9   Posttreatment extraoral/intraoral photographs and panoramic radiograph.

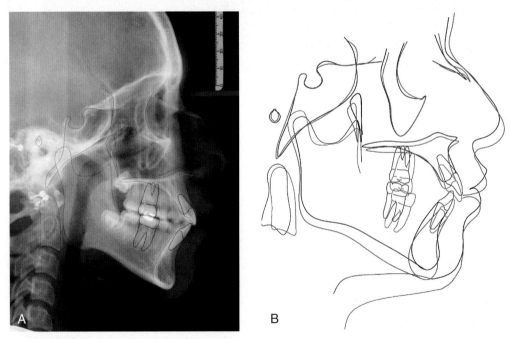

Figure 5-1-10   **A,** Posttreatment lateral cephalogram. **B,** Superimposition. *Black,* pretreatment; *red,* posttreatment.

What are the advantages of the three-piece intrusion arch for retraction of the anterior teeth?

The intrusion retraction appliance is a precise method to deliver a force system tailored to translate the anterior teeth during space closure. The application of an intrusive force by means of a cantilever through the center of resistance of the anterior segment facilitates a translatory movement of these teeth. Also, because the retraction force is applied close to the center of resistance of the anterior segment, bodily movement of the anterior teeth is facilitated.

CASE 5-2
Correction of Bimaxillary Protrusion Using Fiber Reinforced Composite for Space Closure*

A 23-year-old female presented with the chief complaint that "my teeth stick out." Medical and dental histories were noncontributory, and findings from a temporomandibular joint (TMJ) examination were normal with adequate range of jaw movements.

■ PRETREATMENT

Extraoral Analysis (Fig. 5-2-1)

Facial Form	Mesoprosopic
Facial Symmetry	No gross asymmetries noticed
Chin Point	Coincidental with facial midline
Occlusal Plane	Flat
Facial Profile	Convex due to bimaxillary dentoalveolar protrusion
Facial Height	Upper Facial Height/Lower Facial Height: Normal
	Lower Facial Height/Throat Depth: Normal
Lips	Upper: Protrusive; Lower: Protrusive
Nasolabial Angle	Acute
Mentolabial Sulcus	Normal

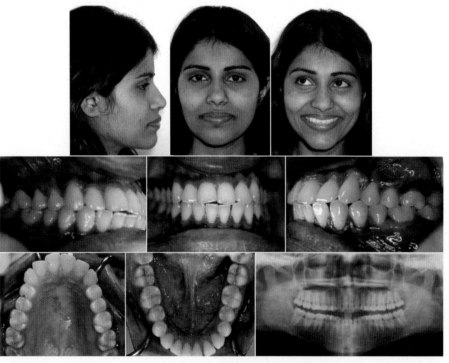

Figure 5-2-1 Initial records of a patient exhibiting bimaxillary dentoalveolar protrusion. Patient shows carious lesion on distal of maxillary right first premolar.

*Portions of Case 5-2 from Uribe F, Nanda R. Treatment of bimaxillary protrusion using fiber-reinforced composite. *J Clin Orthod.* 2007; 41:27-32.

Smile Analysis (Fig. 5-2-2)

Smile Arc	Flat
Incisor Display	Rest: 0 mm
	Smile: 8 mm
Lateral Tooth Display	First molar to first molar
Buccal Corridor	Minimal
Gingival Tissue	Margins: Normal relationship except for mild recession of maxillary left lateral and canine
	Mandibular anteriors have mild recession including left canine
	Recession on maxillary first premolars and left second premolars, as well as mandibular left first premolar
	Papilla: Present in all teeth
Dentition	Tooth size and proportion: Normal
	Tooth shape: Normal
	Axial inclination: Maxillary and mandibular incisors are inclined labially
	Caries of the disto-occlusal surface of maxillary right first premolar
	Connector space and contact area: Closed contacts
Incisal Embrasure	Normal
Dental Midlines	Upper midline is coincidental with facial midline
	Lower midline is shifted to the left by 1 mm as compared with facial midline

Intraoral Analysis (see Fig. 5-2-2)

Teeth Present	87654321/12345678
	87654321/12345678
Molar Relation	Class I bilaterally
Canine Relation	Class I bilaterally
Overjet	0 mm
Overbite	0 mm
Maxillary Arch	U shaped, symmetric
Mandibular Arch	U shaped, symmetric with 1 mm of spacing
Oral Hygiene	Fair

Functional Analysis

Swallowing	Adult
Temporomandibular joint	Normal with adequate range of jaw movements

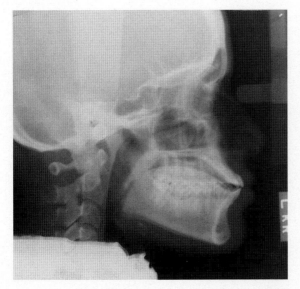

Parameter	Norm	Value
SNA (°)	82	86
SNB (°)	80	84
ANB (°)	2	2
FMA (°)	24	19
MP-SN (°)	32	25
U1-NA (mm/°)	4/22	9/40
L1-NA (mm/°)	4/25	8/38
IMPA (°)	95	117
U1-L1 (°)	130	112
OP-SN (°)	14	10
Upper Lip – E Plane (mm)	−4	0
Lower Lip – E Plane (mm)	−2	2
Nasolabial Angle (°)	103	97

Figure 5-2-2 Pretreatment lateral cephalogram and cephalometric analysis.

Diagnosis and Case Summary

A 23-year-old female patient presented with a convex hard and soft tissue profile due to bimaxillary dentoalveolar protrusion. She had a Class I malocclusion with reduced mandibular plane angle, labially placed and flared maxillary and mandibular anterior teeth, and protrusive upper and lower lips.

PROBLEM LIST			
Pathology/Others	Carious lesion on maxillary right first premolar		
	Mild recession in maxillary left lateral incisor and canine, maxillary first premolars and left second premolars, and mandibular left first premolar		
Alignment	Mandible: Spacing of 1 mm		
Dimension	**Skeletal**	**Dental**	**Soft Tissue**
Anteroposterior	Convex profile due to bimaxillary protrusion	OJ: 0 mm Proclined maxillary and mandibular incisors Acute interincisal angle	Protrusive upper and lower lips Acute nasolabial angle
Vertical	Reduced mandibular plane angle	Flat occlusal plane OB: 0 mm	Reduced incisor display at rest and smile
Transverse		Lower midline 1 mm to the left of facial midline	

OB, overbite; OJ, overjet.

TREATMENT OBJECTIVES			
Pathology/Others	Carious lesion on maxillary first premolar will be addressed (by extraction) as part of the global treatment plan to reduce bimaxillary protrusion		
Alignment	Correction of mandibular spacing by retraction of anterior teeth		
Dimension	**Skeletal**	**Dental**	**Soft Tissue**
Anteroposterior		Improve the proclination of maxillary and mandibular anterior teeth by retraction into the space created by extraction of first premolars	Retraction of maxillary and mandibular incisors to correct lip protrusion
Vertical		Increase OB by extrusion of maxillary and mandibular incisors	Maintain
Transverse		Match lower midline to facial midline	

OB, overbite.

Treatment Options

Correction of maxillary and mandibular incisor inclination and improvement of upper and lower lip protrusion requires 4 premolar extraction. Because the amount of dentoalveolar protrusion is so severe, closure of extraction space entirely by retraction of anterior teeth is desirable, resulting in the necessity to reinforce posterior anchorage. Posterior anchorage can be reinforced by application of differential moments (i.e., promoting bodily mesial movement of the posterior teeth against lingual tipping of the anterior teeth).

The most common way of creating differential moments for extraction space closure is loop mechanics, which is based on the off-center V bend principle. The closer the V bend toward a section of the arch is, the higher the moment is generated and anchorage is reinforced. The retraction force of the anterior teeth is provided by a nickel titanium coil spring instead of a loop.

TREATMENT SEQUENCE AND BIOMECHANICAL PLAN

Maxilla	Mandible
Extraction of first premolars.	Extraction of first premolars.
Splint molars and second premolars with FRC to create a single unit. Bond first molar bracket on first molars. Bond canine to canine. Initial aligning .018 inch NiTi arch wire.	Splint molars and second premolars with FRC to create a single unit. Bond first molar bracket on first molars. Bond canine to canine. Initial aligning .018 inch NiTi arch wire.
Place .018 inch SS arch wire with gable bends about one third of the distance from the first molars to the canines. Place nickel titanium coil springs from molar tube to the canine bracket, applying 150 g of retraction force.	Place .018 inch SS arch wire with gable bends about one third of the distance from the first molars to the canines. Place NiTi coil springs from molar tube to the canine bracket, applying 150 g of retractive force.
Finishing with CNA .016 × .022 inch arch wire.	Finishing with CNA .016 × .022 inch arch wire.
Debond and wrap around retainer.	Debond and fixed retainer.
6-month recall appointment for retention check.	6-month recall appointment for retention check.

CNA, Connecticut new arch wire; *FRC,* fiber reinforced composite; *NiTi,* nickel titanium; *SS,* stainless steel.

■ TREATMENT SEQUENCE

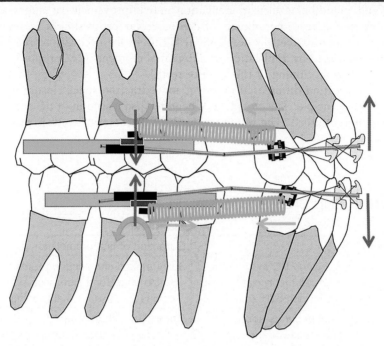

Figure 5-2-3 Diagram depicting the appliance used for en-masse retraction of the upper and lower anterior teeth after extraction of the four first premolars. Fiber reinforced composite was placed in the upper and lower buccal segments at the initial bonding visit. A .018 stainless steel arch wire with a gable bend approximately 4 mm in front of the first molars produces a tip-back moment. The arch wire was engaged anteriorly from canine to canine. The anterior segment was co-ligated together, and nickel titanium retraction springs connected the anterior and posterior segments.

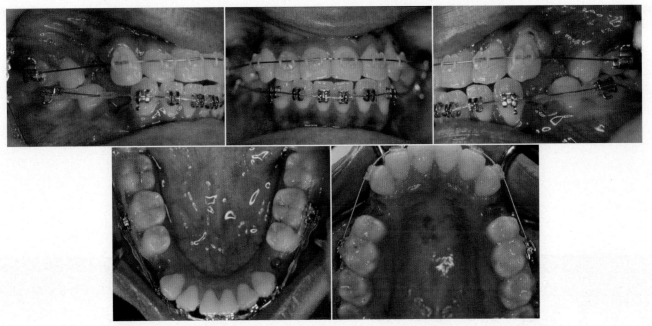

Figure 5-2-4 Initial bonding visit. Fiber reinforced composite is observed in the occlusal slides from the second molars to second premolars in upper and lower arches. Initial nickel titanium aligning arch wire with a light elastic chain from first molar to first molar.

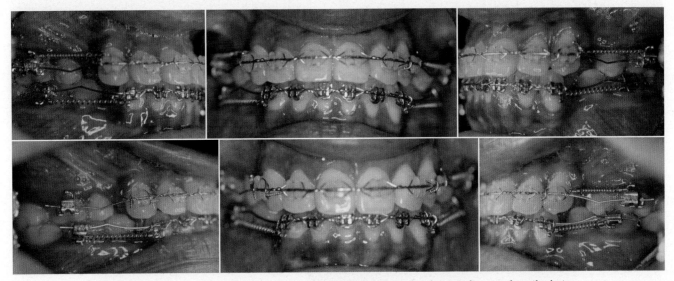

Figure 5-2-5 Images of space closure progression with the appliance described in Figure 5-2-3.

▪ FINAL RESULTS

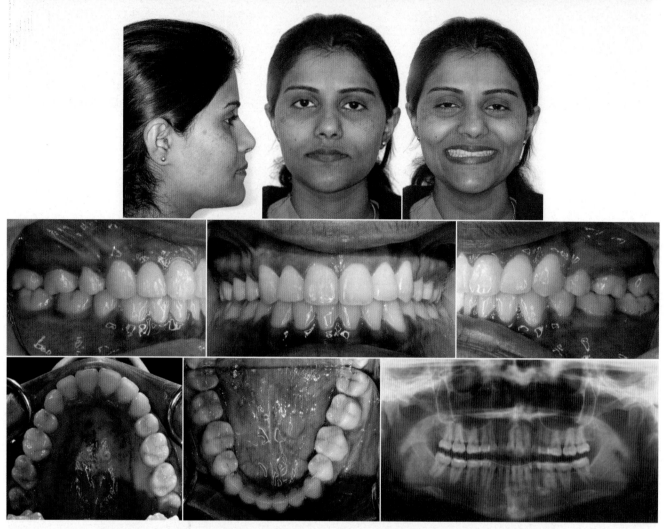

Figure 5-2-6 Posttreatment extraoral/intraoral photographs and panoramic radiograph. Final records showing the maintenance of good occlusion and controlled retraction of the anterior teeth with significant reduction of lip protrusion.

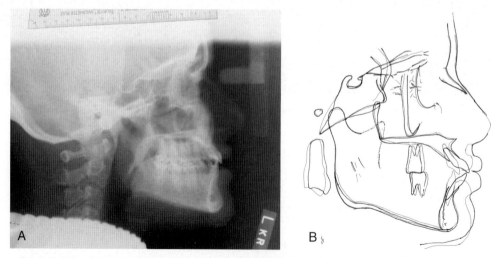

Figure 5-2-7 **A,** Posttreatment lateral cephalogram. **B,** Superimposition. *Black,* pretreatment; *blue,* posttreatment. General superimpositions illustrating good anchorage preservation and significant incisor retraction by controlled tipping.

Why was retraction of anterior teeth performed on round wire?
This method allows for en masse retraction of the anterior teeth during space closure. The method can be incorporated to straight wire mechanics by adding a gable bend to a round stainless steel wire, usually of .018-inch dimension. The bend allows one to control anchorage in the posterior segment and promotes intrusion of the anterior teeth, which, combined with a retraction force from the nickel titanium coil spring, results in tipping of the incisors with the incisal edge moving along the occlusal plane. The cross section of the wire prevents a moment from being generated in the incisors, which could make the force system indeterminate.

CASE 6-1
Anchorage Control with a Cantilever in a Unilateral Class II Malocclusion

A 12-year-old female patient's chief complaint was crowding in her upper and lower front teeth. Medical and dental histories were noncontributory, and findings from a temporomandibular (TMJ) examination were normal with adequate range of jaw movements.

■ PRETREATMENT

Extraoral Analysis (Fig. 6-1-1)

Facial Form	Mesoprosopic
Facial Symmetry	No gross asymmetry noted
Chin Point	Coincidental with facial midline
Occlusal Plane	Normal
Facial Profile	Convex due to a retrognathic mandible
Facial Height	Upper Facial Height/Lower Facial Height: Normal
	Lower Facial Height/Throat Depth: Normal
Lips	Competent, Upper: Normal; Lower: Normal
Nasolabial Angle	Normal
Mentolabial Sulcus	Normal

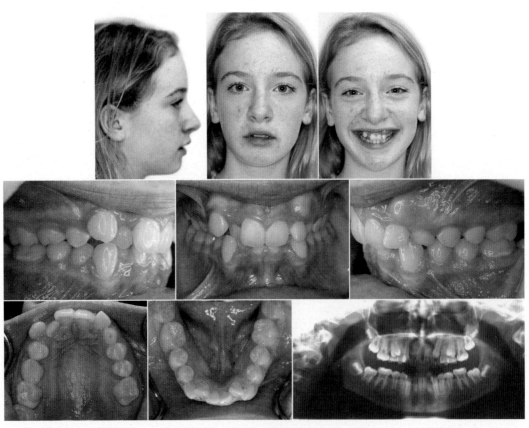

Figure 6-1-1 Pretreatment extraoral/intraoral photographs and panoramic radiograph.

Smile Analysis (Fig. 6-1-2)

Smile Arc	Consonant
Incisor Display	Rest: 4 mm
	Smile: 14 mm (4 mm of gingival display)
Lateral Tooth Display	Maxillary molar to molar
Buccal Corridor	Large
Gingival Tissue	Margins: Uneven heights of maxillary incisors
	Papilla: Present in all teeth
	Localized marginal gingivitis right canines
Dentition	Tooth size and proportion: Normal
	Tooth shape: Normal
	Incisal wear maxillary right lateral incisor
	Axial inclination: Maxillary teeth inclined lingually
	Connector space and contact area: Closed contacts
Incisal Embrasure	Normal
Midlines	Upper and lower dental midlines are coincidental with facial midline

Intraoral Analysis (see Fig. 6-1-2)

Teeth Present	7654321/12C456
	7654321/1234567
Molar Relation	Class II end on right side and Class I on left side
Canine Relation	Class II end on right side and maxillary unerupted on left side
Overjet	3 mm
Overbite	5 mm
Maxillary Arch	Symmetric with crowding
Mandibular Arch	U shaped with crowding and normal curve of Spee
Oral Hygiene	Fair

Functional Analysis

Swallowing	Adult pattern
Temporomandibular joint	Normal with adequate range of jaw movements

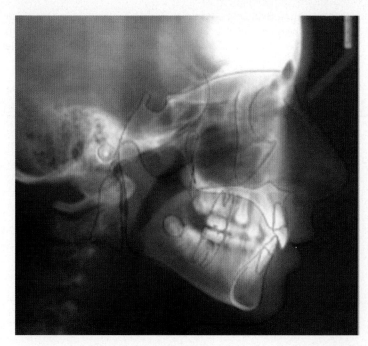

Parameter	Norm	Value
SNA (°)	82	77
SNB (°)	80	73
ANB (°)	2	4
FMA (°)	24	28
MP-SN (°)	32	36
U1-NA (mm/°)	4/22	1.2/10
L1-NA (mm/°)	4/25	2.6/19
IMPA (°)	95	88
U1-L1 (°)	130	147
OP-SN (°)	14	18
Upper Lip – E Plane (mm)	−4	−1
Lower Lip – E Plane (mm)	−2	−1.7
Nasolabial Angle (°)	103	120
Soft Tissue Convexity (°)	135	123

Figure 6-1-2   Pretreatment lateral cephalogram with tracing and cephalometric analysis.

Diagnosis and Case Summary

A 12-year-old female patient had convex soft and hard tissue profiles due to a retrognathic mandible and a dental Class II subdivision right malocclusion. Vertically, an asymmetric anterior deep bite with supraerupted maxillary incisors is present resulting in 4 mm of maxillary gingival display upon smiling.

PROBLEM LIST			
Pathology/Others	Localized marginal gingivitis on right canines Irregular maxillary gingival margins of anterior maxillary teeth Incisal wear maxillary right lateral incisor		
Alignment	8 mm of crowding present in present in maxillary arch and 8 mm of crowding present in mandibular arch Ectopically placed maxillary left canine		
Dimension	**Skeletal**	**Dental**	**Soft Tissue**
Anteroposterior	Class II denture base due to retrognathic mandible	Class II end on molar and canine relation on right side Retroclined maxillary and mandibular incisors Acute interincisal angle	Increased nasolabial angle
Vertical		Anterior deep bite of 5 mm due to extrusion of maxillary incisors	
Transverse			

TREATMENT OBJECTIVES			
Pathology/Others	Reinforce oral hygiene Restore distal aspect of incisal edge of the right maxillary incisor		
Alignment	Align maxillary and mandibular teeth by flaring incisors and utilization of Leeway space present Align maxillary left canine into the arch		
Dimension	**Skeletal**	**Dental**	**Soft Tissue**
Anteroposterior		Correct Class II molar relation on the right side to Class I Flare maxillary and mandibular anterior teeth to correct the incisal inclination, interincisal angle	
Vertical		Intrude maxillary anterior teeth to correct the deep bite	Intrude maxillary anterior teeth to reduce the gingival display upon smiling Level the maxillary gingival margins of anterior segment
Transverse			

Treatment Options

In the maxillary arch, unilateral extraction of the right first/second premolar with distalization of the right canine into Class I and protraction of the right side first molar into full cusp Class II could be an option in the present case. A disadvantage of this option is that space closure could result in further retroclination of maxillary incisors and midline deviation. A second nonextraction option could be distalization of the right side first molar into Class I and utilization of the Leeway space for distalization of right buccal segment into Class I. An advantage of this option is that it is a nonextraction approach.

In the mandibular arch, alignment could be performed by flaring incisors by 3 mm. As incisors are retroclined, a nonextraction approach is best.

The nonextraction option was opted by the patient after discussion of the treatment plan options.

TREATMENT SEQUENCE AND BIOMECHANICAL PLAN

Maxilla	Mandible
Band molars and bond maxillary arch.	Band molars and bond mandibular arch.
Sectional leveling 5-5 with .016, .018, and .016 × .022 inch NiTi arch wires.	Level with .016, .018, and .016 × .022 inch NiTi arch wires.
.017 × .025 inch NiTi intrusion arch tied to sectional .019 × 25 inch SS arch wire (from left first molar to right first premolar) between the central incisors to intrude the incisors and tip back the right first molar.	Continue leveling with .017 × .025 inch NiTi arch wire.
Leveling of the entire arch with .017 × .025 inch NiTi once Class I molar is achieved on the right side.	Continue leveling with .017 × .025 inch NiTi arch wire.
Push coil between right first molar and first premolar with Class II elastics to further distalize the first molar.	Continue leveling with .017 × .025 inch NiTi arch wire.
.016 × .022 inch SS base arch wire with .017 × .025 inch CNA cantilever to hold right molar in place and distalize right buccal segment into Class I.	Continue leveling with .019 × .025 inch NiTi arch wire.
.016 × .025 inch CNA with finishing bends.	.016 × .025 inch CNA with finishing bends.
Debond and wrap around retainer.	Debond and place fixed lingual retainer.
6-month recall appointment for retention check.	6-month recall appointment for retention check.

CNA, Connecticut new arch wire; *NiTi,* nickel titanium; *SS,* stainless steel.

■ TREATMENT SEQUENCE

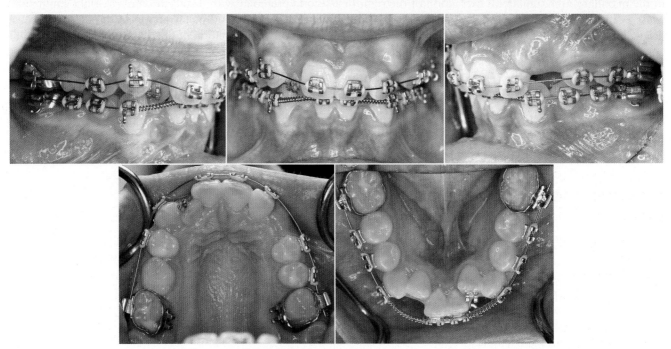

Figure 6-1-3   Initial leveling.

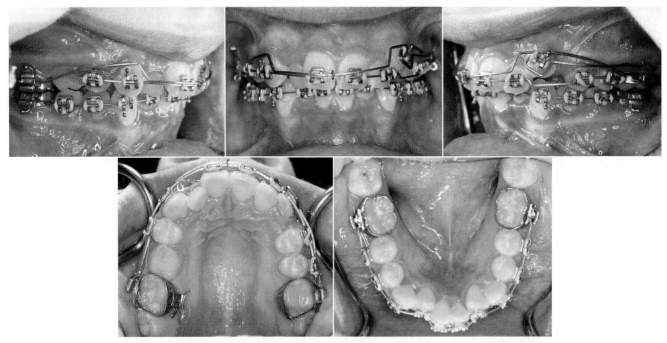

Figure 6-1-4   A Connecticut new arch wire intrusion arch intrudes the maxillary anterior teeth and tips the right first molar distally. A segmental arch wire from maxillary right first premolar to the left first molar counteracts the molar tip-back effect of intrusion arch on the left first molar and any counterclockwise moment due to the intrusion force on the anterior segment.

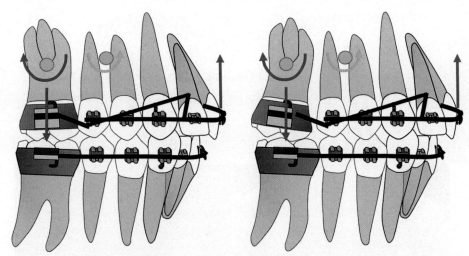

Figure 6-1-5   An intrusion arch results in a clockwise moment and extrusive force on the maxillary right first molar. The anterior base arch from first premolar on right side to the left maxillary first molar acts as anchorage to unite and resist the counterclockwise moment due to the intrusion force on the anterior segment.

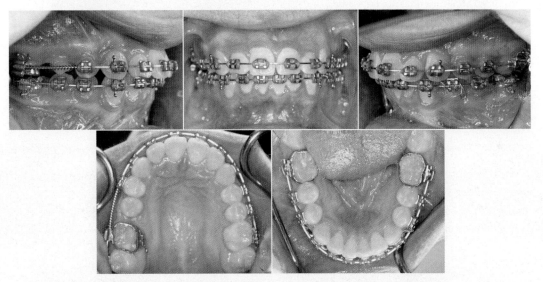

Figure 6-1-6   Push a coil with Class II elastics to further distalize maxillary right side first molar.

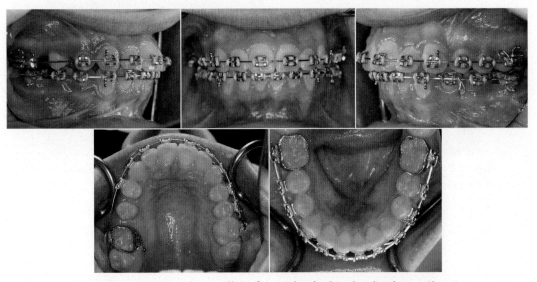

Figure 6-1-7   Right side maxillary first molar further distalized into Class I.

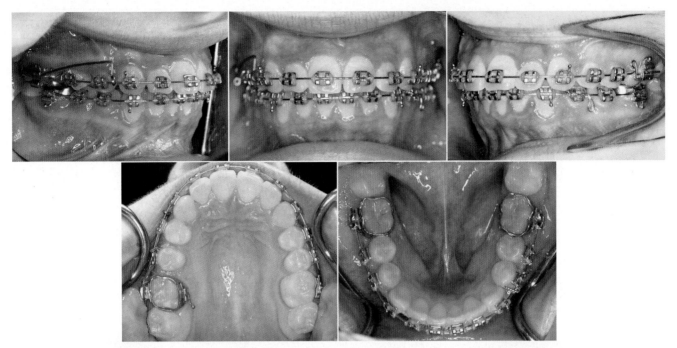

Figure 6-1-8 Cantilever from the maxillary first molar was delivered to maintain Class I occlusion and to reinforce anchorage for retraction of the maxillary right buccal segment into Class I.

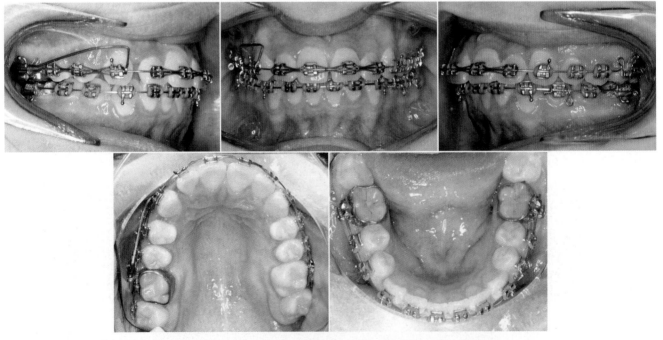

Figure 6-1-9 Retraction of the maxillary right buccal segment into Class I and improvement in the maxillary midline.

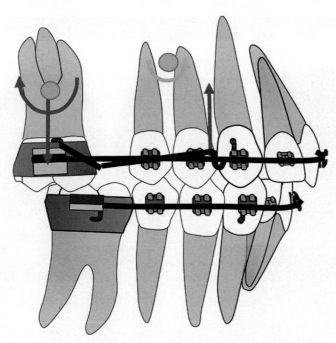

Figure 6-1-10 Cantilever from the right maxillary first molar creates a clockwise moment and extrusive force on the first molar and an intrusion force on the anterior segment. The anterior force passing slightly anterior to the center of resistance of the anterior segment will result in a small counterclockwise moment of the force. A clockwise moment on the right maxillary first molar will reinforce the anchorage for retraction of the maxillary right buccal segment into Class I.

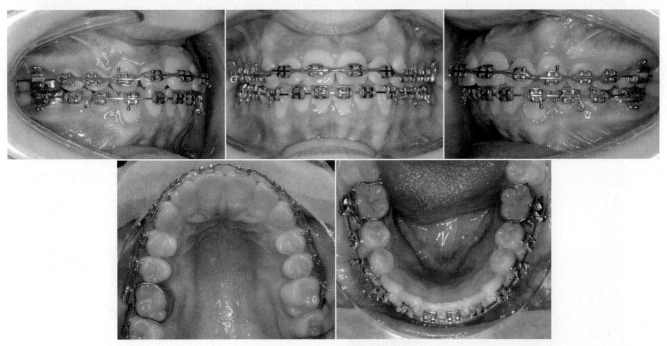

Figure 6-1-11 Finishing phase.

■ FINAL RESULTS

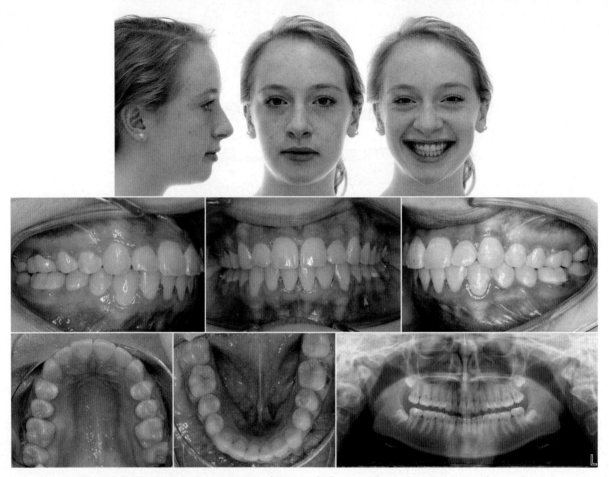

Figure 6-1-12   Posttreatment extraoral/intraoral photographs and panoramic radiograph.

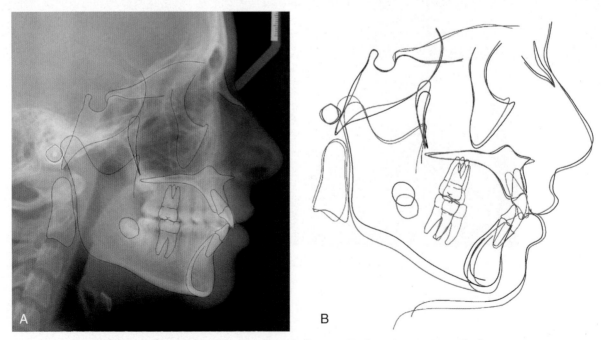

Figure 6-1-13   A, Posttreatment lateral cephalogram. B, Superimposition. *Black,* pretreatment; *red,* posttreatment.

How does a cantilever system correct a Class II molar occlusion?
This force system is usually applied when the Class II molar occlusion is present unilaterally. A one-piece intrusion arch is preferred when both molars need to be tipped back. The force system consists of an anterior intrusive force and a posterior tip back moment that corrects the Class II molar occlusion. Once the molar is tipped back, space mesial to the molar, which is used to retract the anterior teeth, is usually observed. The retraction requires being done in conjunction with Class II elastics to maintain the tip back as the anterior teeth are retracted.

Tip Back–Tip Forward Mechanics for the Correction of the Class II Subdivision

A 14-year-old female patient presented to the orthodontic clinic with a chief complaint of crowding present in the maxillary anterior teeth. Medical and dental histories were noncontributory, and findings from a temporomandibular joint (TMJ) examination were normal with adequate range of jaw movements.

▪ PRETREATMENT

Extraoral Analysis (Fig. 6-2-1)

Facial Form	Mesoprosopic
Facial Symmetry	No gross asymmetries noticed
Chin Point	Coincidental with facial midline
Occlusal Plane	Normal
Facial Profile	Orthognathic
Facial Height	Upper Facial Height/Lower Facial Height: Normal
	Lower Facial Height/Throat Depth: Normal
Lips	Competent, Upper: Retrusive; Lower: Normal
Nasolabial Angle	Obtuse
Mentolabial Sulcus	Normal

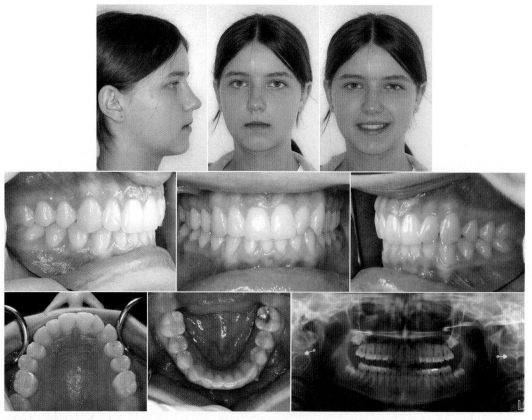

Figure 6-2-1   Pretreatment extraoral/intraoral photographs and panoramic radiograph.

Smile Analysis (Fig. 6-2-2)

Smile Arc	Consonant
Incisor Display	Rest: 3 mm
	Smile: 9 mm
Lateral Tooth Display	Maxillary first premolar to first premolar
Buccal Corridor	Medium
Gingival Tissue	Margins: Regular, slightly higher in the maxillary right lateral incisor
	Papilla: Present in all teeth
Dentition	Tooth size and proportion: Normal
	Tooth shape: Normal
	Axial inclination: Slight tipping of maxillary incisor crowns to the left
	Connector space and contact area: Long connector space with reduced incisal embrasure between central incisors and central to lateral incisors
Incisal Embrasure	Reduced
Midlines	Upper dental midline shifted to the right of facial midline by 1 mm

Intraoral Analysis (see Fig. 6-2-2)

Teeth Present	7654321/1234567 Unerupted 8s
	7654321/1234567
Molar Relation	Left: Class II end on; Right: Class I
Canine Relation	Left: Class II end on; Right: Class I
Overjet	2 mm
Overbite	4 mm
Maxillary Arch	Symmetric with 2 mm of crowding
Mandibular Arch	U shaped with normal curve of Spee
Oral Hygiene	Fair

Functional Analysis

Swallowing	Adult normal pattern
Temporomandibular joint	Normal with adequate range of jaw movements

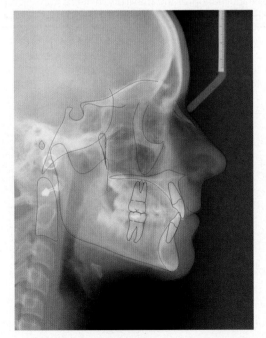

Parameter	Norm	Value
SNA (°)	82	82
SNB (°)	80	80
ANB (°)	2	2
FMA (°)	24	20
MP-SN (°)	32	28
U1-NA (mm/°)	4/22	2/17
L1-NA (mm/°)	4/25	2/19
IMPA (°)	95	90
U1-L1 (°)	130	141
OP-SN (°)	14	14
Upper Lip – E Plane (mm)	−4	−6
Lower Lip – E Plane (mm)	−2	−3.4
Nasolabial Angle (°)	103	115
Soft Tissue Convexity (°)	135	126

Figure 6-2-2   Pretreatment lateral cephalogram with tracing and cephalometric analysis.

Diagnosis and Case Summary

A 14-year-old female patient had a straight soft and hard tissue profile. She had a dental Class II subdivision left malocclusion with retroclined maxillary and mandibular incisors, an increased interincisal angle, and a retrusive upper lip with an obtuse nasolabial angle.

PROBLEM LIST			
Pathology/Others	Slight gingival margin discrepancy between maxillary lateral incisors Reduced incisal embrasures in maxillary anterior teeth		
Alignment	2 mm of maxillary crowding		
Dimension	**Skeletal**	**Dental**	**Soft Tissue**
Anteroposterior		Class II end on molar and canine relation on the left side Retroclined maxillary and mandibular incisors Increased interincisal angle	Obtuse nasolabial angle Retrusive upper lip
Transverse		Maxillary midline shifted to right side by 1 mm Mild mesiodistal crown inclination of the maxillary incisors to the left	
Vertical		OB: 4 mm	

OB, overbite.

TREATMENT OBJECTIVES			
Pathology/Others	Assess gingival heights and incisal embrasures in the maxillary anterior segment after orthodontic treatment.		
Alignment	Relieve maxillary crowding		
Dimension	**Skeletal**	**Dental**	**Soft Tissue**
Anteroposterior		Correct Class II end on molar and canine relation on the left side Correct maxillary and mandibular inclination and interincisor angle by flaring incisors	
Transverse		Shift maxillary midline to the left side by 1 mm Correct the mesiodistal axial inclination of the maxillary incisors	
Vertical		Correct overbite by intruding the maxillary incisors by 1-2 mm	

Treatment Options

Both extraction and nonextraction options were available for this patient. The extraction option consisted of removing the maxillary left first premolar, shifting the maxillary midline toward the left side, and finishing with a Class II molar on left side, Class I molar on the right side, and Class I canine bilaterally.

The nonextraction option entailed the distalization of the maxillary left buccal segment, finishing with a bilateral Class I molar and canine relationship. Distalization could be done with the help of headgear, temporary anchorage devices (TADs), or an intrusion arch. The patient elected a nonextraction approach.

TREATMENT SEQUENCE AND BIOMECHANICAL PLAN

Maxilla	Mandible
Band first molars and bond teeth anterior to first molars.	Band molars and bond mandibular arch.
Sectional leveling 5-5 with .016, .018, and .016 × .022 inch NiTi arch wires.	Level with .016, .018, and .016 × .022 inch NiTi arch wires.
.017 × .025 inch NiTi intrusion arch tied to the base arch wire between the central and lateral incisors to intrude the incisors and tip back the first molars. .032 inch CNA TPA with tip back bend on the left side and tip forward bend on the right side.	Continue leveling with .017 × .025 inch NiTi arch wire.
.016 × .022 inch SS base arch wire from right first molar to left second premolar with .017 × .025 inch CNA cantilever to maintain the first molar tip back and distalize the left buccal segment into Class I. Unilateral Class II elastics to reinforce anchorage on the left.	Continue leveling with .019 × .025 inch NiTi arch wire.
.016 × .025 inch CNA with finishing bends.	.016 × .025 inch CNA with finishing bends.
Debond and wrap around retainer.	Debond and place fixed lingual retainer.
6-month recall appointment for retention check.	6-month recall appointment for retention check.

CNA, Connecticut new arch wire; *NiTi,* nickel titanium; *SS,* stainless steel; *TPA,* transpalatal arch.

■ TREATMENT SEQUENCE

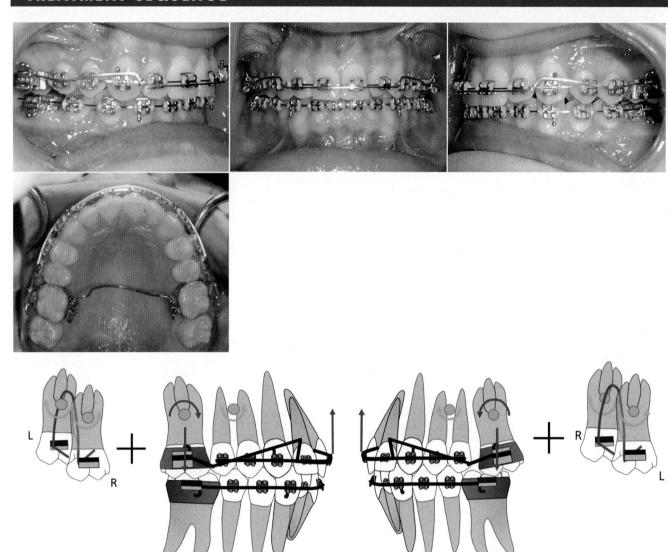

Figure 6-2-3 Intrusion arch tied to the maxillary incisors, resulting in intrusion of the maxillary incisors and tip back of the first molars. Transpalatal arch (TPA) with tip back bend on the left side and tip forward bend on the right side. Tip back moments on the left side due to TPA and intrusion arch result in a synergistic effect on the left side and cancel out each other on the right, resulting in tipping back of the left first molar only.

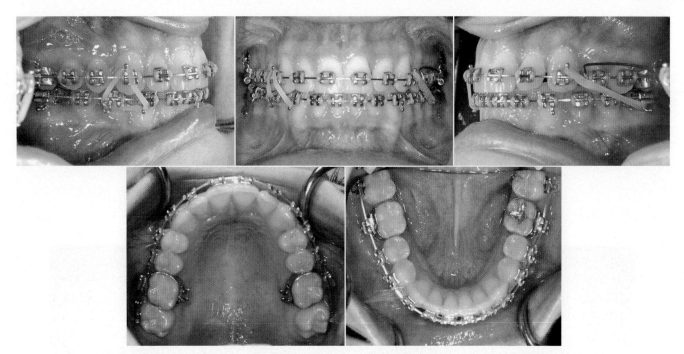

Figure 6-2-4 Connecticut new arch wire .017 × .025 inch cantilever to hold the maxillary left first molar in place and Class II elastics to reinforce anchorage during the distalization of the buccal segment into Class I.

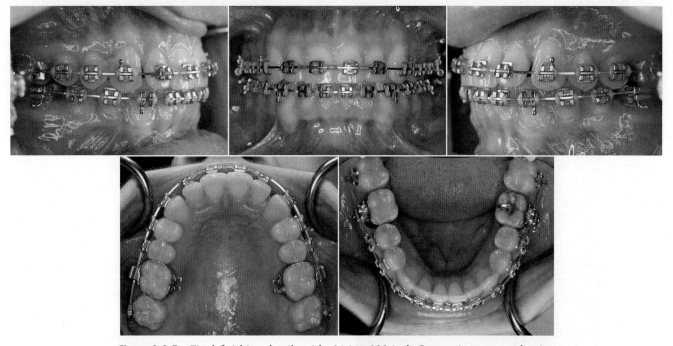

Figure 6-2-5 Final finishing details with .016 × .022 inch Connecticut new arch wire.

■ FINAL RESULTS

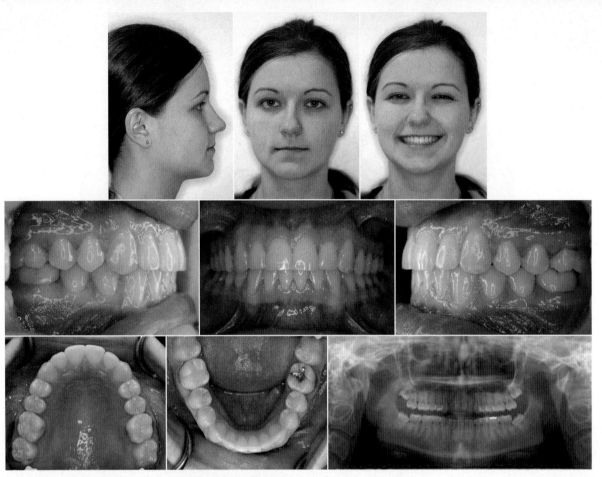

Figure 6-2-6   Posttreatment extraoral/intraoral photographs and panoramic radiograph.

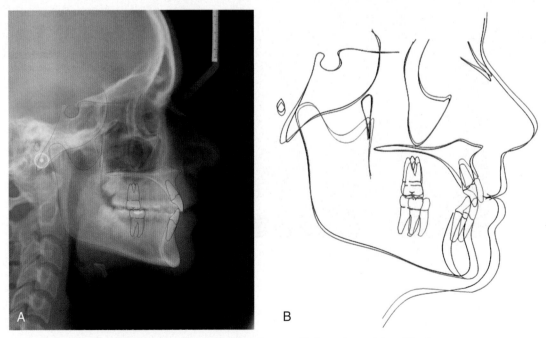

Figure 6-2-7   **A,** Posttreatment lateral cephalogram. **B,** Superimposition. *Black,* pretreatment; *red,* posttreatment.

What is the advantage of a tip back–tip forward approach?
The tip back–tip forward approach is a biomechanical force system that is useful in the correction of Class II subdivision malocclusions. The side where tip back is desired, the molar, receives a tip back moment from the intrusion arch and from the transpalatal arch in a synergistic tandem effect. On the other hand, on the Class I side, the molar receives a tip back moment from the intrusion arch, which is counteracted with the tip forward moment of the transpalatal arch, resulting in no net movement. A patient who requires incisor intrusion is further benefited from this force system.

CASE 6-3
Use of a Fixed Functional Appliance for Class II Correction

A 13-year-old pubertal male patient was referred by his general dentist for assessment of the anterior deep bite. Medical and dental histories were noncontributory, and findings from the temporomandibular joint (TMJ) examination were normal with adequate range of jaw movements.

▪ PRETREATMENT

Extraoral Analysis (Fig. 6-3-1)

Facial Form	Mesoprosopic
Facial Symmetry	No gross asymmetries noticed
Chin Point	Coincidental with the facial midline
Occlusal Plane	Normal
Facial Profile	Slightly convex because of a retrognathic mandible
Facial Height	Upper Facial Height/Lower Facial Height: Normal
	Lower Facial Height/Throat Depth: Normal
Lips	Competent, Upper: Normal; Lower: Normal
Nasolabial Angle	Obtuse
Mentolabial Sulcus	Normal

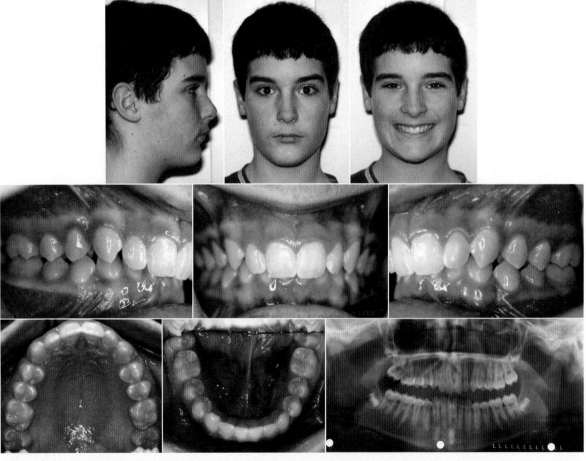

Figure 6-3-1 Pretreatment extraoral/intraoral photographs and panoramic radiograph.

Smile Analysis (Fig. 6-3-2)

Smile Arc	Consonant
Incisor Display	Rest: 3 mm
	Smile: 10 mm
Lateral Tooth Display	Second premolar to second premolar
Buccal Corridor	Normal
Gingival Tissue	Margins: Maxillary incisor margins are more incisal as compared with the canines matching incisal edge discrepancy
	Papilla: Present
Dentition	Tooth size and proportion: Reduced mesiodistal width of maxillary lateral incisors
	Tooth shape: Sharp incisal edge of the maxillary canines; rounded incisal edge of lateral incisors
	Axial inclination: Maxillary and mandibular teeth inclined lingually
	Connector space and contact area: Long connector between the maxillary central incisors displacing the papilla gingivally
Incisal Embrasure	Large between maxillary lateral incisors and canines due to incisal edge morphology of the canines
Midlines	Maxillary and mandibular midlines are coincidental with facial midline

Intraoral Analysis (see Fig. 6-3-2)

Teeth Present	7654321/1234567
	7654321/1234567 (Unerupted 8s)
Molar Relation	Class II bilaterally
Canine Relation	Class II bilaterally
Overjet	4 mm
Overbite	8 mm
Maxillary Arch	U shaped, symmetric with extruded maxillary incisors
Mandibular Arch	U shaped with deep curve of Spee
Oral Hygiene	Fair

Functional Analysis

Swallowing	Normal adult pattern
Temporomandibular joint	Normal with adequate range of jaw movements

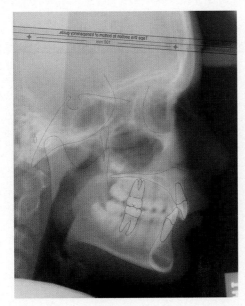

Parameter	Norm	Value
SNA (°)	82	81
SNB (°)	80	77
ANB (°)	2	4
FMA (°)	24	22
MP-SN (°)	32	28
U1-NA (mm/°)	4/22	1/12
L1-NA (mm/°)	4/25	2/19
IMPA (°)	95	94
U1-L1 (°)	130	143
OP-SN (°)	14	13
Upper Lip – E Plane (mm)	−4	−2
Lower Lip – E Plane (mm)	−2	−1
Nasolabial Angle (°)	103	131
Witt's appraisal (mm)	−1	4

Figure 6-3-2 Pretreatment lateral cephalogram with tracing and cephalometric analysis.

Diagnosis and Case Summary

A 13-year-old pubertal male patient presented with a convex skeletal and soft tissue profile mainly due to retrognathic mandible. He had a Class II malocclusion with lingually inclined maxillary and mandibular incisors, a deep overbite, an increased interincisal angle, and an obtuse nasolabial angle.

PROBLEM LIST			
Pathology/Others	Sharp incisal edge morphology of maxillary incisors Reduce mesiodistal width of maxillary lateral incisors		
Alignment			
Dimension	**Skeletal**	**Dental**	**Soft Tissue**
Anteroposterior	Convex skeletal profile due to a retrognathic mandible	OJ: 4 mm Class II molar and canine relationship Upper and lower incisors are lingually inclined Obtuse interincisal angle	Convex soft tissue profile Obtuse nasolabial angle
Transverse			
Vertical	Low mandibular plane angle	OB: 8 mm (100%)	

OB, overbite; *OJ,* overjet.

TREATMENT OBJECTIVES			
Pathology/Others	Assess incisal embrasure between maxillary lateral incisors and canines after orthodontic treatment for possible composite buildups on lateral incisors and incisal tip reduction of the canines Slenderize slightly the mandibular anterior teeth to normalize the Bolton relation associated with the reduced mesiodistal width of the maxillary lateral incisors		
Alignment			
Dimension	**Skeletal**	**Dental**	**Soft Tissue**
Anteroposterior	Improve the skeletal convexity with the fixed functional appliance	Improve the inclination of maxillary and mandibular incisor, interincisal angle Improve overjet by advancing the mandibular dental arch mesially with a fixed functional appliance	Correct the convex soft tissue profile by improving the position of mandibular arch
Transverse			
Vertical		Improve the anterior overbite by leveling the arches	

Treatment Options

Two options were available for this patient.

The first option involved the correction of the Class II malocclusion and increased overjet with a fixed functional appliance such as the Herbst Appliance, Forsus appliance, or Twin Force Bite Corrector (TFBC).

The second option entailed the extraction of the maxillary first premolars and retraction of the maxillary anterior teeth to improve the overjet. The disadvantage of this option is the difficulty of correcting the deep overbite and controlling the incisor inclination during space closure as these teeth were already retroclined.

Patient selected a nonextraction treatment option (option 1).

TREATMENT SEQUENCE AND BIOMECHANICAL PLAN

Maxilla	Mandible
Band molars, bond maxillary arch, level with .016 inch NiTi arch wire.	Band molars and bond mandibular arch. Level with .016 inch NiTi arch wire.
Continue leveling with .016 × .022 inch NiTi arch wire. Place .017 × .025 inch CNA intrusion arch tied over the main archwire in the incisors to level the arch (Fig. 6-3-4).	Continue leveling with .016 × .022 inch NiTi arch wire.
Continue leveling with .017 × .025 inch NiTi arch wire.	Continue leveling with .017 × .025 inch NiTi arch wire.
Continue leveling with .019 × .025 inch NiTi arch wire.	Continue leveling with .019 × .025 inch NiTi arch wire.
Place .019 × .025 inch SS arch wire and attach Place Twin Force Bite Corrector to the arch.	Place .019 × .025 inch SS arch wire and attach Twin Force Bite Corrector to the arch.
.016 × .022 CNA with finishing bends.	.016 × .022 CNA with finishing bends.
Debond and wrap around retainer.	Debond and place fixed lingual retainer.
6-month recall appointment for retention check.	6-month recall appointment for retention check.

CNA, Connecticut new arch wire; NiTi, nickel titanium; SS, stainless steel.

■ TREATMENT SEQUENCE

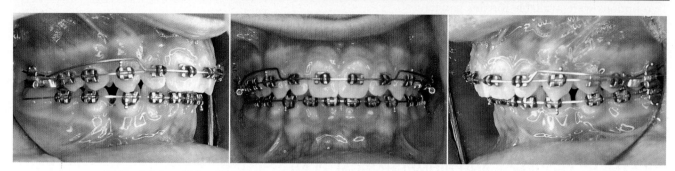

Figure 6-3-3 .016 × .022 inch nickel titanium wire with .017 × .025 inch Connecticut new arch wire intrusion arch tied in the maxillary anterior teeth for leveling of the maxillary arch.

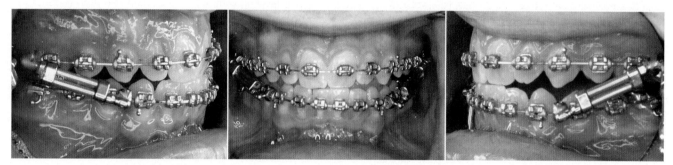

Figure 6-3-4 Insertion of the Twin Force Bite Corrector (fixed functional appliance).

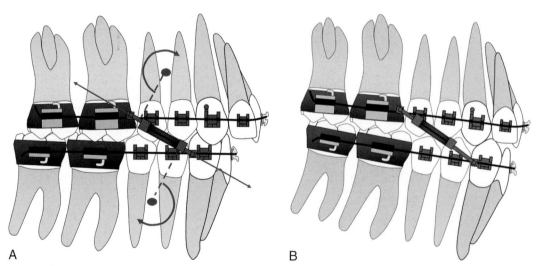

Figure 6-3-5 **A,** Twin Force Bite Corrector exerts a distal and upwards force on maxillary arch and mesial and downward force on the mandibular arch. **B,** Resulting clockwise rotation of both arches results in steepening of the occlusal plane.

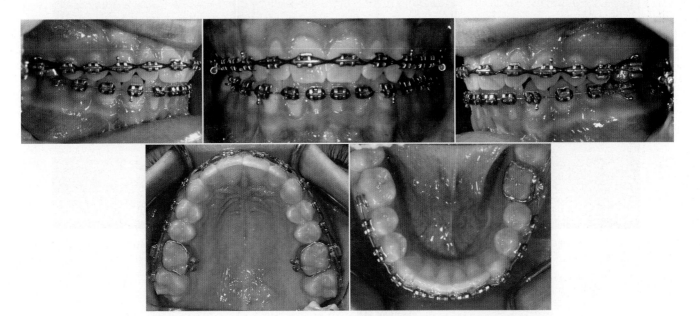

Figure 6-3-6   Finishing stage, .016 × .022 inch Connecticut new arch wire.

FINAL RESULTS

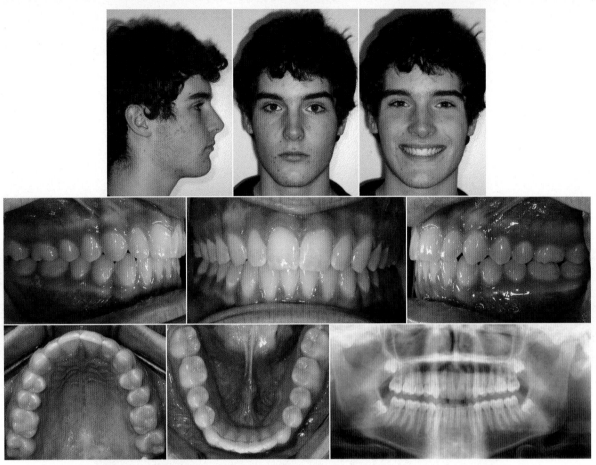

Figure 6-3-7   Posttreatment extraoral/intraoral photographs and panoramic radiograph.

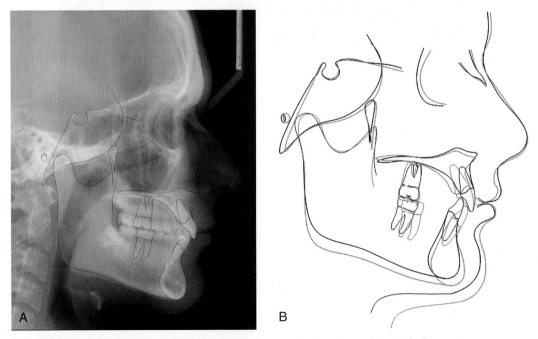

Figure 6-3-8   **A,** Posttreatment lateral cephalogram. **B,** Superimposition. *Black,* pretreatment; *green,* posttreatment.

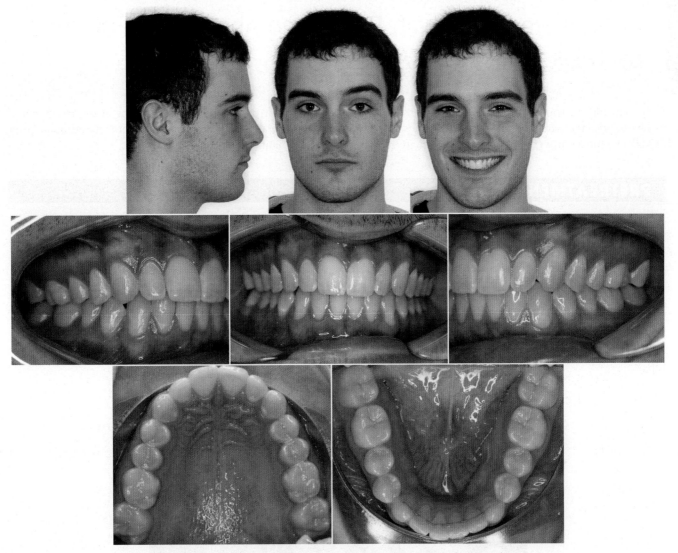

Figure 6-3-9   Six-year postretention extraoral/intraoral photographs.

? Why was a Twin Force Bite Corrector (TFBC) used in this case instead of a Herbst?
Both are similar types of appliances for the correction of the Class II malocclusion.
The advantage of the TFBC is that it is a fixed functional appliance that does not
require laboratory fabrication. This is important when breakage occurs; replacement
of parts can be easily accomplished without needing a new impression to be sent to
a laboratory. Furthermore, the TFBC is easily added to fixed appliance therapy.
Typically it is left intraorally for 3 to 4 months and then removed. Class II elastics
are prescribed thereafter to maintain the correction during the finishing stage.

**What important biomechanic considerations are necessary when using the TFBC for
Class II correction?**
It is important to add a transpalatal arch (TPA) while using the TFBC because it
prevents the first molars from tipping labially. This can be easily accomplished by
adding a .032-inch Connecticut new arch wire or stainless steel arch wire to soldered
tubes on the lingual of the first molars. A tight cinch of the lower arch wire is also
required to prevent spaces from opening.

Class II Treatment with Distalizing Appliances Followed by TADs to Maintain Anchorage

A 16-year-old postpubertal female patient came with a chief complaint of irregular teeth present in the front region of her upper jaw. Medical and dental histories were noncontributory, and findings from a temporomandibular joint (TMJ) examination were normal with adequate range of jaw movements.

■ PRETREATMENT

Extraoral Analysis (Fig. 6-4-1)

Facial Form	Mesoprosopic
Facial Symmetry	No gross asymmetry noticed
Chin Point	Coincidental with facial midline
Occlusal Plane	Normal
Facial Profile	Convex due to prognathic maxilla
Facial Height	Upper Facial Height/Lower Facial Height: Normal
	Lower Facial Height/Throat Depth: Normal
Lips	Competent, Upper: Protrusive; Lower: Normal
Nasolabial Angle	Obtuse
Mentolabial Sulcus	Normal

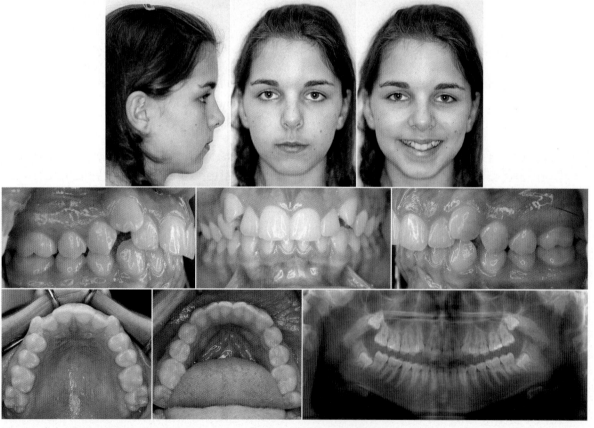

Figure 6-4-1   Pretreatment extraoral/intraoral photographs and panoramic radiograph.

Smile Analysis (Fig. 6-4-2)

Smile Arc	Consonant
Incisor Display	Rest: 4 mm
	Smile: 8 mm
Lateral Tooth Display	Second premolar to second premolar
Buccal Corridor	Small
Gingival Tissue	Margins: Canine margins are high
	Papilla: Present
Dentition	Tooth size and proportion: Normal
	Tooth shape: Normal
	Axial inclination: Maxillary teeth inclined lingually
	Connector space and contact area: No contact between lateral incisor and canine
Incisal Embrasure	Normal
Midlines	Upper shifted to right by 2 mm and lower dental midline is on with facial midline

Intraoral Analysis (see Fig. 6-4-2)

Teeth Present	7654321/1234567 Unerupted 8s
	7654321/1234567
Molar Relation	Class II bilaterally
Canine Relation	Class II bilaterally
Overjet	4 mm
Overbite	4 mm
Maxillary Arch	U shaped, symmetric with crowding of 8 mm
Mandibular Arch	U shaped, with crowding of 2 mm and normal curve of Spee
Oral Hygiene	Fair

Functional Analysis

Swallowing	Normal
Temporomandibular joint	Normal with normal range of jaw movements

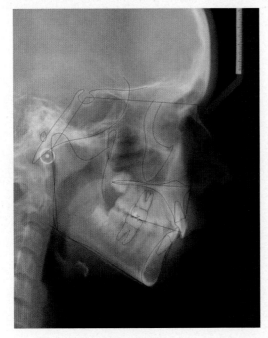

Parameter	Norm	Value
SNA (°)	82	84
SNB (°)	80	80
ANB (°)	2	4
FMA (°)	24	24
MP-SN (°)	32	30
U1-NA (mm/°)	4/22	1.5/15
L1-NA (mm/°)	4/25	4.6/30
IMPA (°)	95	90
U1-L1 (°)	130	130
OP-SN (°)	14	15
Upper Lip – E Plane (mm)	−4	0.7
Lower Lip – E Plane (mm)	−2	1.6
Nasolabial Angle (°)	103	115
Soft Tissue Convexity (°)	135	125

Figure 6-4-2 Pretreatment lateral cephalogram with tracing and cephalometric analysis.

Diagnosis and Case Summary

A 16-year-old postpubertal female patient presented with skeletal and dental Class II malocclusion with convex soft tissue profile mainly due to prognathic maxilla and normal mandible. Maxillary canines are ectopically placed buccally and gingivally.

PROBLEM LIST			
Pathology/Others			
Alignment	8-mm crowding in maxillary arch and 2 mm in mandibular arch		
Dimension	**Skeletal**	**Dental**	**Soft Tissue**
Anteroposterior	Class II denture base due to prognathic maxilla	Full cusp Class II molar and canine relation OJ: 4 mm	Obtuse nasolabial angle
Vertical		50% overbite	
Transverse		Maxillary midline 2 mm left of the facial midline	

OJ, overjet.

TREATMENT OBJECTIVES			
Pathology/Others			
Alignment	Align maxillary and mandibular arch to relieve crowding (maxillary arch to be aligned after distalization of buccal segment)		
Dimension	**Skeletal**	**Dental**	**Soft Tissue**
Anteroposterior	Camouflage the skeletal Class II denture base by dental correction	Correct Class II molar and canine relation to Class I relationship by maxillary molar distalization and maintaining incisor position Slight flaring of lower incisors with alignment and leveling of lower curve of Spee	
Vertical		Decrease overbite by leveling curve of Spee	
Transverse		Improve maxillary midline to match facial midline	

Treatment Options

Correction of Class II dental relationship and alignment of buccally and gingivally placed canines can be performed by either extraction of the maxillary first premolars or distalization of the maxillary dentition. In case of extraction, molars must be finished in Class II relationship and canines in Class I. In case of distalization, maxillary molars must be sequentially distalized with the anterior maxillary dentoalveolar segment as an anchor. During retraction of premolars (for correction of buccal segment), molars must be stabilized by temporary anchorage devices (TADs)/headgear. Although both procedures are expected to provide the same aesthetic results, distalization of the maxillary arch can lead to longer duration of treatment time.

This patient opted for a nonextraction treatment with a two-phase distalization approach. The maxillary molars were to be distalized by a distal jet appliance and maintained in that position with TADs for retraction of the anterior teeth.

TREATMENT SEQUENCE AND BIOMECHANICAL PLAN

Maxilla	Mandible
Pick up impression for distal jet appliance.	Band molars and bond mandibular arch.
Band molars, bond maxillary arch, place distal jet appliance for distalization of maxillary molars (Fig. 6-4-3).	Level with .016 inch NiTi arch wire.
Continue with distal jet appliance (Fig. 6-4-4).	Continue leveling with .016 × .022 inch NiTi arch wire.
Continue with distal jet appliance (Fig. 6-4-5).	Continue leveling with .017 × .025 inch NiTi arch wire.
Discontinue distal jet appliance after molar relation becomes super Class I. Place TAD just mesial to root of first maxillary molar bilaterally. Stabilize both first molars with TADs with .019 × .025 inch SS wire section. Retract maxillary first and second premolar using elastomeric chain from TADs. Level with .016 inch NiTi arch wire (Fig. 6-4-6).	Continue leveling with .017 × .025 inch NiTi arch wire.
Retract maxillary first and second premolars using elastomeric chain from first molars. Continue leveling using .016 × .022 inch NiTi arch wire.	Continue leveling with .019 × .025 inch NiTi arch wire.
Engage canines with leveling wire; continue leveling with .016 × .022 inch NiTi arch wire (Fig. 6-4-7).	Continue leveling with .019 × .025 inch NiTi arch wire.
Continue leveling with .019 × .025 inch NiTi arch wire.	.016 × .025 inch CNA with finishing bends.
.017 × .025 inch CNA with finishing bends (Fig. 6-4-8).	.017 × .025 inch CNA with finishing bends.
Debond and wrap around retainer (Fig. 6-4-9).	Debond and deliver Hawley retainer.
6-month recall appointment for retention check.	6-month recall appointment for retention check.

CNA, Connecticut new arch wire; *NiTi,* nickel titanium; *SS,* stainless steel; *TAD,* temporary anchorage device.

■ TREATMENT SEQUENCE

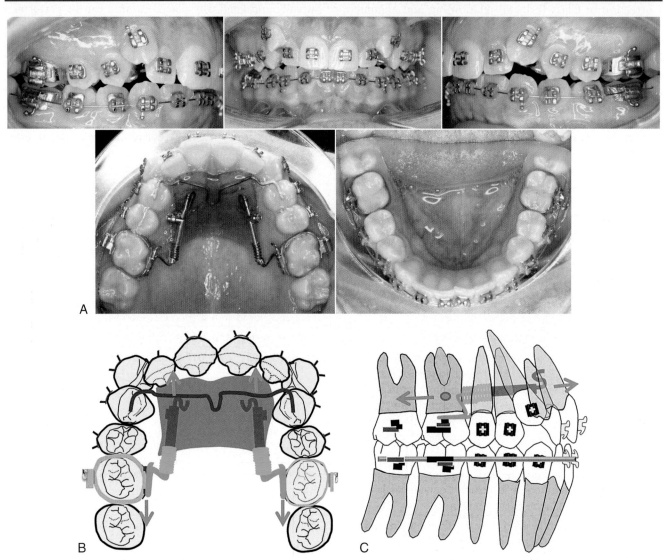

Figure 6-4-3 **A,** Intraoral photographs with distal jet appliance. **B,** Distal jet appliance produces a distal force on the molars and mesial force on the anterior dentoalveolar segment. **C,** Line of action of the distal force passes through center of resistance of the molars, reducing distal tipping of the molars.

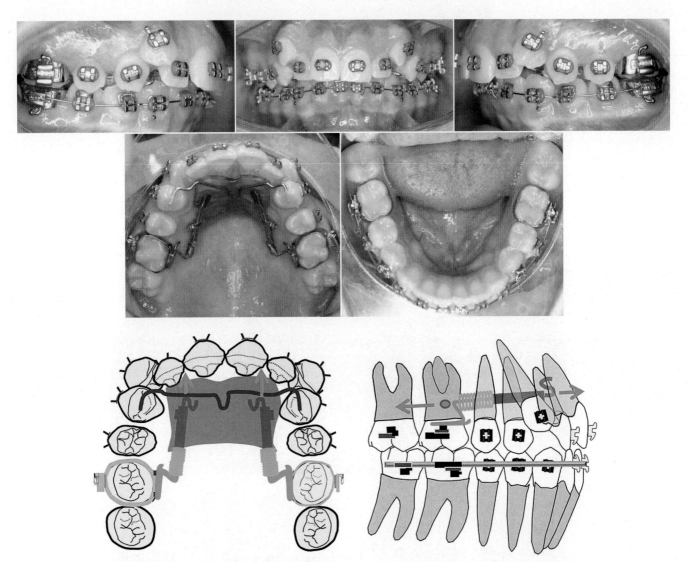

Figure 6-4-4 Distalization of maxillary molars and opening up of spaces in premolar region.

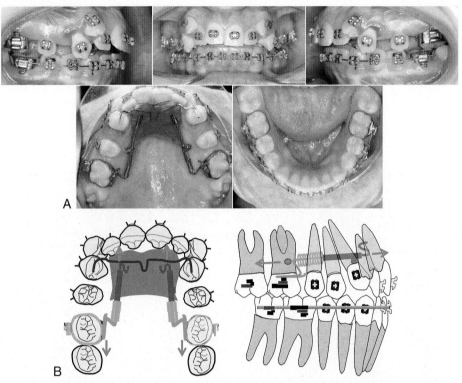

Figure 6-4-5 **A,** Clinical photos depicting further distalization of maxillary molars and opening up of spaces in the premolar region. **B,** Diagram representing the force system of a distal jet appliance.

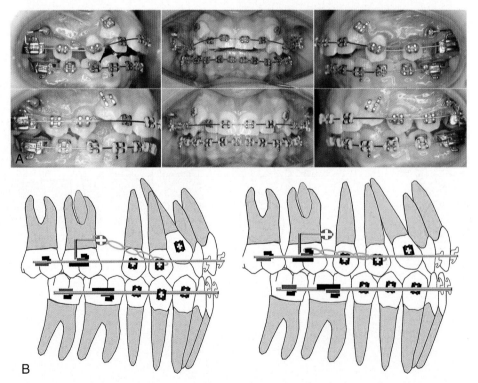

Figure 6-4-6 **A,** Distal jet activation discontinues. A temporary anchorage device (TAD) is placed mesial to the maxillary first molar, which is stabilized with a TAD. An elastomeric chain is used to retract the first and second premolars. **B,** Diagram depicting further retraction of the premolars with help of an elastomeric chain from the first molar.

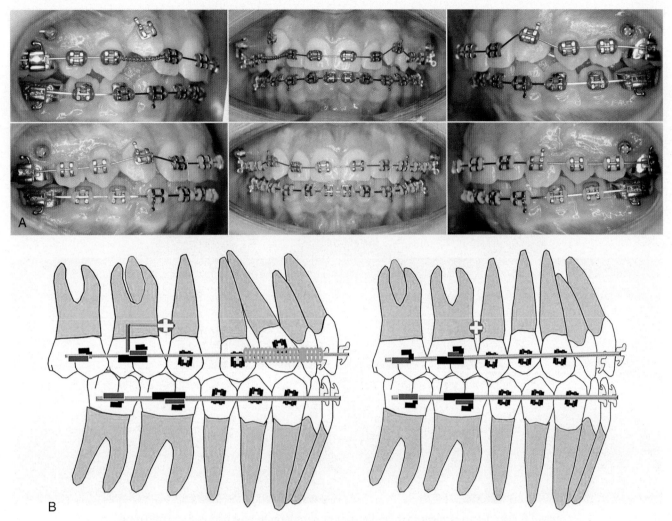

Figure 6-4-7 **A,** Opening of space with a push coil. **B,** Leveling of the maxillary arch.

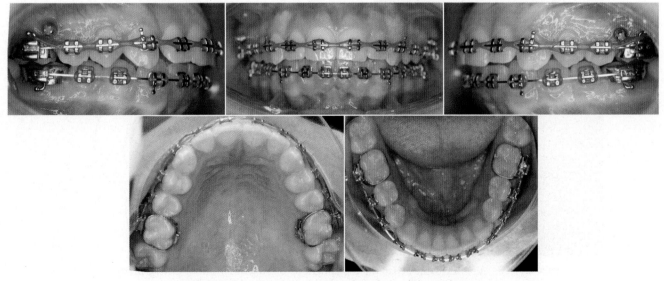

Figure 6-4-8 Finishing stage and settling of the occlusion.

■ FINAL RESULTS

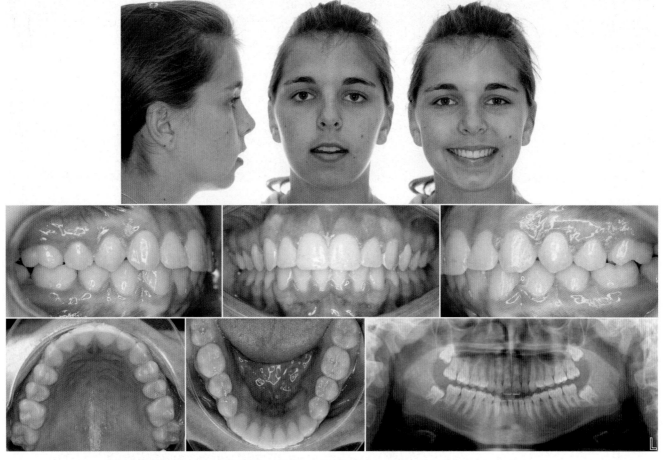

Figure 6-4-9   Posttreatment extraoral/intraoral photographs and panoramic radiograph.

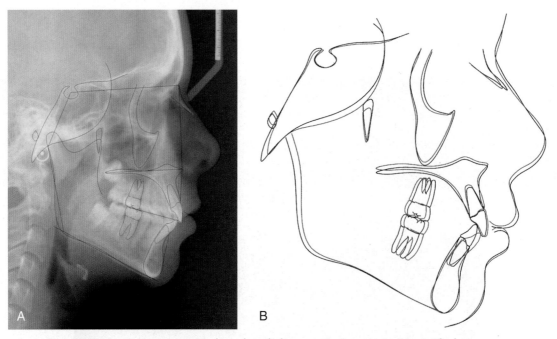

Figure 6-4-10   **A,** Posttreatment lateral cephalogram. **B,** Superimposition. *Black,* pretreatment; *red,* posttreatment.

What is the advantage of a distal jet appliance over other intramaxillary distalizers?
As the line of the force passes through the center of resistance of maxillary molars, the tendency to distally tip the maxillary molar is reduced during distalization.

Why is a temporary anchorage device (TAD) placed during retraction of premolars?
During retraction of premolars, it is necessary to minimize mesial movement of molars, thus necessitating a stable posterior anchorage.

Why not distalize from the beginning with a TAD-supported distal jet?
This would be another approach that would likely reduce the "round tripping" of the maxillary incisors with non-TAD-supported distalization. However, this method incorporates TADs in an area (interradicular space) that has ease of placement and can be used for direct and indirect anchorage without the need of replacing the TADs.

CASE 7-1
Two-Phase Palatal Mini-Implant–Supported Class III Correction

A 13-year-old female patient was referred by her general dentist for assessment of an anterior crossbite. Medical and dental histories were noncontributory, and findings from a temporomandibular joint (TMJ) examination were normal with adequate range of jaw movements.

◼ PRETREATMENT

Extraoral Analysis (Fig. 7-1-1)

Facial Form	Mesoprosopic
Facial Symmetry	No gross asymmetries noticed
Chin Point	Coincidental with facial midline
Occlusal Plane	Normal
Facial Profile	Slightly concave due to prognathic mandible
Facial Height	Upper Facial Height/Lower Facial Height: Increased lower facial height compared with upper facial height
	Lower Facial Height/Throat Depth: Normal
Lips	Competent, Upper: Protrusive; Lower: Protrusive
Nasolabial Angle	Acute
Mentolabial Sulcus	Normal

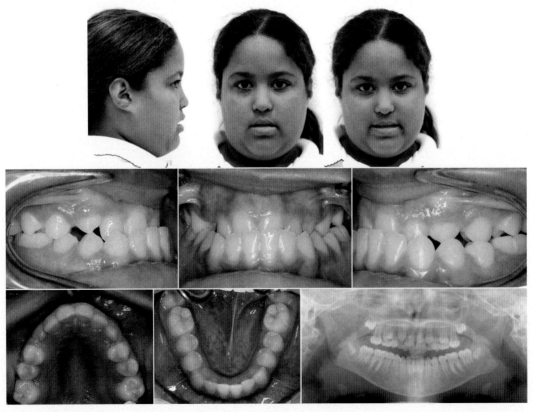

Figure 7-1-1   Pretreatment extraoral/intraoral photographs and panoramic radiograph.

Smile Analysis (Fig. 7-1-2)

Smile Arc	Straight
Incisor Display	Rest: 3 mm
	Smile: 4 mm (guarded smile)
Lateral Tooth Display	Maxillary: Premolar to premolar (guarded smile)
Buccal Corridor	Small
Gingival Tissue	Margins: Irregular due to lingual position of maxillary lateral incisors and canines incompletely erupted
	Papilla: Present in all teeth
Dentition	Tooth size and proportion: Normal
	Tooth shape: Normal
	Axial inclination: Maxillary teeth inclined lingually
	Connector space and contact area: Closed contacts
Incisal Embrasure	Normal
Midlines	Lower dental midline 1 mm to the left with the upper dental midline coincidental with the facial midline

Intraoral Analysis (see Fig. 7-1-2)

Teeth Present	654321/123456 (Unerupted maxillary 7s and mandibular 8s. Missing maxillary 8s.)
	7654321/1234567
Molar Relation	Class III bilaterally full cusp
Canine Relation	Class III bilaterally end on
Overjet	–2 mm
Overbite	3 mm
Maxillary Arch	U shaped
Mandibular Arch	U shaped with normal curve of Spee
Oral Hygiene	Fair
Transverse	Crossbite on left premolar area

Functional Analysis

Swallowing	Adult pattern
Temporomandibular joint	Normal with adequate range of jaw movements

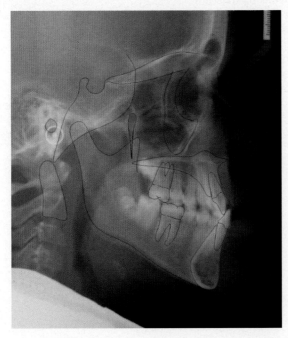

Parameter	Norm	Value
SNA (°)	82	83
SNB (°)	80	84
ANB (°)	2	−1
FMA (°)	24	29
MP-SN (°)	32	36
U1-NA (mm/°)	4/22	3/17
L1-NA (mm/°)	4/25	4/20
IMPA (°)	95	79
U1-L1 (°)	130	143
OP-SN (°)	14	14
Upper Lip – E Plane (mm)	−4	1
Lower Lip – E Plane (mm)	−2	3
Nasolabial Angle (°)	103	92
Soft Tissue Convexity (°)	135	146

Figure 7-1-2 Pretreatment lateral cephalogram with tracing and cephalometric analysis.

Diagnosis and Case Summary

A 13-year-old female patient presented with a concave hard and soft tissue profile mainly due to a normal maxilla and a prognathic mandible and a full-cusp Class III malocclusion with negative overjet and a dental crossbite on the left side.

PROBLEM LIST			
Pathology/Others	Missing maxillary third molars		
Alignment			
Dimension	**Skeletal**	**Dental**	**Soft Tissue**
Anteroposterior	Mild concavity Class III denture base due to prognathic mandible	Full cusp Class III molar and half cusp canine relationship OJ: –2 mm Retroclined mandibular incisors Obtuse interincisal angle	Protrusive upper and lower lip Acute nasolabial angle Concave soft tissue profile
Transverse		Maxillary first premolar in crossbite. Lower dental midline 1 mm to the left of the facial midline	
Vertical		Increased LFH	Uneven anterior maxillary gingival margins

LFH, lower facial height; *OJ,* overjet.

TREATMENT OBJECTIVES			
Pathology/Others			
Alignment			
Dimension	**Skeletal**	**Dental**	**Soft Tissue**
Anteroposterior		Correction of Class III molar and canine relation through protraction of maxillary dentition Correct negative OJ by flaring maxillary incisors slightly and lingual retraction of mandibular incisors Correct interincisal angle	
Transverse		Correct crossbite of maxillary first premolars through anteroposterior correction and dental expansion	
Vertical			Evaluate gingival margins in the maxillary anterior region after finishing for possible gingivectomies as needed

OJ, overjet.

Treatment Options

Because the patient had reached puberty, a reverse face mask therapy for correction of skeletal Class III relation would likely be limited in achieving skeletal correction. Therefore the best option at this stage is to correct the dental Class III relation with camouflage treatment and inform the patient and parent about the possibility of continuation of mandibular growth and the potential need of surgical treatment in the future.

Mechanically, for the protraction of the maxillary dentition, one can use a reverse face mask, Class III elastics, or temporary anchorage devices (TADs), which have the advantage of being compliance free. The patient chose to use TADs to protract the entire maxilla.

TREATMENT SEQUENCE AND BIOMECHANICAL PLAN

Maxilla	Mandible
Band molars and bond maxillary arch.	Band molars and bond mandibular arch bypassing incisors.
Leveling with .016, .018, .016 × .022 inch NiTi arch wires.	Level with .016, .018 inch NiTi arch wires.
.017 × .022 inch SS arch wire with push coil distal to the lateral incisors to achieve positive OJ.	.20 inch SS arch wire.
Place TADs in palate, TPA form first molar to first molar. Stabilize the maxillary incisors with the TADs (splinted with acrylic) and place NiTi closed coil for protraction of posterior teeth.	Bond lower incisors and incorporate these teeth into arch wire.
CNA .016 × .022 inch finishing arch wire.	CNA .016 × .022 inch finishing arch wire.
Debond and wrap around retainer.	Debond and bond a lingual 3-3 retainer.
6-month recall appointment for retention check.	6-month recall appointment for retention check.

CNA, Connecticut new arch wire; *NiTi,* nickel titanium; *OJ,* overjet; *SS,* stainless steel; *TAD,* temporary anchorage device; *TPA,* transpalatal arch.

■ TREATMENT SEQUENCE

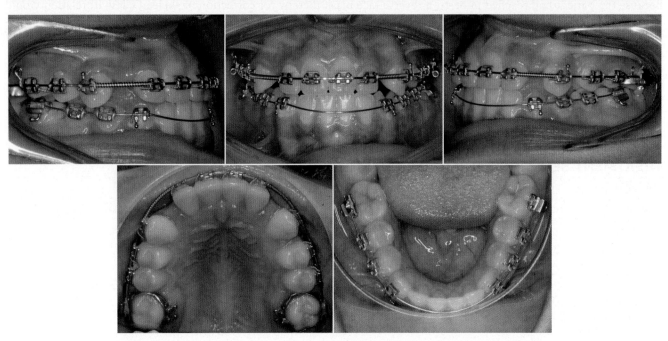

Figure 7-1-3   Initial leveling with push coil and correction of anterior crossbite.

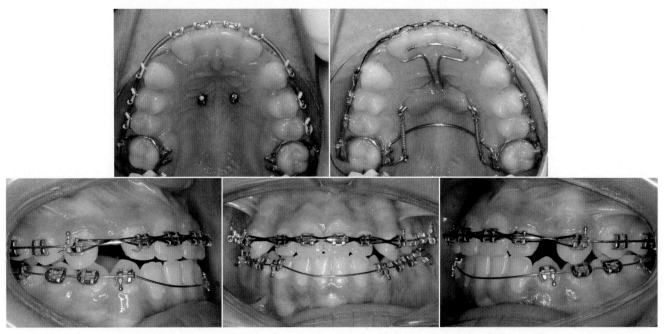

Figure 7-1-4   Protraction appliance. Two temporary anchorage devices placed in the palate and splinted by acrylic. Arms extended from the acrylic to receive the nickel titanium coils delivering the force from the transpalatal arch.

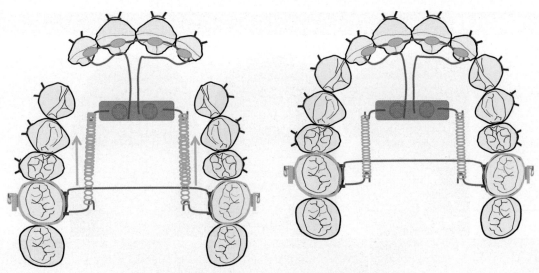

Figure 7-1-5   Biomechanics of the protraction appliance.

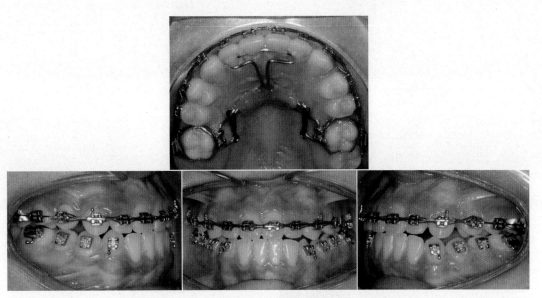

Figure 7-1-6   Protraction of posterior teeth complete.

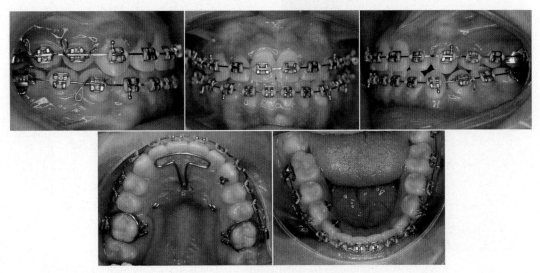

Figure 7-1-7   Finishing of the occlusion.

■ FINAL RESULTS

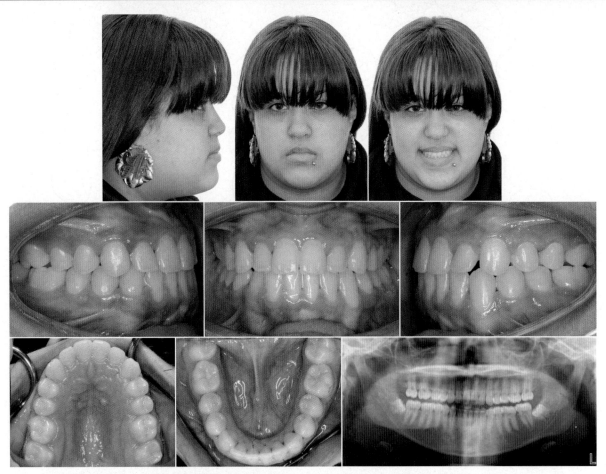

Figure 7-1-8   Posttreatment extraoral/intraoral photographs and panoramic radiograph.

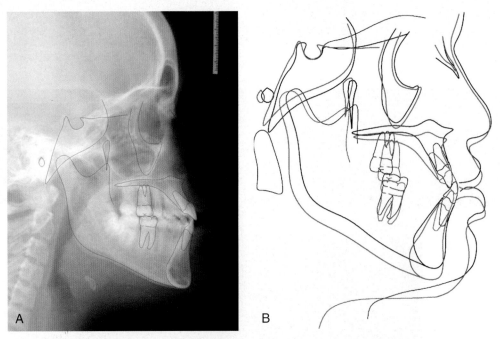

Figure 7-1-9   **A,** Posttreatment lateral cephalogram. **B,** Tracing and radiographic superimposition *Black* (pretreatment); *red* (posttreatment).

Why was a two-phase protraction used?
A single phase of full protraction of the maxilla could be complex to properly control the tooth movement three-dimensionally. A two-phase approach allows the overjet to be normalized initially, and then a second phase protracts the posterior buccal segments in a controlled manner.

CASE 7-2
Miniplate-Supported Nonextraction Class III Correction

A 17-year-old female patient's chief complaint was that her lower teeth were in front of the upper teeth. Medical and dental histories were noncontributory, and findings from a temporomandibular (TMJ) examination were normal with adequate range of jaw movements.

■ PRETREATMENT

Extraoral Analysis (Fig. 7-2-1)

Facial Form	Mesoprosopic
Facial Symmetry	No gross asymmetries noticed
Chin Point	On with the facial midline
Occlusal Plane	Normal
Facial Profile	Orthognathic
Facial Height	Upper Facial Height/Lower Facial Height: Normal
	Lower Facial Height/Throat Depth: Normal
Lips	Competent, Upper: Protrusive; Lower: Protrusive.
Nasolabial Angle	Acute
Mentolabial Sulcus	Deep

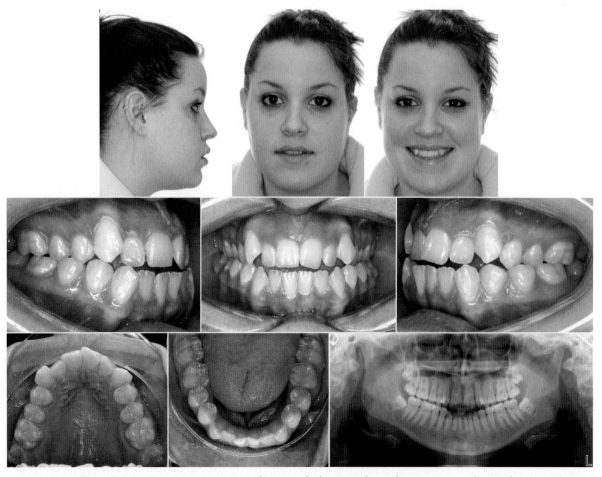

Figure 7-2-1   Pretreatment extraoral/intraoral photographs and panoramic radiograph.

Smile Analysis (Fig. 7-2-2)

Smile Arc	Flat
Incisor Display	Rest: 4 mm
	Smile: 9 mm
Lateral Tooth Display	First molar to first molar
Buccal Corridor	Normal
Gingival Tissue	Margins: Maxillary canine margins are more apical than normal, and lateral incisors are more incisal than normal
	Papilla: Present in all anterior teeth; displaced gingivally between maxillary central incisors due to large interproximal connector
Dentition	Tooth size and proportion: Normal
	Tooth shape: Sharp incisal tip on maxillary canines
	Inclination: Normal
	Axial inclination: Maxillary teeth inclined lingually
	Connector space and contact area: Long between maxillary central incisors
Incisal Embrasure	Increased between maxillary lateral incisors and canines due to morphology of canines
Midlines	Lower dental midline 1 mm to the left with the upper dental midlines coincidental with the facial midline

Intraoral Analysis (see Fig. 7-2-2)

Teeth Present	7654321/1234567 (Unerupted 8s)
	7654321/1234567
Molar Relation	Class III bilaterally
Canine Relation	Class III bilaterally
Overjet	0 mm
Overbite	−2 mm
Maxillary Arch	U shaped, asymmetric with constricted right first and second premolars and 3 mm of crowding
Mandibular Arch	U shaped with crowding of 3 mm and flat curve of Spee
Oral Hygiene	Fair

Functional Analysis

Swallowing	Normal adult pattern
Temporomandibular joint	Normal with adequate range of jaw movements

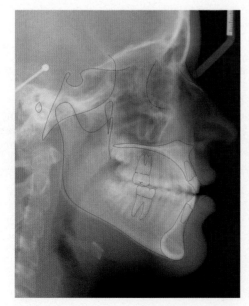

Parameter	Norm	Value
SNA (°)	82	83
SNB (°)	80	80
ANB (°)	2	3
FMA (°)	24	28
MP-SN (°)	32	40
U1-NA (mm/°)	4/22	4/17
L1-NA (mm/°)	4/25	7/26
IMPA (°)	95	86
U1-L1 (°)	130	132
OP-SN (°)	14	17
Upper Lip – E Plane (mm)	−4	−2
Lower Lip – E Plane (mm)	−2	0
Nasolabial Angle (°)	103	98
Witt's Appraisal (mm)	−1	−3

Figure 7-2-2   Pretreatment lateral cephalogram with tracing and cephalometric analysis.

Diagnosis and Case Summary

A 17-year-old female patient presented with a straight hard and soft tissue profile, an increased mandibular plane angle, and a long lower facial height. She had a Class III malocclusion with negative overjet (OJ), an anterior open bite, and labially placed and retroclined mandibular incisors with first and second premolars in crossbite.

PROBLEM LIST			
Pathology/Others	Thin biotype on labial of mandibular incisors with slight recession on right central incisors Sharp incisal tip of maxillary canines		
Alignment	3 mm of maxillary and mandibular crowding		
Dimension	**Skeletal**	**Dental**	**Soft Tissue**
Anteroposterior		OJ: –3 mm Retroclined lower incisors Class III molar and canine relationship	Straight soft tissue profile Protrusive upper and lower lips
Transverse		First and second premolars in crossbite Mandibular midline shifted to the right side by 1 mm	

Vertical	High mandibular plane
	   angle
	Long lower facial
	   height
		OB: –2	Uneven gingival heights in
			   anterior maxillary region
			   with canine margins
			   more apically positioned
			   and lateral incisor
			   margins more coronal

OB, overbite; *OJ,* overjet

TREATMENT OBJECTIVES			
Pathology/Others	Extract all the third molars		
Alignment	Relieve the maxillary and mandibular crowding by flaring the incisors		
Dimension	**Skeletal**	**Dental**	**Soft Tissue**

Anteroposterior		Correct the reverse overjet by flaring maxillary
		   incisors and retracting mandibular incisors and
		   dental arch distally with help of TADs
		Improve the molar and canine relation by
		   distalization with help of TADs
			Reduce lower lip protrusion

Transverse		Correct the maxillary first and second premolar
		   lingual crossbite by expanding the maxillary
		   arch in the premolar region with help of the
		   arch wires
		Shift the mandibular midline 1 mm to the left	

Vertical		Improve the anterior open bite by extruding the
		   lower incisors
			Evaluate gingival margins in
			   anterior maxillary region
			   posttreatment for esthetic
			   periodontal procedures

TAD, temporary anchorage device.

Treatment Options

Four possible treatment options were available:

The first option consisted of extraction of the lower first premolars and retraction of the mandibular anterior teeth. The disadvantage of this option is that it does not address the anterior open bite.

The second alternative included the extraction of the mandibular third molars and distalization of the complete lower arch distally with the help of temporary anchorage devices (TADs). By distalizing the mandibular arch with TADs in the retromolar area, the Class III relationship and the anterior open bite are addressed simultaneously with the retraction force.

The third option relied on the extraction of all the first premolars to relieve crowding and perform group B space closure in the maxillary arch and group A space closure in the mandibular arch to correct molar and canine relationship.

The fourth option consisted of orthognathic surgery; however, the skeletal disharmony was not as severe to indicate this approach.

Patient chose the second option.

TREATMENT SEQUENCE AND BIOMECHANICAL PLAN

Maxilla	Mandible
Band first molars, bond the rest of the arch, and initiate leveling with .016, .018, .016 × .022 inch NiTi arch wires.	Band first molars, bond the rest of the mandibular arch, place .032 inch SS lower lingual holding arch, and initiate leveling with .016, .018, .016 × .022 inch NiTi arch wires.
Continue leveling with .017 × .025 inch NiTi arch wire, push coil between maxillary lateral incisors and first premolars to create space for the canines.	Continue leveling with .017 × .025 inch NiTi arch wire. Place miniplates in the buccal shelf next to the mandibular first molars. Start distalization of the maxillary dental arch by connecting the miniplates to the canines and premolars with elastomeric chains. Place 200 g of distalization force.
Continue leveling with .019 × .025 inch NiTi arch wire. .019 × .25 inch SS arch wire.	Continue leveling with .019 × .025 inch NiTi arch wire. .019 × .25 inch SS arch wire and continue distalization force.
.016 × .022 inch CNA with finishing bends.	.016 × .022 inch CNA with finishing bends.
Debond and wrap around retainer.	Debond and wrap around retainer and remove the miniplates.
6-month recall appointment for retention check.	6-month recall appointment for retention check.

CNA, Connecticut new arch wire; *NiTi,* nickel titanium; *SS,* stainless steel.

■ TREATMENT SEQUENCE

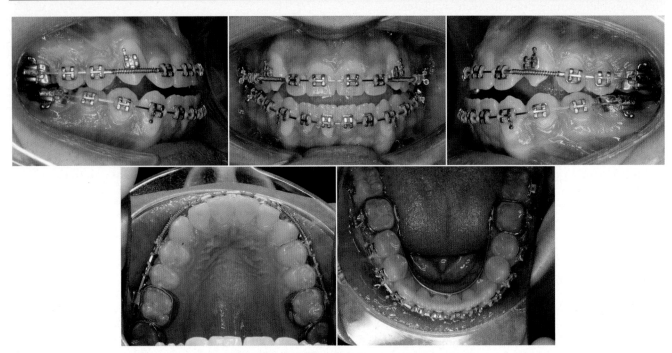

Figure 7-2-3   Initial leveling in progress.

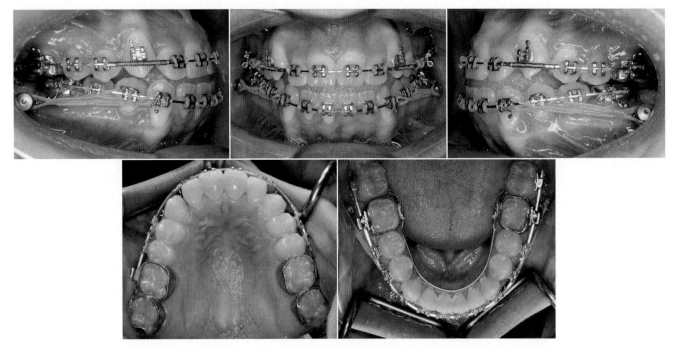

Figure 7-2-4   Mandibular arch distalization by placing 200 g of retraction force from the miniplates plates to the lower arch with the help of an elastomeric chain.

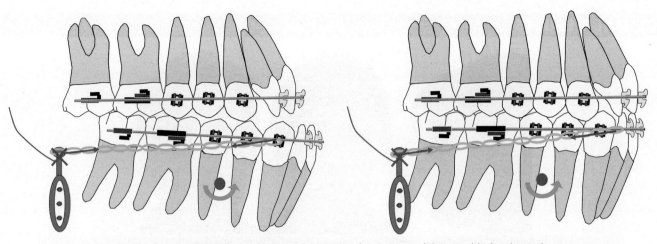

Figure 7-2-5 Distalization force above the center of resistance of the mandibular dentoalveolar arch causes counterclockwise moment of the lower arch, resulting in distalization and closure of anterior open bite.

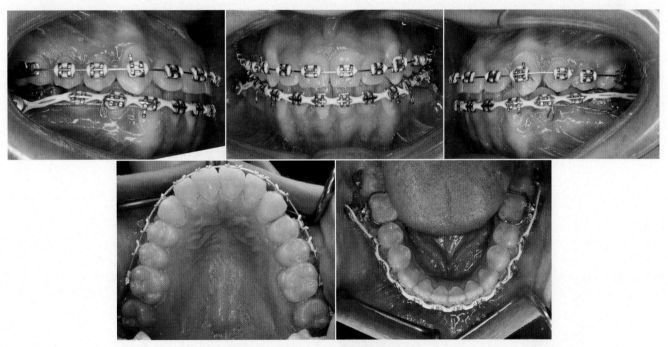

Figure 7-2-6 Finishing and settling of the occlusion.

■ FINAL RESULTS

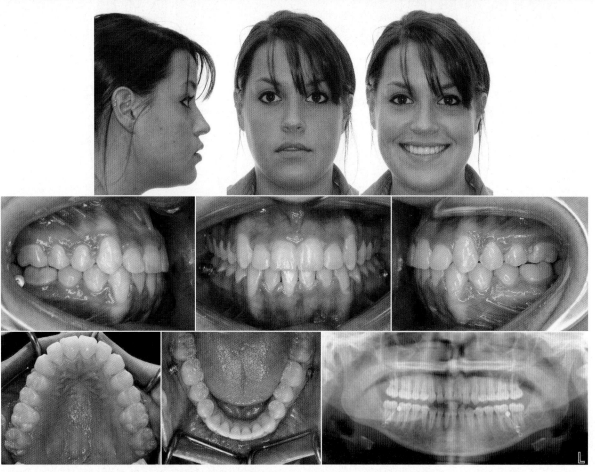

Figure 7-2-7 Posttreatment extraoral/intraoral photographs and panoramic radiograph. Note periapical lesions on the mandibular anterior segment as a result of an automobile accident.

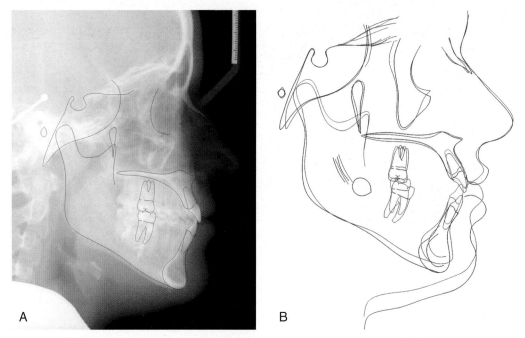

A   B

Figure 7-2-8   A, Posttreatment lateral cephalogram. **B,** Superimposition. *Black,* pretreatment; *red,* posttreatment.

Why use a miniplate and not a mini-implant for distalization of the mandibular arch?
A miniplate has been the more common approach in the literature for distalization
of the buccal segments in the mandible. A mini-implant in the buccal ridge is another
alternative from which anchorage can be drawn for the delivery of the same force
system. Usually miniplates have a slightly better success rate than mini-implants, but
a surgical procedure is necessary for both insertion and removal of the hardware.
From a biomechanical perspective, the force system is the same if both types of TADs
are placed in the same location.

Unilateral Mandibular Premolar Extraction for Midline Correction and Unilateral Maxillary Canine Substitution

A 45-year-old male's chief complaint was that "I want to take care of my teeth and close all spaces." Medical and dental histories were noncontributory, and findings from a temporomandibular (TMJ) examination were normal with adequate range of jaw movements.

■ PRETREATMENT

Extraoral Analysis (Fig. 7-3-1)

Facial Form	Mesoprosopic
Facial Symmetry	Slight mandibular asymmetry to the left side
Chin Point	Slightly left of facial midline
Occlusal Plane	Normal
Facial Profile	Orthognathic
Facial Height	Upper Facial Height/Lower Facial Height: Normal
	Lower Facial Height/Throat Depth: Slightly increased
Lips	Competent, Upper: Normal, Lower: Normal
Nasolabial Angle	Obtuse
Mentolabial Sulcus	Normal

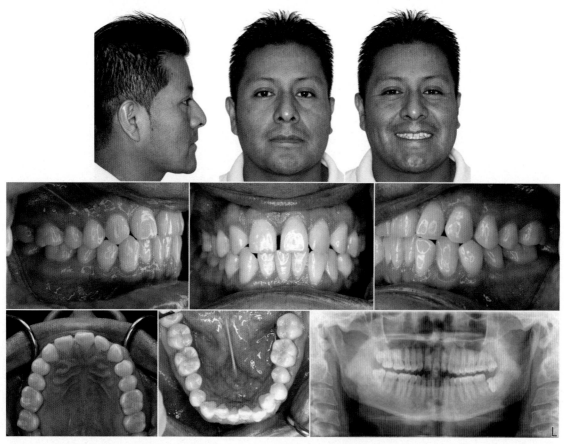

Figure 7-3-1   Pretreatment extraoral/intraoral photographs and panoramic radiograph.

Smile Analysis

Smile Arc	Reverse
Incisor Display	Rest: 0 mm
	Smile: 5 mm (50%)
Lateral Tooth Display	Second premolar to second premolar
Buccal Corridor	Narrow
Gingival Tissue	Margins: Maxillary canine margins are more incisal than incisors
	Gingival recession of maxillary left central and lateral incisor, mandibular right central and left lateral incisors, and mandibular right first premolar. Gingival recession with erosion on mandibular left first premolar.
	Papilla: Present in all anterior teeth. Displaced gingivally between maxillary central incisors due to large interproximal connector.
Dentition	Tooth size and proportion: Long left maxillary lateral incisor
	Tooth shape: Normal
	Axial inclination: Normal
	Connector space and contact area: Long between left maxillary central incisor and lateral incisor. Not present between central incisors (diastema).
Incisal Embrasure	Normal between maxillary left central and lateral incisor. Not present between central incisors (diastema) and large between right maxillary central incisor and canine because of absence of right lateral incisor.
Midlines	Maxillary dental midline is shifted to right side by 1 mm and mandibular midline shifted to left by 3 mm as compared with facial midline

Intraoral Analysis

Teeth Present	8765431/12345678
	87654321/1234567 (Impacted mandibular left 8)
Molar Relation	Class I bilaterally
Canine Relation	Class I bilaterally
Overjet	1 mm edge to edge on left lateral incisors and maxillary right central incisor and mandibular canine
Overbite	1 mm
Maxillary Arch	U shaped asymmetric with congenitally missing right lateral incisor (1 mm of spacing)
Mandibular Arch	U shaped with 4 mm of crowding and normal curve of Spee
Oral Hygiene	Fair

Functional Analysis

Swallowing	Normal adult pattern
Temporomandibular joint	Normal with adequate range of jaw movements

Diagnosis and Case Summary

A 45-year-old male had an orthognathic soft and hard tissue profile, as well as a Class I malocclusion with congenitally missing maxillary right lateral incisor, anterior crossbite and open bite tendencies, and deviation of maxillary midline to the right side by 1 mm and mandibular midline to the left side by 3 mm.

PROBLEM LIST			
Pathology/ Others	Congenitally missing maxillary right lateral incisor		
	Mild to moderate bone loss with respect to mandibular anterior teeth		
	Horizontally impacted mandibular left third molar		
	Partially erupted maxillary right third molar		
	5 mm probing depth distal mandibular left second molar, subgingival calculus/bleeding between mandibular right canine and lateral incisor		
	Gingival recession of maxillary left central and lateral incisor, mandibular right central and left lateral incisors, and mandibular right first premolar		
	Gingival recession with erosion on left mandibular left first premolar		
Alignment	Spacing (1 mm approx) in maxillary arch		
	4 mm of crowding present in mandibular arch		

Dimension	**Skeletal**	**Dental**	**Soft Tissue**
Anteroposterior		Reduced OJ due to missing tooth maxillary right lateral incisor	Obtuse nasolabial angle
		Lingually inclined lower incisors, edge-to-edge occlusion between left lateral incisors and maxillary right central incisor and mandibular canine	
Transverse	Slight mandibular asymmetry to the left side	Edge-to-edge maxillary left canine and mandibular left first premolar	
		Maxillary dental midline shifted to right side by 2 mm	
		Mandibular midline shifted to left side by 3 mm midline	
		Lingually inclined mandibular second molars	
Vertical	Slightly long lower facial height	OB: 1 mm	Uneven gingival margins in maxillary anterior region due to recession and missing right lateral incisor
		Edge-to-edge left lateral incisors	
		Reversed smile arch and decreased incisor display at smile	

OB, overbite; *OJ*, overjet.

TREATMENT OBJECTIVES			
Pathology/ Others	Extraction of all third molars		
	Scaling and root planning and clearance from periodontist to start orthodontic treatment		
	Periodontal maintenance every 4 months during orthodontic treatment		
	Consider gingival grafts in areas of recession after orthodontic treatment		
	Contour maxillary right canine to the shape of a lateral incisor		
Alignment	Close maxillary spacing and relieve mandibular crowding by extracting mandibular right first premolar and retracting canine distally		

Dimension	**Skeletal**	**Dental**	**Soft Tissue**
Anteroposterior		Improve overjet and edge-to-edge anterior relationship by retracting mandibular anterior teeth	
		Correct "canine relationship" on the right by retracting distally the mandibular canine to occlude with maxillary first premolar (substitute for canine)	
Transverse		Improve maxillary midline by IPR on the left side	
		Improve mandibular midline by retracting teeth toward right side by extracting lower right first premolar	
		Improve buccolingual inclination of second molars	
Vertical		Improve overbite and smile arc by extruding maxillary incisors	Evaluate gingival margins after orthodontic treatment and consider esthetic periodontal procedures

IPR, interproximal reduction.

Treatment Options

1. Extraction of the mandibular right first premolar and substitution of the maxillary right canine for the missing maxillary right lateral incisor. Interproximal reduction on the maxillary left side to improve the maxillary midline.
2. Open space for an implant on the right lateral incisor site with the extraction of the right mandibular first premolar. This entails a risk of significantly flaring maxillary incisors and moving the maxillary midline to the left side unless a maxillary first premolar is extracted on the right or the right buccal segment is distalized with temporary anchorage devices, in conjunction with the extraction of the mandibular right first premolar.
3. Extraction of a mandibular incisor while maintaining the maxillary right canine substitution for the lateral incisor. The disadvantage of a mandibular incisor extraction is the potential open gingival embrasure (black triangle) after space closure, especially with the already reduced periodontium in the anterior mandibular region.
4. Interproximal reduction in the lower arch while maintaining the occlusal relationship on the buccal segments. Address anterior aesthetics with space appropriation and restoration of the anterior teeth. Although this option would result in the shortest treatment time, it does not address the significant midline deviation.

After discussing with patient, Option 1 was selected as the patient wanted to reduce expenses involved with implant placement.

TREATMENT SEQUENCE AND BIOMECHANICAL PLAN

Maxilla	Mandible
Refer the patient to the periodontist for full mouth root planing and attain disease-free state. Extract third molars.	Refer the patient to the periodontist for full mouth root planing and attain disease-free state. Extract mandibular right first premolar and third molars.
Bond maxillary arch. Contour right canine to the shape of lateral incisor.	Bond mandibular arch. Place segment of .016 × .022 inch CNA wire from mandibular right second molar to second premolar and retract mandibular right canine distally with a T loop (.017 × .025 inch CNA).
Sequentially align with .016, .018, and .016 × .022 inch NiTi arch wires.	Leveling with .016 × .022 inch CNA continuous arch wire.
Continue leveling with .019 × .025 inch SS arch wire. Elastomeric chain to close the remaining spaces.	Continue leveling with .017 × .025 inch SS arch wire.
Maxillary right first premolar substituted as maxillary right canine and right maxillary canine substituted as right maxillary lateral incisor. IPR maxillary left segment to correct maxillary midline.	Continue leveling with .019 × .025 inch SS arch wire. Elastomeric chain to close the remaining spaces.
Finish the occlusion with .016 × .022 inch CNA.	Finish the occlusion with .016 × .022 inch CNA. Converge roots of mandibular central incisors to reduce the black triangles. Contour incisal edges of central incisors.
Debond and wrap around retainer.	Debond and place a canine to canine lingual bonded retainer canine to canine retainer.
6-month recall appointment for retention check.	6-month recall appointment for retention check.

CNA, Connecticut new arch wire; IPR, interproximal reduction; NiTi, nickel titanium; SS, stainless steel.

■TREATMENT SEQUENCE

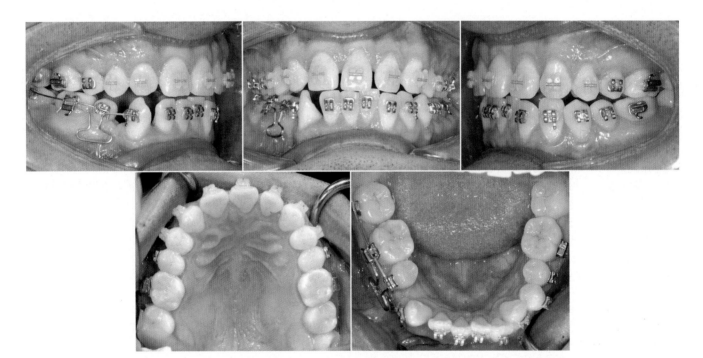

Figure 7-3-2   Segmental retraction of mandibular right canine with a T loop.

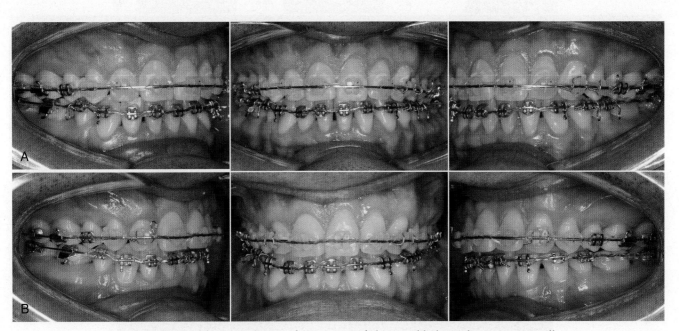

Figure 7-3-3   **A,** After completion of retraction of the mandibular right canine. Maxillary right first premolar was substituted for the maxillary right canine, and right maxillary canine was substituted for the right maxillary lateral incisor. **B,** For the black triangle to be reduced between the mandibular central incisors, roots of the mandibular anterior teeth were converged with vertical "Z" bends.

FINAL RESULTS

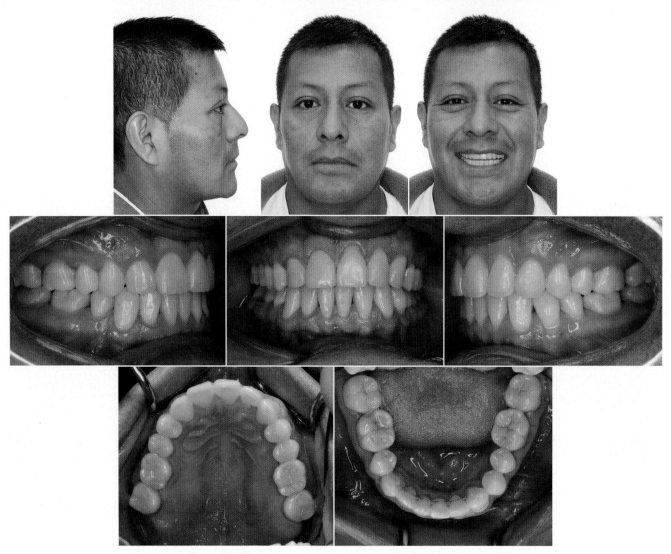

Figure 7-3-4   Posttreatment extraoral/intraoral photographs.

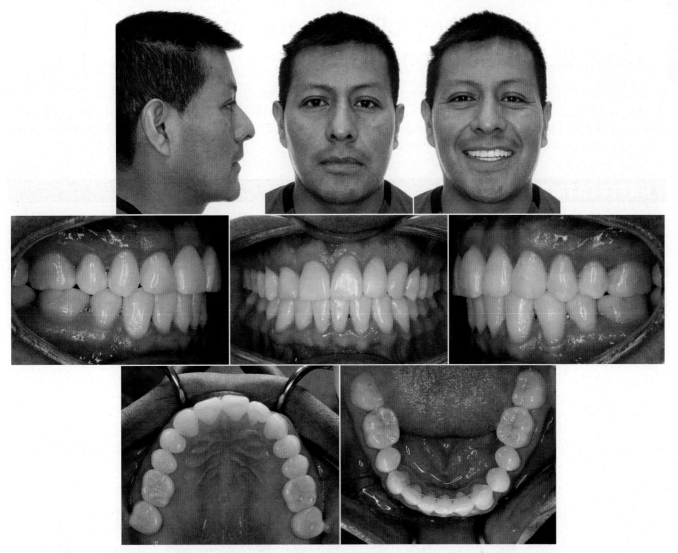

Figure 7-3-5 Postretention extraoral/intraoral photographs after external tooth bleaching.

Why was a T loop used for canine retraction?
The anchorage needs were high on the right side. A segmental approach with a T loop allows one to properly apply a differential moment technique for maximum anchorage during retraction. Preactivation bends and loop positioning maximizes the retraction of the canine with minimum anchorage loss. No arch wire was placed in the adjacent teeth during canine retraction as drift of these teeth was expected to correct the dental midlines.

How was the morphology of the maxillary right lateral incisor replicated from the canine?
The first indication for canine substitution is that the morphology of the canine resembles partially that of the lateral incisor. Important anatomic considerations are that the incisogingival height of the canine is small, the labial surface is relatively flat, and the tooth shade is light instead of opaque. Finally, lingual root torque is important to reduce the prominence of the canine root.

CASE 7-4
Conventional Orthognathic Surgery in a Severe Class III Malocclusion

A 20-year-old male patient presented with a chief complaint that his lower teeth were in front of the upper teeth. Medical and dental histories were noncontributory, and findings from a temporomandibular joint (TMJ) examination were normal with adequate range of jaw movements.

▪ PRETREATMENT

Extraoral Analysis (Fig. 7-4-1)

Facial Form	Leptoprosopic
Facial Symmetry	No gross asymmetry noticed
Chin Point	Coincidental with facial midline
Occlusal Plane	Flat
Facial Profile	Concave due to maxillary deficiency and prognathic mandible
Facial Height	Upper Facial Height/Lower Facial Height: Reduced
	Lower Facial Height/Throat Depth: Increased
Lips	Competent, Upper: Normal, Lower: Normal
Nasolabial Angle	Normal
Mentolabial Sulcus	Shallow
Malar Prominences	Deficient

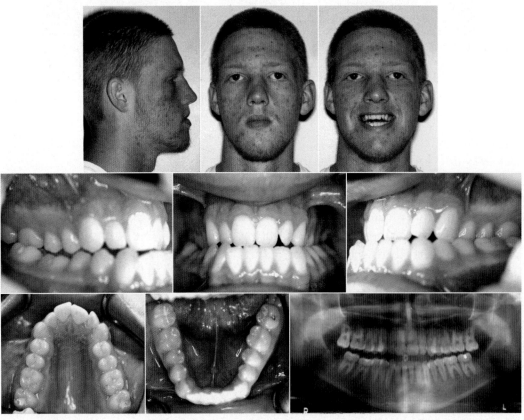

Figure 7-4-1 Pretreatment extraoral/intraoral photographs and panoramic radiograph.

Smile Analysis (Fig. 7-4-2)

Smile Arc	Flat
Incisor Display	Rest: 0 mm
	Smile: 9 mm
Lateral Tooth Display	Second premolar to second premolar
Buccal Corridor	Wide (especially on right side)
Gingival Tissue	Margins: Adequate height relationships
	Papilla: Present
Dentition	Tooth size and proportion: Normal
	Tooth shape: Normal
	Axial inclination: Maxillary teeth inclined labially, mandibular teeth retroclined
	Connector space and contact area: Normal
Incisal Embrasure	Normal except for increased incisal embrasure between maxillary right central and lateral incisor due to the rotation of the lateral
Midlines	Lower midline shifted to the left side by 2 mm as compared with the facial midline

Intraoral Analysis (see Fig. 7-4-2)

Teeth Present	7654321/1234567
	7654321/1234567
Molar Relation	Class III (full tooth) bilaterally
Canine Relation	Class III (full tooth) bilaterally
Overjet	−3 mm
Overbite	0 mm
Maxillary Arch	U shaped, symmetric, constricted, posterior crossbite
Mandibular Arch	U shaped with crowding of 3 mm and normal curve of Spee
Oral Hygiene	Fair

Functional Analysis

Swallowing	Normal adult pattern
Temporomandibular joint	Normal with adequate range of jaw movements

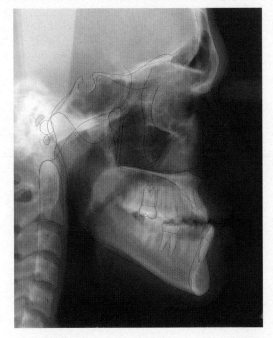

Parameter	Norm	Value
SNA (°)	82	84
SNB (°)	80	89
ANB (°)	2	−5
FMA (°)	24	23
MP-SN (°)	32	26
U1-NA (mm/°)	4/22	7/27
L1-NA (mm/°)	4/25	3/17
IMPA (°)	95	81
U1-L1 (°)	130	140
OP-SN (°)	14	4
Upper Lip – E Plane (mm)	−4	−8
Lower Lip – E Plane (mm)	−2	−2
Nasolabial Angle (°)	103	102
Witt's Appraisal (mm)	−1	−7

Figure 7-4-2 Pretreatment lateral cephalogram with tracing and cephalometric analysis.

Diagnosis and Case Summary

A 20-year-old male patient presented with concave soft and hard tissue profiles due to a combination of maxillary deficiency and mandibular prognathism. He had a Class III relationship with reduced mandibular plane angle, negative overjet, flared maxillary incisors, retroclined mandibular incisors, and bilateral skeletal crossbite due to constricted maxilla.

PROBLEM LIST			
Pathology/Others			
Alignment	3 mm of crowding present in mandibular arch 4 mm of crowding in maxillary arch		
Dimension	**Skeletal**	**Dental**	**Soft Tissue**
Anteroposterior	Concave profile due to maxillary deficiency and mandibular prognathism Witts appraisal: –7 mm	OJ: –3 mm Slight proclination of maxillary incisors Retroclined lower incisors Class III molars and canines	Concave soft tissue profile Retrusive upper lip
Transverse	Skeletal crossbite due to constricted maxilla and anteroposterior relationship	Maxillary dental arch in crossbite Mandibular buccal segments inclined lingually Mandibular midline shifted to the left side by 2 mm	
Vertical	Reduced upper facial height Reduced mandibular plane angle	Reduced incisor display at rest Flat smile arc Occlusal plane angle is reduced	

OJ, overjet.

TREATMENT OBJECTIVES			
Pathology/Others			
Alignment	Relieve the mandibular crowding by flaring the incisors and maxillary crowding with expansion		
Dimension	**Skeletal**	**Dental**	**Soft Tissue**
Anteroposterior	Advance the maxilla to improve the deficiency Set back the mandible to improve the skeletal Class III relationship	Correct the reverse overjet Correct the maxillary and mandibular incisor inclination during the presurgical stage	Correct the concave soft tissue profile and retrusive upper lip by surgical correction of the skeletal discrepancy
Transverse	Correct crossbite by advancing the maxilla and setting back the mandible	Shift the mandibular midline 2 mm to the right	
Vertical	Downfracture the maxilla to improve the upper facial height and improve the mandibular plane angle	Clockwise rotation of the occlusal plane to improve the smile arc	Improve incisal display at rest and smile

Treatment Options

Orthognathic surgery is indicated for the correction of severe skeletal facial concavity, paranasal deficiency, and Class III malocclusion. In the present case, the upper facial height and the amount of incisor show are reduced. Moreover, occlusal plane is nearly parallel to the sella-nasion (SN) plane. Two treatment options are available for this patient.

The first option is a maxillary downfracture to increase the upper facial height and increase the amount of incisor show along with mandibular set back to reduce the mandibular prognathism.

The second option is a maxillary downfracture and mandibular setback along with clockwise rotation of maxillary mandibular complex. The advantage of this approach over the first approach is that it will improve the paranasal flattening, improve the amount of incisor show, increase the upper facial height, improve the smile arc, and enhance the total amount of mandibular setback possible. The patient chose this second option.

TREATMENT SEQUENCE AND BIOMECHANICAL PLAN

Maxilla	Mandible
Band molars, bond maxillary arch, leveling with .018, .016 × .022, .019 × .025 inch NiTi arch wires. Place .019 × .025 SS arch wire before placement of surgical wire.	Band molars, bond mandibular arch, leveling with .018, .016 × .022, .019 × .025 inch NiTi arch wires. Place .019 × .025 SS arch wire before placement of surgical wire.
Crimp surgical hooks on to the .019 × .025 inch SS arch wire. Recall patients after 4 weeks for presurgical impressions.	Crimp surgical hooks on to the .019 × .025 inch SS arch wire. Recall patient after 4 weeks for presurgical impressions.
Take impression and face bow transfer for surgical stent fabrication.	Take impression and face bow transfer for surgical stent fabrication.
Orthognathic surgery.	Orthognathic surgery.
Two weeks after the surgery, remove the stent and check for appliance breakages, remove the surgical wires, replace all the debonded brackets, place .016 × .022 inch NiTi arch wires and ligate securely. Wear intermaxillary elastics to seat the occlusion.	Two weeks after the surgery, remove the stent and check for appliance breakages, remove the surgical wires, replace all the debonded brackets, place .016 × .022 inch NiTi arch wires and ligate securely. Wear intermaxillary elastics to seat the occlusion.
Continue with .017 × .025 inch NiTi arch wire.	Continue with .017 × .025 inch NiTi arch wire.
Continue with .019 × .025 inch NiTi arch wire.	Continue with .019 × .025 inch NiTi arch wire.
.016 × .022 inch CNA with finishing bends.	.016 × .022 inch CNA with finishing bends.
Debond and wrap around retainer.	Debond and bond lingual canine to canine retainer.
6-month recall appointment for retention check.	6-month recall appointment for retention check.

CNA, Connecticut new arch wire; *NiTi,* nickel titanium; *SS,* stainless steel.

TREATMENT SEQUENCE

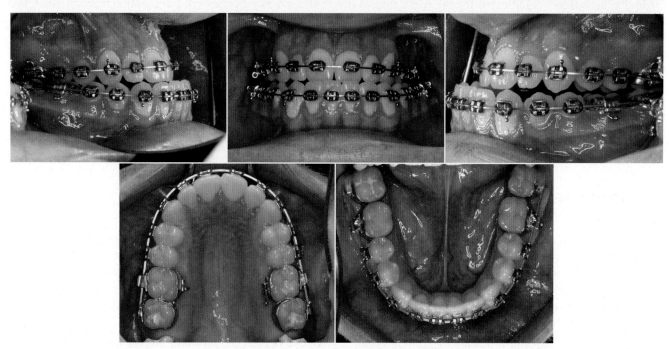

Figure 7-4-3   Presurgical alignment with .019 × .025 inch nickel titanium arch wire.

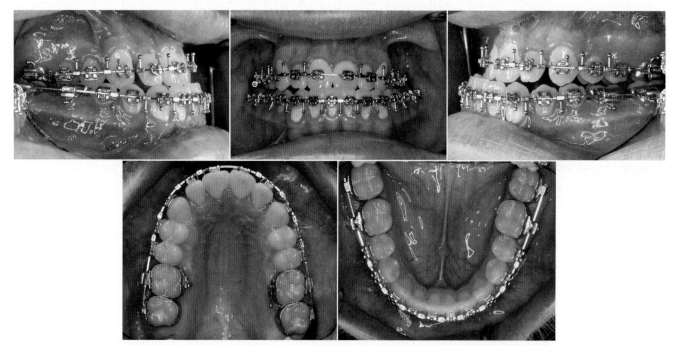

Figure 7-4-4   Presurgical stage with .019 × .025 inch stainless steel arch wire with surgical hooks crimped on it.

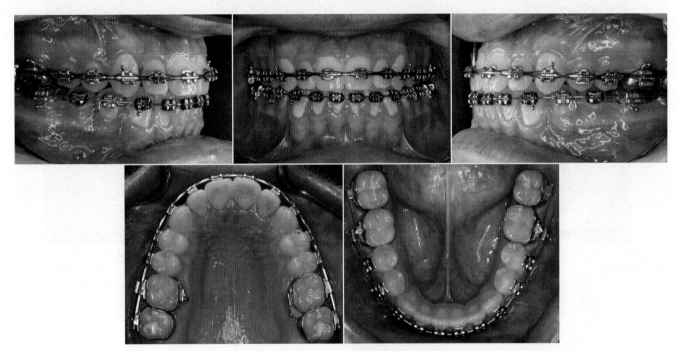

Figure 7-4-5 One month after the surgery.

■ FINAL RESULTS

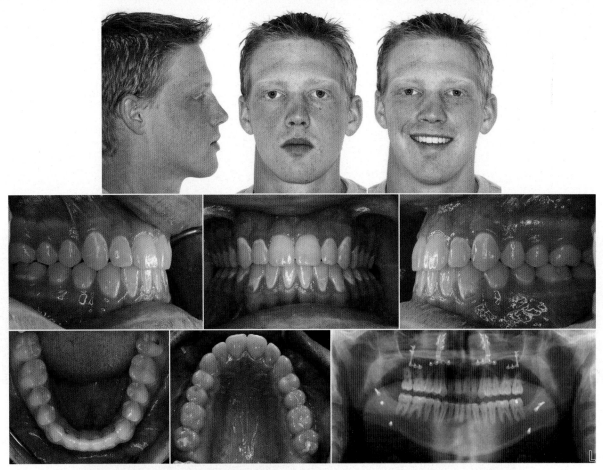

Figure 7-4-6 Posttreatment extraoral/intraoral photographs and panoramic radiograph.

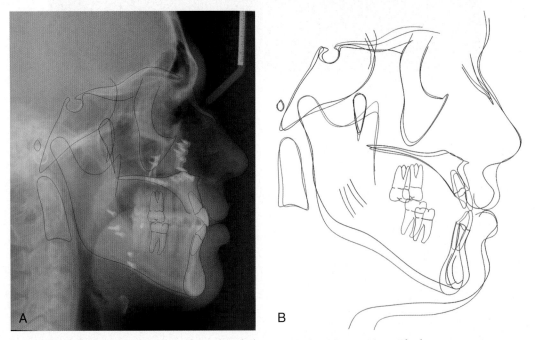

Figure 7-4-7 **A,** Posttreatment lateral cephalogram. **B,** Superimposition. *Black,* pretreatment; *red,* posttreatment.

How does clockwise rotation of the maxillomandibular complex result in improvement of smile arc and enhance the amount of mandibular setback possible?
The clockwise rotation of the maxillomandibular complex is a favorable approach for patients with maxillary deficiency, mandibular prognathism, flat occlusal plane, and normal to short anterior facial height. This rotation improves the projection of the paranasal area, creates a consonant smile arc by increasing the steepness of the occlusal plane, and improves the incisor display at rest and smile.

Why not treat this patient with Surgery First Approach?
This patient was treated before Surgery First had become a more common treatment alternative in orthognathic surgery. Although the esthetic and occlusal outcome were excellent, currently, this patient would have been treated with the Surgery First approach as all the characteristics for this surgical approach were present. Some of these characteristics are the minimal maxillary and mandibular crowding and adequate maxillary incisal anteroposterior inclination.

One of the advantages of Surgery First is that treatment duration is usually shorter. This could have benefited this patient since significant amount of white spot lesions were evident at the end of treatment.

Section 3

Transverse Problems

CASE 8-1
Maxillary Expansion and Stop Advance Wire for the Correction of a Mild Class III Malocclusion

A 12-year-old prepubertal male patient was referred by his general dentist for assessment of anterior and posterior crossbite. Medical and dental histories were noncontributory, and findings from a temporomandibular joint (TMJ) examination were normal with adequate range of jaw movements.

▪ PRETREATMENT

Extraoral Analysis (Fig. 8-1-1)

Facial Form	Mesoprosopic
Facial Symmetry	No gross asymmetries noticed
Chin Point	Coincidental with facial midline
Occlusal Plane	Steep
Facial Profile	Straight
Facial Height	Upper Facial Height/Lower Facial Height: Normal
	Lower Facial Height/Throat Depth: Increased throat depth
Lips	Competent, Upper: Normal; Lower: Protrusive
Nasolabial Angle	Obtuse
Mentolabial Sulcus	Shallow

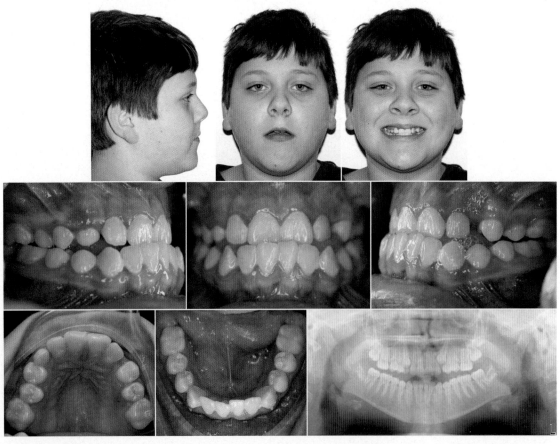

Figure 8-1-1   Pretreatment extraoral/intraoral photographs and panoramic radiograph.

Smile Analysis (Fig. 8-1-2)

Smile Arc	Flat
Incisor Display	Rest: 2 mm
	Smile: 8 mm
Lateral Tooth Display	Maxillary: Molar to molar
Buccal Corridor	Normal
Gingival Tissue	Margins: Regular
	Papilla: Present in all teeth
	Thin biotype on labial of lower incisors
	Generalized marginal gingivitis
Dentition	Tooth size and proportion: Normal
	Tooth shape: Normal
	Axial inclination: Mandibular incisors are inclined lingually
	Connector space and contact area: Contact area displaced gingivally between left central and lateral incisor
Incisal Embrasure	Normal except between maxillary left central and lateral incisor (open embrasure)
Midlines	Maxillary dental midline 2 mm left of facial midline

Intraoral Analysis (see Fig. 8-1-2)

Teeth Present	654C21/12456
	7654321/1234567 Unerupted 8s, U7s, and 3s
Molar Relation	Class III bilaterally
Canine Relation	Not evaluated as maxillary canines are unerupted
Overjet	−3 mm
Overbite	2 mm
Maxillary Arch	U shaped, symmetric with 7 mm of crowding
Mandibular Arch	U shaped with 3 mm of crowding and deep curve of Spee
Oral Hygiene	Poor

Functional Analysis

Swallowing	Normal adult pattern
Temporomandibular joint	Normal with adequate range of jaw movements

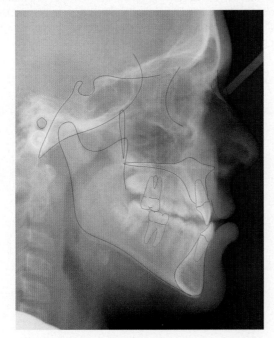

Parameter	Norm	Value
SNA (°)	82	76
SNB (°)	80	74
ANB (°)	2	−2
FMA (°)	24	27
MP-SN (°)	32	38
U1-NA (mm/°)	4/22	3/18
L1-NA (mm/°)	4/25	3/21
IMPA (°)	95	83
U1-L1 (°)	130	143
OP-SN (°)	14	20
Upper Lip – E Plane (mm)	−4	−4
Lower Lip – E Plane (mm)	−2	0
Nasolabial Angle (°)	103	116

Figure 8-1-2 Pretreatment lateral cephalogram with tracing and cephalometric analysis.

Diagnosis and Case Summary

A 12-year-old prepubertal male patient had a straight soft and hard tissue profile. He had a vertically, steep mandibular plane angle with a long lower facial height and steep occlusal plane, as well as a Class III malocclusion with retroclined mandibular incisors, anterior and posterior crossbite, and obtuse nasolabial angle.

PROBLEM LIST			
Pathology/Others	Poor oral hygiene Over-retained maxillary deciduous right canine		
Alignment	Maxillary crowding: 7 mm, blocked out Mandibular crowding: 3.019 × .025 inch SS arch wire with short Class III elastics to seat occlusion		
Dimension	**Skeletal**	**Dental**	**Soft Tissue**
Anteroposterior	Skeletal Class III	Class III molar relation OJ: –3 mm Retroclined mandibular incisors	Protrusive lower lip Obtuse nasolabial angle
Transverse	Narrow maxilla	Maxillary midline 2 mm to the left of facial midline Posterior crossbite bilaterally	
Vertical	Increased mandibular plane angle Long lower facial height	Steep occlusal plane	

OJ, overjet; *SS,* stainless steel.

TREATMENT OBJECTIVES			
Pathology/Others	Provide specific instructions for oral hygiene prior to appliance placement and carefully evaluate home care during treatment Extract over-retained right maxillary deciduous canine		
Alignment	Create space for canines by flaring maxillary incisors to relieve crowding Flare mandibular incisors to relieve crowding		
Dimension	**Skeletal**	**Dental**	**Soft Tissue**
Anteroposterior		Flare maxillary incisors to correct anterior crossbite Improve Class III molar relation with Class III elastics Flare mandibular incisors to improve incisor inclination	Improve nasolabial angle by flaring maxillary incisors
Transverse	Expand maxilla	Expand maxillary arch to correct the posterior crossbite Correct upper midline by opening space for maxillary left canine	
Vertical			

Treatment Options

Two treatment alternatives were available for the correction of the anterior crossbite.

The first option involves maxillary expansion with an RME (rapid maxillary expander) appliance and face mask therapy. This therapy is indicated for this specific patient because the skeletal discrepancy is mild. In this type of patient, face mask therapy results in normalization of the skeletal growth, as well as correction of the Class III relationship. The only disadvantage would be the potential further increase in the mandibular plane angle.

The second option also involves maxillary expansion with an RME appliance. However, instead of orthopedics, orthodontic treatment would address the occlusal discrepancy by flaring the maxillary incisors to attain positive overbite. Because the skeletal discrepancy is minimal, this approach would yield positive occlusal results with favorable growth. The disadvantage of this option is the potential significant flaring of the maxillary incisors with excessive mandibular growth.

The patient chose the second option.

TREATMENT SEQUENCE AND BIOMECHANICAL PLAN

Maxilla	Mandible
Fit bands on first molars, take a pick-up impression for fabrication of RME. Cement RME appliance and initiate palatal expansion for correction of posterior crossbite.	
.016, .08 inch SS stop advance arch wires to align and flare maxillary incisors.	Band molars and bond mandibular arch, initiate leveling with .016, .018, .016 × .022 inch NiTi arch wire.
Attain positive overjet and continue leveling with .019 × .025 inch NiTi arch wire.	Continue leveling with .019 × .025 inch NiTi arch wire.
.019 × .025 inch SS arch wire with short Class III elastics to seat occlusion.	.016 × .022 inch SS arch wire with short Class III elastics to seat occlusion.
Finish with .016 × .022 inch CNA.	Finish with .016 × .022 inch CNA.
Debond and wrap around retainer.	Debond and deliver Hawley retainer.
6-month recall appointment for retention check.	6-month recall appointment for retention check.

CNA, Connecticut new arch wire; *NiTi,* nickel titanium; *RME,* rapid maxillary expander; *SS,* stainless steel.

■TREATMENT SEQUENCE

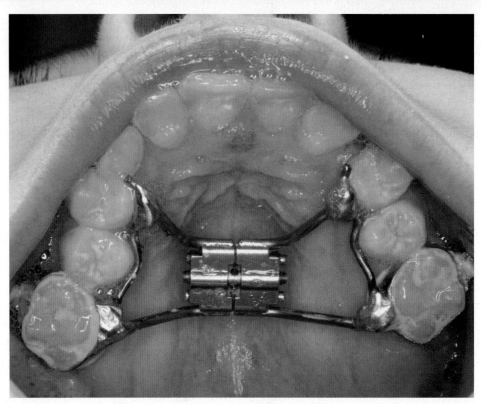

Figure 8-1-3   Rapid palatal appliance cemented in place for expansion of the maxillary dental arch for correction of the posterior crossbite.

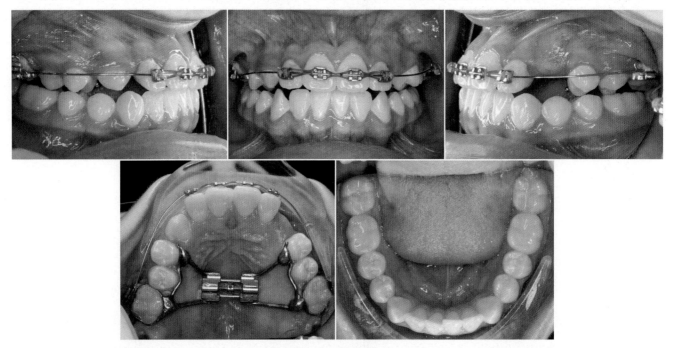

Figure 8-1-4   A .016 inch stainless steel arch wire with a stop advance arch wire to flare maxillary incisors to create space for the maxillary canines.

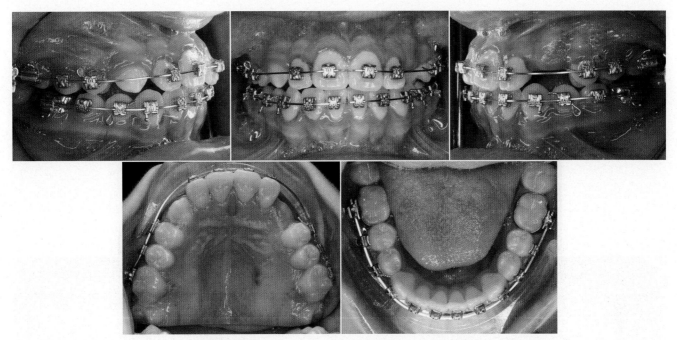

Figure 8-1-5   Maxillary and mandibular arch leveling.

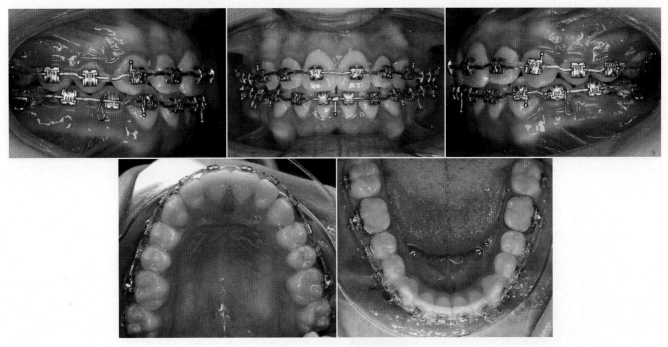

Figure 8-1-6   Finishing stage.

■ FINAL RESULTS

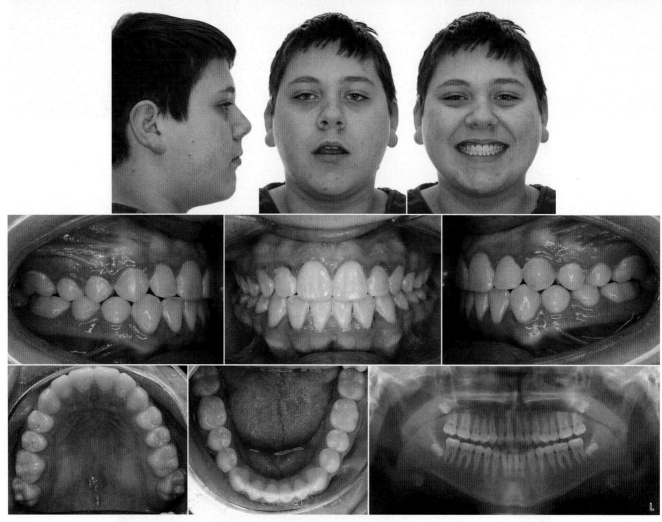

Figure 8-1-7   Posttreatment extraoral/intraoral photographs and panoramic radiograph.

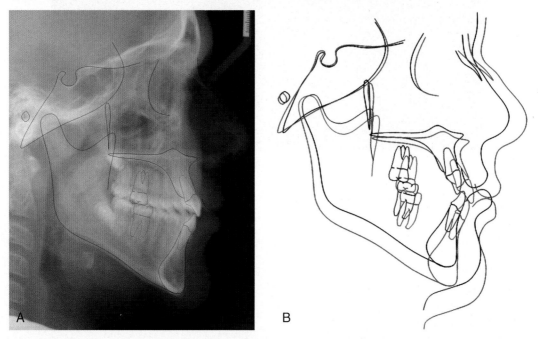

A   B

Figure 8-1-8   **A,** Posttreatment lateral cephalogram. **B,** Superimposition. *Black,* pretreatment; *red,* posttreatment.

How does the stop advance wire help in flaring of the maxillary incisors?
A stop advance wire produces an equal and opposite force system. In this patient, the maxillary incisors needed to be tipped labially to correct the overjet. This was one of the main objectives in this patient. The side effect of this labial force is distalization of the buccal segment in a Class III occlusion. For this side effect to be minimized, Class III elastics are required. In this patient favorable facial growth contributed to the correction and prevented further tipping of the incisors.

CASE 8-2
Bidimensional Distraction for Maxillary Unilateral Crossbite and Canine Retraction*

A 16-year-old female patient presented with a chief complaint of irregular teeth in the maxillary anterior region. Findings from a temporomandibular joint (TMJ) examination were normal with adequate range of jaw movements.

■ PRETREATMENT

Extraoral Analysis (Fig. 8-2-1)

Facial Form	Mesoprosopic
Facial Symmetry	No gross asymmetry noticed
Chin Point	Coincidental with facial midline
Occlusal Plane	Normal
Facial Profile	Straight
Facial Height	Upper Facial Height/Lower Facial Height: Normal
	Lower Facial Height/Throat Depth: Normal
Lips	Competent, Upper: Protrusive; Lower: Protrusive
Nasolabial Angle	Acute
Mentolabial Sulcus	Normal

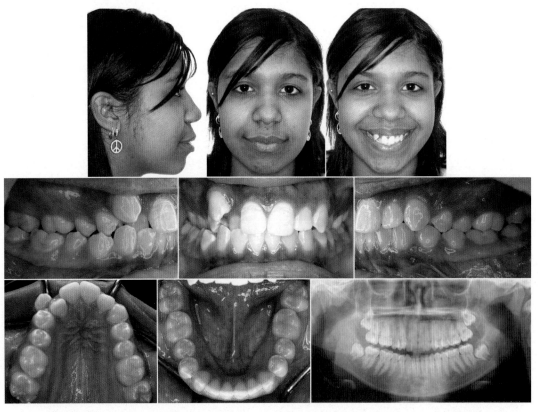

Figure 8-2-1 Pretreatment extraoral/intraoral photographs and panoramic radiograph.

*Portions of Case 8-2 from Uribe F, Agarwal S, Janakiraman N, Shafer D, Nanda R. Bidimensional dentoalveolar distraction osteogenesis for treatment efficiency. *Am J Orthod Dentofacial Orthop.* 2013;144:290-298.

Smile Analysis (Fig. 8-2-2)

Smile Arc	Consonant
Incisor Display	Rest: 1 mm
	Smile: 9 mm
Lateral Tooth Display	First molar to first molar
Buccal Corridor	Wide on the right side
Gingival Tissue	Margins: Maxillary right lateral incisor and canine margins are irregular due to crowding
	Papilla: Present
Dentition	Tooth size and proportion: Normal
	Tooth shape: Normal
	Axial inclination: Maxillary and mandibular teeth inclined labially
	Connector space and contact area: Normal
Incisal Embrasure	Normal
Midlines	Upper and lower midlines are coincidental with facial midline

Intraoral Analysis (see Fig. 8-2-2)

Teeth Present	7654321/1234567
	7654321/1234567 (Unerupted 8s)
Molar Relation	Class I on the left side and Class II on the right side
Canine Relation	Class I on the left side and Class II on the right side
Overjet	2 mm
Overbite	2 mm
Maxillary Arch	U shaped, asymmetric with 9 mm of crowding, labially placed right canine and lingually placed right lateral incisor
Mandibular Arch	U shaped, symmetric, well aligned with normal curve of Spee
Oral Hygiene	Good

Functional Analysis

Swallowing	Anterior tongue posture for seal during swallowing
Temporomandibular joint	Normal with normal range of jaw movements, no CR-CO discrepancy

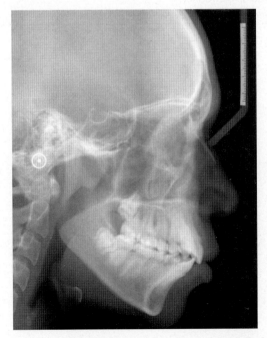

Parameter	Norm	Value
SNA (°)	85	87
SNB (°)	81	82
ANB (°)	4	5
FMA (°)	28	26
MP-SN (°)	38	34
U1-NA (mm/°)	7/22	12/28
L1-NA (mm/°)	9/33	16/40
IMPA (°)	98	104
U1-L1 (°)	119	105
OP-SN (°)	16	12
Upper Lip – E Plane (mm)	0	4
Lower Lip – E Plane (mm)	4	7
Nasolabial Angle (°)	90	95

Figure 8-2-2 Pretreatment lateral cephalogram and cephalometric analysis.

Diagnosis and Case Summary

A 16-year-old female patient had a straight soft and convex hard tissue profile and a Class II subdivision malocclusion. The maxillary right canine is blocked labially out of the arch, the maxillary right lateral incisor is in anterior crossbite, and a unilateral crossbite is present on the right side. The maxillary and mandibular anterior teeth are proclined, resulting in an acute interincisal angle and protrusive upper and lower lips with an acute nasolabial angle.

PROBLEM LIST

Pathology/Others

Alignment		9 mm of crowding present in maxillary arch Labially blocked out maxillary right canine	
Dimension	**Skeletal**	**Dental**	**Soft Tissue**
Anteroposterior	Convex profile	Class II molar and canine relation on right side Proclined maxillary and mandibular incisors Acute interincisal angle Anterior crossbite of maxillary right lateral incisor	Convex profile Protrusive upper and lower lips Acute nasolabial angle
Transverse	Maxillary constriction	Right side unilateral buccal crossbite Left premolars in crossbite tendency	
Vertical		Slightly reduced incisor display at rest	

TREATMENT OBJECTIVES

Pathology/Others

Alignment		Align the maxillary arch after creating space on the right side by extraction of the right first premolar	
Dimension	**Skeletal**	**Dental**	**Soft Tissue**

Anteroposterior		Maintain the Class II molar on right and distalize the
		    right canine into Class I with dentoalveolar
		    distraction
		Correct crossbite of maxillary right lateral incisor	

Transverse	Expand right buccal
	    segment surgically
		Expand right buccal segment by means of
		    dentoalveolar distraction	

Vertical			

Treatment Options

The malocclusion in this patient was evident in two planes of space, sagittal and transverse. The traditional approach would be to address the transverse dimension early in treatment by means of a surgically assisted rapid palatal expansion, followed by extraction of the maxillary right first premolar to align the labially placed right maxillary canine. Total treatment time was expected to be around 20 to 24 months.

The second alternative was to simultaneously perform surgically assisted unilateral rapid palatal expansion and distraction of the labially placed right maxillary canine into the extraction space of the right first premolar, taking anchorage from a skeletal anchorage device.

The third alternative would entail a four-premolar extraction treatment to reduce the incisor inclination in conjunction with the first or second option. This option would also require distalization of the maxillary right buccal segment (aided by skeletal anchorage) in order to move the incisors lingually without affecting the maxillary midline.

The patient chose the second option over a conventional approach because the total treatment time estimated was around 12 to 15 months.

TREATMENT SEQUENCE AND BIOMECHANICAL PLAN

Maxilla	Mandible
Dentoalveolar segmental osteotomy for transverse dentoalveolar distraction of the maxillary right side buccal segment to correct the right unilateral crossbite and for distraction of the maxillary right canine after extraction of the right maxillary canine (Fig. 8-2-5). Place skeletal anchorage plate on the right side of the maxilla to connect the canine distractor. Place rapid palatal expander and canine distractor.	
Continue palatal expansion and canine distraction at the rate of 4 turns/day.	Band 6s and 7s, place .032 × .032 inch CNA lingual arch, segmental .019 × .025 inch SS wire connecting right 6s and 7s.
Bond 5-5 and align the arch with .016 × .022, .019 × .025 inch NiTi arch wires.	Bond 5-5 and align the arch with .016 × .022, .019 × .025 inch NiTi arch wires.
.016 × .022 inch CNA with finishing bends and seating elastics.	.016 × .022 inch CNA with finishing bends and seating elastics.
Debond and wrap around retainer. Remove the bone plate.	Debond and place 3-3 lingual fixed retainer.
6-month recall appointment for retention check.	6-month recall appointment for retention check.

CNA, Connecticut new arch wire; NiTi, nickel titanium; SS, stainless steel.

■ TREATMENT SEQUENCE

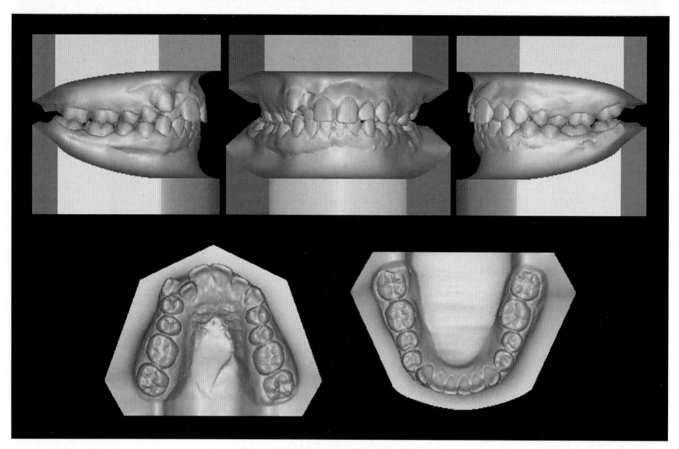

Figure 8-2-3   Pretreatment dental cast.

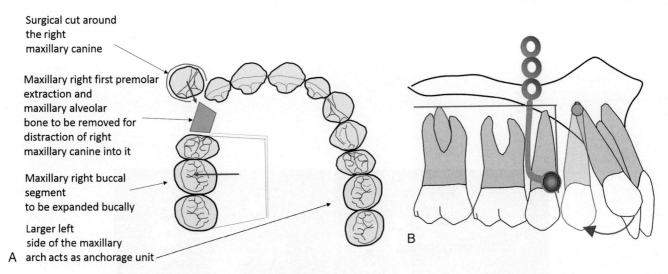

Surgical cut around
the right
maxillary canine

Maxillary right first premolar
extraction and
maxillary alveolar
bone to be removed for
distraction of right
maxillary canine into it

Maxillary right buccal
segment
to be expanded bucally

Larger left
side of the maxillary
A arch acts as anchorage unit

B

Figure 8-2-4   Surgical plan. **A,** Maxillary occlusal view showing the intended skeletal and dental movement. **B,** Right maxillary canine to be distracted into the extraction space of the right first premolar.

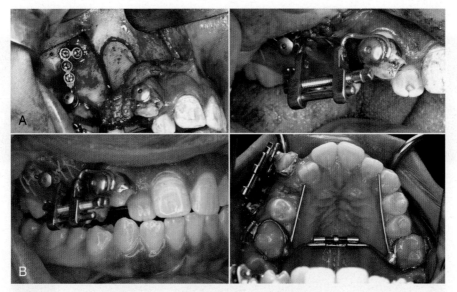

Figure 8-2-5   A, Osteotomies for unilateral dentoalveolar expansion and canine retraction, respectively. **B,** Trial mounting of the distraction appliance during surgery to confirm mobility of the osteotomized dentoalveolar right maxillary buccal segment and canine.

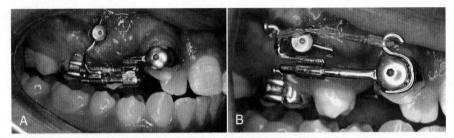

Figure 8-2-6   **A,** Right buccal view showing the new distractor in place after fracture of the first canine distraction device. Bending of the miniplate in mesial-lingual direction is evident. **B,** Right buccal view showing a change of the canine retraction distractor device to a sliding yoke appliance attached from the skeletal miniplate to the canine, allowing orthodontic retraction of the right maxillary canine.

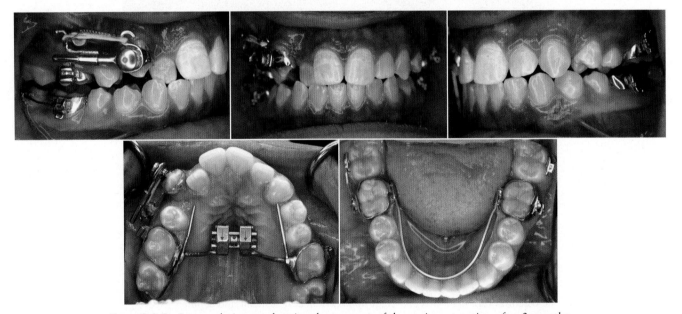

Figure 8-2-7   Intraoral pictures showing the progress of the canine retraction after 2 months.

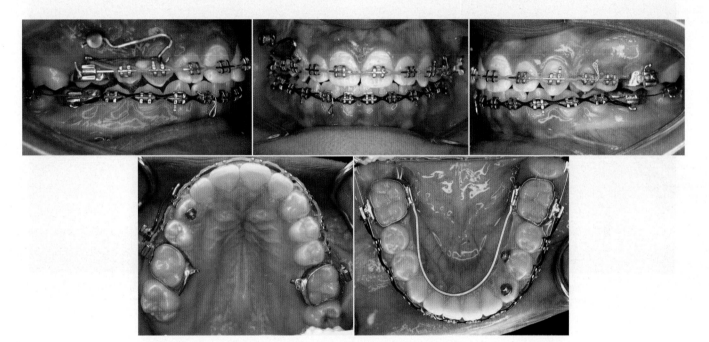

Figure 8-2-8 Intraoral photographs showing finishing and settling of occlusion.

■ FINAL RESULTS

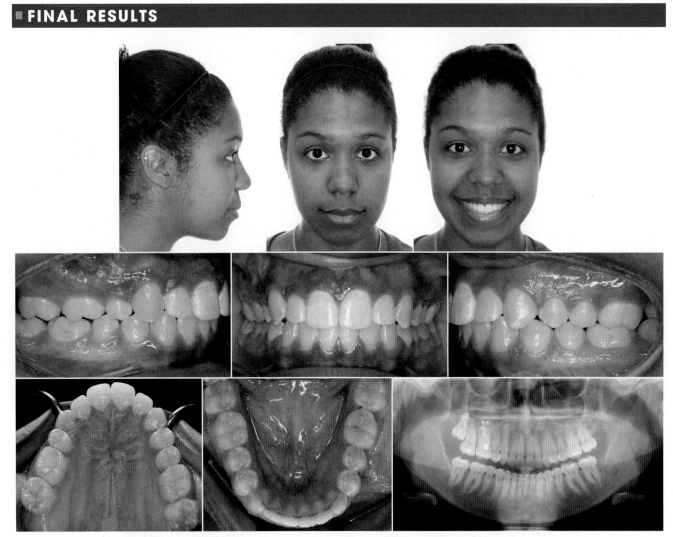

Figure 8-2-9 Posttreatment extraoral/intraoral photographs and panoramic radiograph after 13 months of treatment.

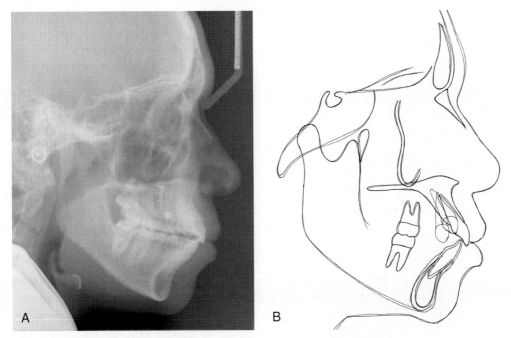

Figure 8-2-10 **A,** Posttreatment lateral cephalogram. **B,** Superimposition. *Blue,* pretreatment; *red,* posttreatment.

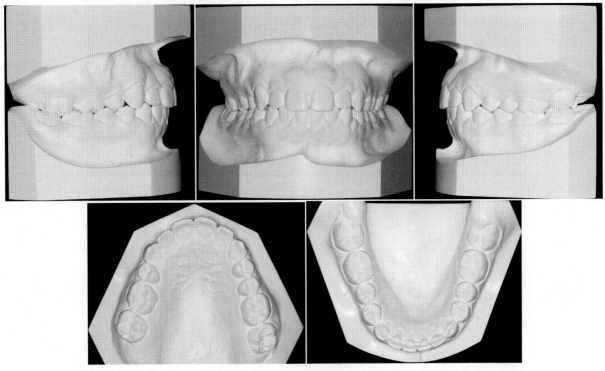

Figure 8-2-11 Posttreatment dental casts.

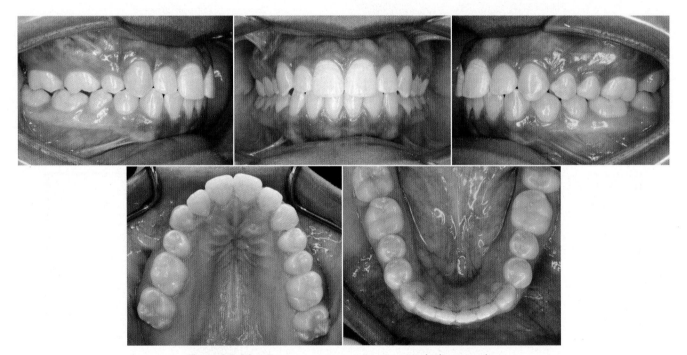

Figure 8-2-12   One-year postretention intraoral photographs.

Why was the anteroposterior dentoalveolar distraction of the maxillary right canine performed from a mini-plate instead of the maxillary molar?
The maxillary first molar was to be distracted laterally for the correction of the unilateral crossbite. Thus this segment was also receiving an osteotomy with mobilization. Drawing anchorage from this mobilized segment would have resulted in mesial tipping of the segment, which required maximum anteroposterior anchorage control. Thus a miniplate was placed in the maxilla to distract the canine distally with maximum retraction of this tooth and no anchorage loss.

What is the prognosis of vitality of the distracted canine?
The prognosis of the vitality of the canine after receiving an osteotomy is usually favorable in the long term. Some temporary loss of sensitivity may be found after surgery. In this patient, however, temperature tests revealed possible loss of vitality of the pulpal tissue. The patient is being monitored by an endodontist for any symptoms that have not yet occurred.

CASE 9-1
Correction of a Canted Maxillary Incisal Plane with Different Approaches to a One-Couple System

A 12-year-old male patient's chief complaint was crowding in his upper and lower front teeth. Medical and dental histories were noncontributory, and findings from a temporomandibular joint (TMJ) examination were normal with adequate range of jaw movements.

■ PRETREATMENT

Extraoral Analysis (Fig. 9-1-1)

Facial Form	Mesoprosopic
Facial Symmetry	No gross asymmetry noted
Chin Point	Coincidental with facial midline
Occlusal Plane	Normal
Facial Profile	Convex due to retrognathic mandible
	Facial Height: Upper Facial Height/Lower Facial Height: Slightly reduced
	Lower Facial Height/Throat Depth: Normal
Lips	Competent, Upper: Normal; Lower: Normal
Nasolabial Angle	Obtuse
Mentolabial Sulcus	Normal

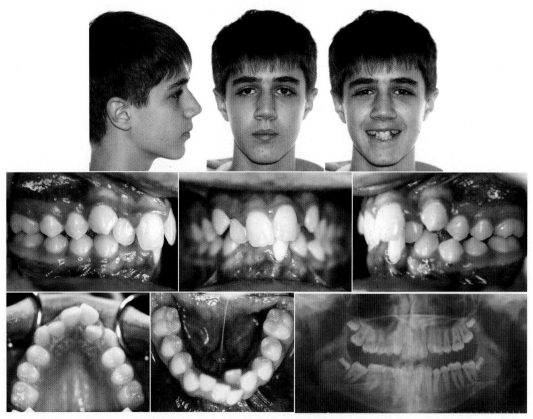

Figure 9-1-1 Pretreatment extraoral/intraoral photographs and panoramic radiograph.

Smile Analysis (Fig. 9-1-2)

Smile Arc	Consonant
Incisor Display	Rest: 3 mm
	Smile: 8 mm (asymmetric incisal display)
Lateral Tooth Display	Maxillary second premolar to second premolar
Buccal Corridor	Normal
Gingival Tissue	Margins: Uneven heights of maxillary incisors due to incisal plane cant
	Papilla: Present in all teeth
	Recession of mandibular left central incisor with reduced attached gingival width
Dentition	Tooth size and proportion: Normal
	Tooth shape: Rounded incisal edge of maxillary lateral incisors
	Prominent root of mandibular left central incisor
	Axial inclination: Upright maxillary and mandibular incisors
	Maxillary central incisor crowns are tipped to the left
	Connector space and contact area: Long between maxillary central incisors displacing the papilla gingivally
Incisal Embrasure	Increased between maxillary right central and lateral incisor
Midlines	Upper dental midline shifted to the left side by 2 mm with respect to the facial midline

Intraoral Analysis (see Fig. 9-1-2)

Teeth Present	654321/123456
	654321/123456 (Unerupted 7 and 8s)
Molar Relation	Class II on right and Class I left
Canine Relation	Class II end on bilaterally
Overjet	4 mm
Overbite	7 mm
Maxillary Arch	V shaped with 4 mm of crowding and lingually blocked-out left lateral incisor
Mandibular Arch	V shaped with 8 mm of crowding, lingually blocked-out left lateral incisor and normal curve of Spee
Oral Hygiene	Fair

Functional Analysis

Swallowing	Normal adult pattern
Temporomandibular joint	Normal with adequate range of jaw movements

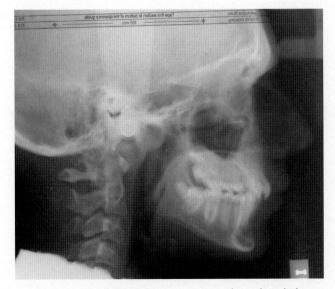

Parameter	Norm	Value
SNA (°)	82	82
SNB (°)	80	78
ANB (°)	2	4
FMA (°)	24	26
MP-SN (°)	32	34
U1-NA (mm/°)	4/22	4/26
L1-NA (mm/°)	4/25	3/22
IMPA (°)	95	90
U1-L1 (°)	130	135
OP-SN (°)	14	13
Upper Lip – E Plane (mm)	−4	−3
Lower Lip – E Plane (mm)	−2	0
Nasolabial Angle (°)	103	108

Figure 9-1-2 Pretreatment lateral cephalogram and cephalometric analysis.

Diagnosis and Case Summary

A 12-year-old male patient had convex soft and hard tissue profiles due to a retrognathic mandible Class II subdivision right malocclusion. Vertically, he had an asymmetric anterior deep bite with supraerupted maxillary incisors and maxillary and mandibular arch crowding.

PROBLEM LIST			
Pathology/Others	Irregular maxillary gingival margins of anterior maxillary teeth Recession of mandibular left central incisor with reduced attached gingiva width and prominent root		
Alignment	Maxillary arch crowding: 4 mm Mandibular arch crowding: 8 mm Lingually placed maxillary and mandibular left lateral incisor		
Dimension	**Skeletal**	**Dental**	**Soft Tissue**
Anteroposterior	Convex profile due to retrognathic mandible	Class II end canine relation bilaterally	Increased nasolabial angle
Vertical		Anterior deep bite of 7 mm due to supraerupted maxillary incisors Maxillary incisal cant	
Transverse		Maxillary midline shifted to left side by 2 mm with tipped crowns of the central incisors to the left	

TREATMENT OBJECTIVES			
Pathology/Others	Level the maxillary anterior teeth to level the gingival margins Monitor recession and correct root prominence of the left mandibular central incisor		
Alignment	Align maxillary and mandibular teeth by flaring of the incisors and expansion of the arches		
Dimension	**Skeletal**	**Dental**	**Soft Tissue**
Anteroposterior		Correct Class II canine relation bilaterally	
Vertical		Asymmetric intrusion of maxillary anterior teeth to correct the deep bite Level the lower arch	Level the maxillary gingival margins of maxillary anterior segment
Transverse		Asymmetric intrusion of maxillary anterior teeth to correct the maxillary midline	

Treatment Options

Two options were presented:
1. Extraction of four premolars to relieve crowding
2. Nonextraction option with expansion of the arches

The patient selected a nonextraction option. For correction of the asymmetric overjet due to the supraerupted maxillary incisors with a cant, intrusion was to be approached with a one-couple system.

TREATMENT SEQUENCE AND BIOMECHANICAL PLAN

Maxilla	Mandible
Band molars and bond maxillary incisors.	
Sectional leveling central incisors and right lateral incisor with .016, .018, and .016 × .022 inch NiTi, .016 × .022 inch SS arch wires.	
Spot weld a crosstube on to the main arch wire distal to the right lateral incisor bracket. .017 × .025 inch CNA cantilever from the crosstube with hook next to the right first molar, with extrusive force acting at the posterior segment and intrusive force with a clockwise moment acting on the anterior segment. Place 25 g of force.	
Continue asymmetric anterior intrusion with a .017 × .025 inch NiTi intrusion arch tied to the right lateral incisor.	Band molars and bond mandibular arch. Continue leveling with .016, .018, .016 × .022, and .017 × .025 inch NiTi arch wires.
Continue leveling with .019 × .025 inch SS arch wire. Push coil between left central incisor and first premolar to open up the space for blocked left lateral incisor.	Continue leveling with .017 × .025 inch SS arch wire. Push coil between left central incisor and first premolar to open up the space for the blocked left lateral incisor.
Continue leveling with .019 × .025 inch SS arch wire.	Continue leveling with .019 × .025 inch SS arch wire.
.016 × .025 inch CNA with finishing bends.	.016 × .025 inch CNA with finishing bends.
Debond and wrap around retainer.	Debond and bond a lingual canine to canine retainer.
6-month recall appointment for retention check.	6-month recall appointment for retention check.

CNA, Connecticut new arch wire; *NiTi,* nickel titanium; *SS,* stainless steel.

▪TREATMENT SEQUENCE

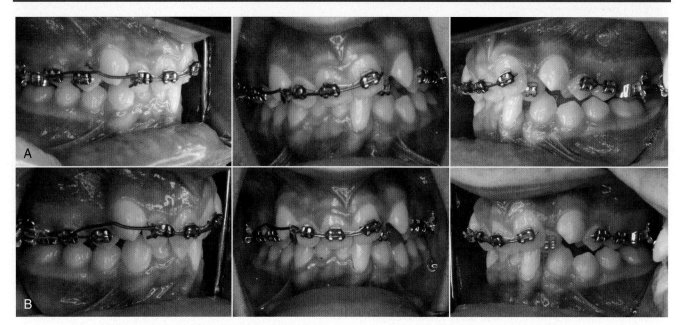

Figure 9-1-3 **A,** .017 × .025 inch Connecticut new arch wire cantilever from the crosstube with hook next to the right first molar, with extrusive force acting at posterior segment and intrusive force acting at the anterior. **B,** Improvement in anterior deep bite and correction of axial inclination of maxillary anterior teeth, as well as maxillary midline.

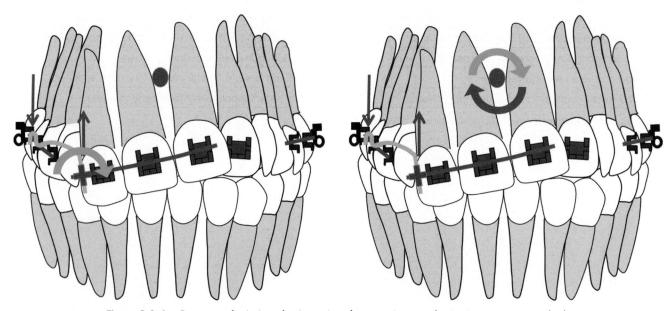

Figure 9-1-4 Cartoons depicting the intrusion force acting on the incisor segment, which results in clockwise moment. In addition, the moment of the one-couple system provides another clockwise moment. This force system results in intrusion, as well as correction of the axial inclination of the incisors.

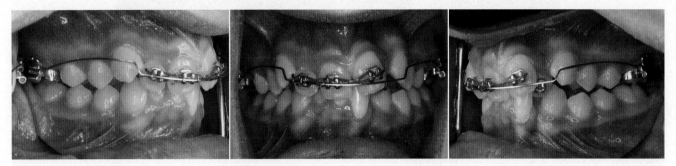

Figure 9-1-5 Nickel titanium intrusion arch tied asymmetrically to the left lateral incisor, resulting in further correction of the anterior deep bite and axial inclination of incisors.

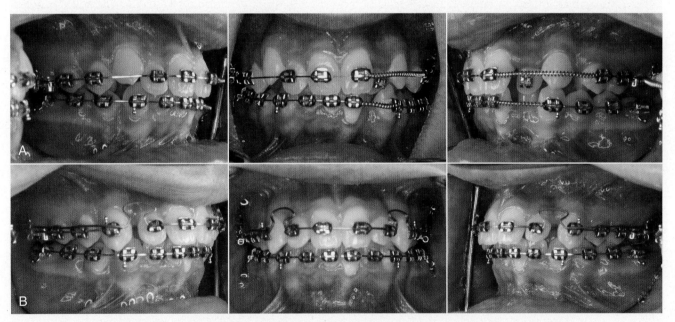

Figure 9-1-6 **A,** Push coil in maxillary and mandibular aches to create space for the blocked out left lateral incisor. **B,** Mushroom loop arch wire for incisor retraction.

■ FINAL RESULTS

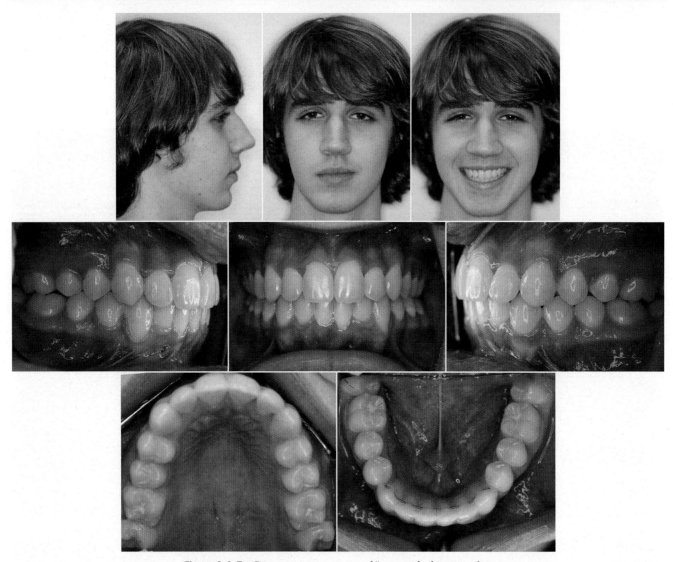

Figure 9-1-7   Posttreatment extraoral/intraoral photographs.

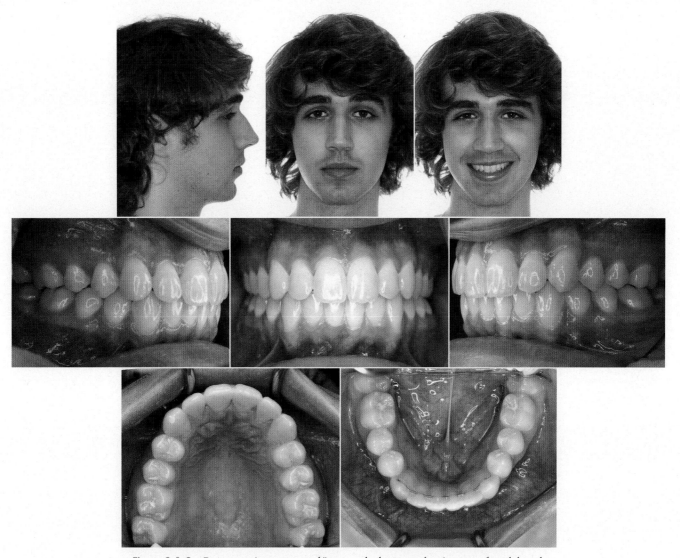

Figure 9-1-8   Postretention extraoral/intraoral photographs 6 years after debond.

Why use a one-couple system to correct the maxillary incisor cant?
A one-couple system is a predictable and versatile appliance in orthodontics. In this patient both components of this system were used to correct the maxillary incisal cant: the force and the moment. For the moment to be delivered in the system, the wire was required to be engaged on a tube. This was accomplished in this patient through the crosstube placed on the anterior segment next to the maxillary right lateral incisor. On the other hand, the force delivered on the other end of the system was attached on top of the segment (single-point contact) that included the maxillary first molar to the first premolar. After initial intrusion and clockwise rotation of the anterior segment, the one-couple system was reversed to conform to a typical intrusion arch configuration, which extended from the molar anteriorly. It was tied asymmetrically on the anterior segment to achieve the necessary intrusion and clockwise rotation of this segment.

Section 4

Impacted Teeth

CASE 10-1
Maxillary Impacted Canine and Anterior Restorations for Microdontic Lateral Incisors

A 23-year-old female patient presented with a chief complaint of spacing in the maxillary anterior region. Medical and dental histories were noncontributory, and findings from a temporomandibular joint (TMJ) examination were normal with adequate range of jaw movements.

PRETREATMENT

Extraoral Analysis (Fig. 10-1-1)

Facial Form	Mesoprosopic
Facial Symmetry	No gross asymmetries noticed
Chin Point	Coincidental with facial midline
Occlusal Plane	Normal
Facial Profile	Normal
Facial Height	Upper Facial Height/Lower Facial Height: Normal
	Lower Facial Height/Throat Depth: Normal
Lips	Competent, Upper: Slightly protrusive, Lower: Protrusive
Nasolabial Angle	Normal
Mentolabial Sulcus	Slightly deep

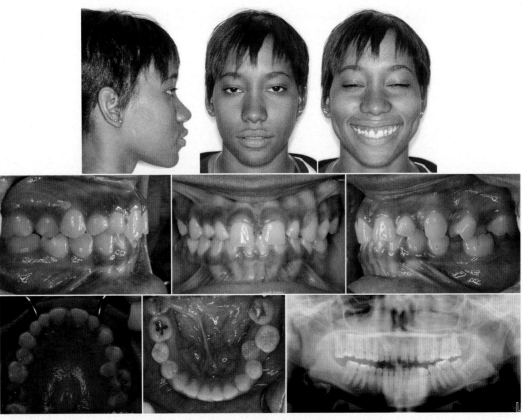

Figure 10-1-1　Pretreatment extraoral/intraoral photographs and panoramic radiograph.

Smile Analysis (Fig. 10-1-2)

Smile Arc	Consonant
Incisor Display	Rest: 4 mm
	Smile: 4 mm of gingival display
Lateral Tooth Display	First molar to first molar
Buccal Corridor	Absent
Gingival Tissue	Margins: Maxillary right canine margin is low (primary tooth), altered passive eruption on maxillary central incisors
	Papilla: Present in teeth with closed contacts
	Low insertion of the labial frenum between the maxillary central incisors
Dentition	Tooth size and proportion: Maxillary lateral incisors smaller in size (primarily in length). Maxillary central incisors short in length due to altered passive eruption.
	Tooth shape: Normal
	Axial inclination: Maxillary and mandibular incisors are labially placed and flared
	Connector space and contact area: No contact between maxillary anterior teeth
Incisal Embrasure	Not present in maxillary central incisors due to diastema; absent between maxillary central incisors and laterals
Midlines	Upper and lower midline are coincidental with the facial midline

Intraoral Analysis (see Fig. 10-1-2)

Teeth Present	87654C21/124567
	7654321/12345678
	Maxillary right third molar supraerupted without antagonist
Molar Relation	Class I on the right side and Class III on left side
Canine Relation	Class III on the left side and not applicable on the right side
Overjet	2 mm
Overbite	5 mm
Maxillary Arch	U shaped with impacted right canine, over-retained deciduous right canine, midline diastema of 3 mm, space of 3 mm distal to right lateral incisor, left second premolar lingually placed, left first molar labially placed, and supraerupted maxillary right third molar
Mandibular Arch	U shaped with 4 mm of crowding, lingually placed left second premolar and molar and labially placed left first molar, and normal curve of Spee
Oral Hygiene	Fair

Functional Analysis

Swallowing	Normal adult pattern
Temporomandibular joint	Normal with adequate range of jaw movements

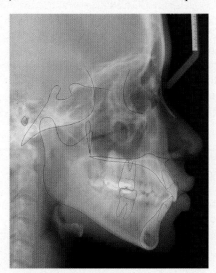

Parameter	Norm	Value
SNA (°)	85	83
SNB (°)	81	80
ANB (°)	4	3
FMA (°)	28	30
MP-SN (°)	38	38
U1-NA (mm/°)	7/22	6/21
L1-NA (mm/°)	9/33	8/30
IMPA (°)	98	91
U1-L1 (°)	119	125
OP-SN (°)	16	20
Upper Lip – E Plane (mm)	0	1.3
Lower Lip – E Plane (mm)	4	2.3
Nasolabial Angle (°)	90	90

Figure 10-1-2 Pretreatment lateral cephalogram with tracing and cephalometric analysis.

Diagnosis and Case Summary

A 23-year-old female patient had a normal hard and convex soft tissue profile. She had a Class III subdivision left malocclusion with flared maxillary and mandibular anterior teeth, impacted right maxillary canine, over-retained right deciduous maxillary canine, maxillary midline diastema of 3 mm, maxillary left first premolar and molar in labial crossbite, and maxillary second premolars in lingual crossbite. Aesthetically in the maxilla, an altered passive eruption is observed in the central incisors, as well as excessive gingival display in the anterior region and small lateral incisors.

PROBLEM LIST

Pathology/ Others	Over-retained right maxillary deciduous canine
	Altered passive eruption with respective to the maxillary central incisors
	Maxillary lateral incisors small in size
	Thick labial frenum between maxillary central incisors
Alignment	Impacted right maxillary canine
	Maxillary midline diastema of 3 mm
	3 mm of space distal to maxillary left lateral incisor
	4 mm of crowding present in mandibular arch with buccolingual displacement of the left buccal segments

Dimension	Skeletal	Dental	Soft Tissue
Anteroposterior		Class III molar relation on the left side	Slightly protrusive upper and lower lips
		Class III canine relation on the left side	
Transverse		Lingually placed left second premolars and mandibular left second molar	
		Labially placed left first molar	
		Dental crossbite (lingual) of right second premolars and between maxillary left first premolar and mandibular second premolar (buccal)	
		Dental cross bite between maxillary left second premolar and mandibular first molar (lingual) and between maxillary left first molar and mandibular second molar (labial)	
Vertical		Supraerupted maxillary right third molar	Increased gingival display upon smiling
			Irregular heights of maxillary anterior gingival margins
			Narrow band of attached gingiva on labial aspect of the anterior mandibular dentition

TREATMENT OBJECTIVES

Pathology/ Others	Extraction of retained right maxillary deciduous canine and supraerupted maxillary right third molar
	Gingivectomy/crown-lengthening procedure respective to the maxillary central incisors
	Frenectomy maxillary labial frenum between central incisors
	Level maxillary anterior gingival margins and build up small maxillary lateral incisors
Alignment	Erupt impacted maxillary right canine into the arch
	Close maxillary midline diastema and space distal to maxillary left lateral incisor
	Align buccolingually displaced teeth on the left buccal segments
	Relieve mandibular crowding

Dimension	Skeletal	Dental	Soft Tissue
Anteroposterior		Maintain Class III molar relation on the left side	
		Correct Class III canine to Class I canine relation on left side	
Transverse		Align the palatally placed maxillary right canine	
		Correct dental crossbites on both buccal segments	
Vertical			Gingivectomy/crown lengthening procedure/leveling of gingival margins of maxillary anterior teeth

Treatment Options

Three treatment options were offered to this patient.

With the first option, the left first or second premolars in both the maxillary and mandibular arch could be extracted and space closed by mesializing the molars. This option will result in a Class I molar and canine relation on both sides at the end of treatment but will have high anchorage demands on the maxillary left first and second molars.

The second option offered was the distalization in mandibular left first and second molars to align the second premolar. This option will also result in Class I molar and a canine relation in both sides at the end of treatment but will require skeletal anchorage to distalize these teeth.

The third option offered was to extract the mandibular left first premolar and proceed with space closure finishing Class I canine bilaterally, Class I molar on the right side, and Class III molar on the left side.

All treatment options included the extraction of maxillary left primary canine and the supraerupted right maxillary third molar and extruding the impacted canine to the arch. In addition, veneers would be placed on the lateral incisors after a crown lengthening/gingivectomy procedure and frenectomy of the labial frenum in the anterior maxilla. The patient chose the third option.

TREATMENT SEQUENCE AND BIOMECHANICAL PLAN

Maxilla	Mandible
Refer the patient to the periodontist for extraction of over-retained left maxillary deciduous canine and bonding of gold chain on the impacted canine for orthodontic eruption. Refer patient to general dentist/oral surgeon for extraction of maxillary right third molar.	Refer patient to general dentist/oral surgeon for extraction of mandibular left first premolar.
Band molars, bond maxillary arch, start alignment with .016 inch NiTi arch wire, bypassing the lateral incisors. Push coil between left first molar and left first premolar to create space for alignment of the left second premolar. Place TPA connecting first molars. Solder a cantilever made out of .017 × .025 inch CNA to the TPA for forced eruption of maxillary right canine. Vertical eruption with 25 g of force.	Band molar and bond rest of the arch, start alignment and leveling with .016 and .016 × .022 inch NiTi arch wires.
Place of .017 × .025 inch CNA cantilever from right first molar to direct the right canine labially and occlusally.	Continue leveling with a .017 × .025 inch CNA.
Bond the lateral incisors and finish space closure and space appropriation for the buildups.	Place .017 × .025 inch SS arch wire and close the extraction space.
Finish the occlusion with .016 × .022 inch CNA.	Finish the occlusion with .016 × .022 inch CNA.
Debond and deliver wrap around retainer.	Debond and deliver Hawley retainer.
Refer to periodontist for crown lengthening/gingivectomy of anterior segment and frenectomy of the labial frenum. Build up restorations of lateral incisors. 6-month recall appointment for retention check.	6-month recall appointment for retention check.

CNA, Connecticut new arch wire; *NiTi,* nickel titanium; *SS,* stainless steel; *TPA,* transpalatal arch.

▪ TREATMENT SEQUENCE

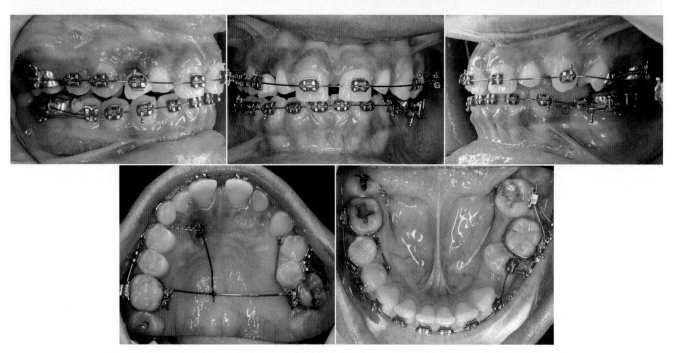

Figure 10-1-3   Cantilever from transpalatal arch for eruption of the right maxillary impacted canine.

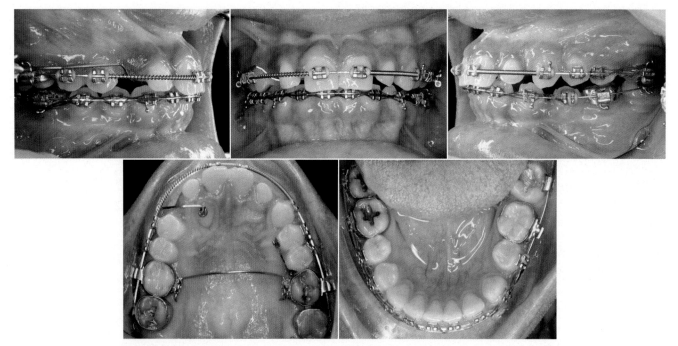

Figure 10-1-4   Cantilever from the maxillary right first molar directing the right maxillary impacted canine labially and occlusally.

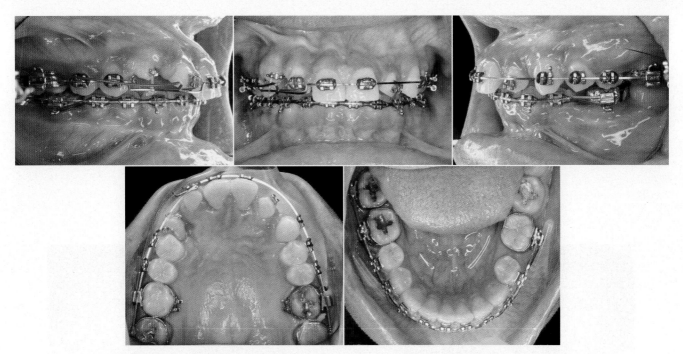

Figure 10-1-5 Cantilevers from the maxillary right first molar for lingual root torque of the maxillary right lateral incisor.

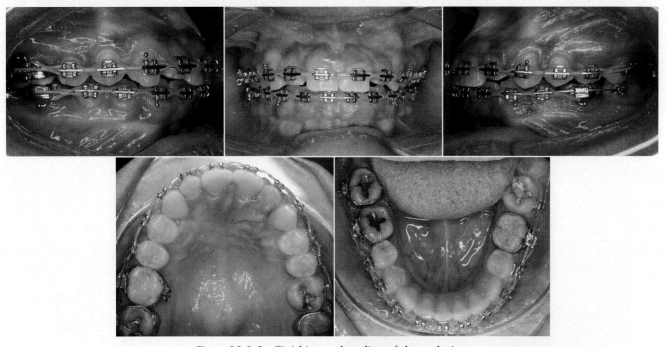

Figure 10-1-6 Finishing and settling of the occlusion.

■ FINAL RESULTS

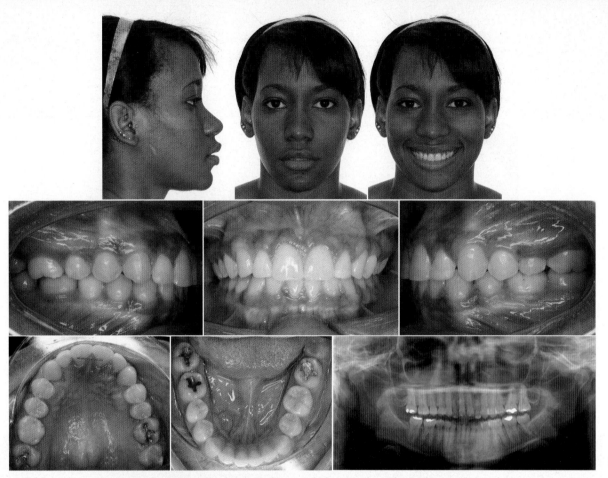

Figure 10-1-7   Posttreatment extraoral/intraoral photographs and panoramic radiograph.

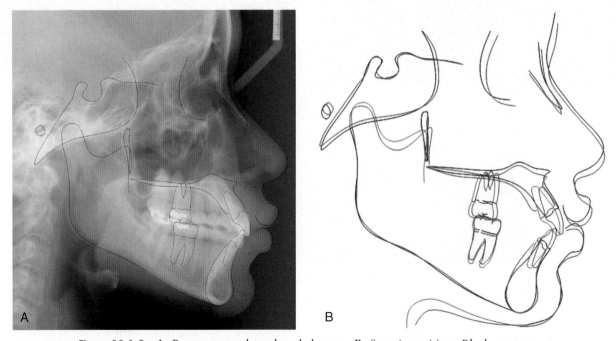

Figure 10-1-8   **A,** Posttreatment lateral cephalogram. **B,** Superimposition. *Black,* pretreatment; *red,* posttreatment.

Why was the impacted canine brought into the arch from a transpalatal arch?
An eruptive force was necessary for the canine that was on the palate. The force was provided by a cantilever that was welded to the transpalatal arch. This allowed for delivering a precise directional force that extruded the canine and displaced it in a labial direction. In addition, this force system allows testing for movement of a potentially ankylosed canine. The primary canine had not been extracted until movement of the impacted canine was confirmed.

Cantilever-Based Eruption of Impacted Maxillary Canines

A 16-year-old postpubertal female patient presented with a chief complaint of gaps present between her maxillary front teeth. Medical and dental histories were noncontributory, and findings from a temporomandibular joint (TMJ) examination were normal with adequate range of jaw movements.

■ PRETREATMENT

Extraoral Analysis (Fig. 10-2-1)

Facial Form	Mesoprosopic
Facial Symmetry	No gross asymmetries noticed
Chin Point	Coincidental with facial midline
Occlusal Plane	Normal
Facial Profile	Straight
Facial Height	Upper Facial Height/Lower Facial Height: Normal
	Lower Facial Height/Throat Depth: Normal
Lips	Competent, Upper: Retrusive; Lower: Retrusive
Nasolabial Angle	Obtuse
Mentolabial Sulcus	Normal

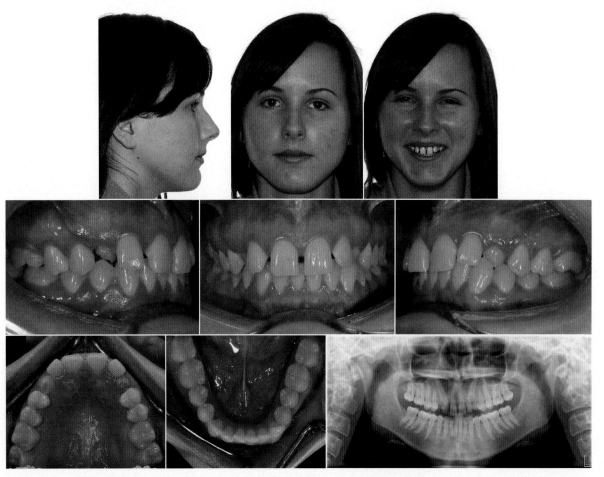

Figure 10-2-1 Pretreatment extraoral/intraoral photographs and panoramic radiograph.

Smile Analysis (Fig. 10-2-2)

Smile Arc	Consonant
Incisor Display	Rest: 7 mm
	Smile: 10 mm
Lateral Tooth Display	First premolar to first premolar
Buccal Corridor	Narrow
Gingival Tissue	Margins: Canine margins are low (primary canines)
	Papilla: Present
	Narrow band of attached gingiva on lower dentition; thin biotype on labial aspect of mandibular incisors
Dentition	Tooth size and proportion: Slightly narrow and long maxillary incisors
	Tooth shape: Normal
	Axial inclination: Maxillary and mandibular teeth inclined lingually
	Connector space and contact area: No contact between maxillary anterior teeth
Incisal Embrasure	Cannot be assessed because contacts on anterior maxillary teeth are absent
Midlines	Upper coincidental with facial midline and lower dental midline is shifted to the left by 2 mm compared with the facial midline

Intraoral Analysis (see Fig. 10-2-2)

Teeth Present	7654C21/12C4567
	7654321/1234567 (Impacted maxillary 3s; 8s not present)
Molar Relation	Class I bilaterally
Canine Relation	Not applicable
Overjet	2 mm
Overbite	4 mm
Maxillary Arch	U shaped, symmetric with 4 mm of spacing and impacted canines bilaterally
Mandibular Arch	U shaped with crowding of 2 mm and normal curve of Spee
Oral Hygiene	Fair

Functional Analysis

Swallowing	Normal adult pattern
Temporomandibular joint	Normal with normal range of jaw movements

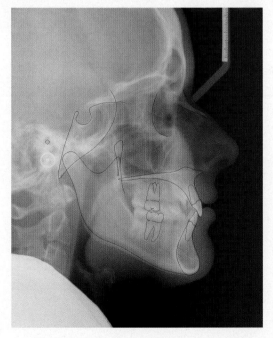

Parameter	Norm	Value
SNA (°)	82	82
SNB (°)	80	79
ANB (°)	2	3
FMA (°)	24	28
MP-SN (°)	32	37
U1-NA (mm/°)	4/22	2/12
L1-NA (mm/°)	4/25	3/22
IMPA (°)	95	86
U1-L1 (°)	130	142
OP-SN (°)	14	18
Upper Lip – E Plane (mm)	−4	−6.8
Lower Lip – E Plane (mm)	−2	−4.7
Nasolabial Angle (°)	103	134
Soft Tissue Convexity (°)	135	124

Figure 10-2-2 Pretreatment lateral cephalogram with tracing and cephalometric analysis.

Diagnosis and Case Summary

A 16-year-old postpubertal female patient had an orthognathic soft and hard tissue profile and obtuse nasolabial angle. She had a Class I malocclusion with over-retained maxillary deciduous canines, bilaterally impacted maxillary canines, and diastemas in the anterior maxillary dentition.

PROBLEM LIST			
Pathology/Others	Congenitally missing third molars Thin gingival biotype in the labial of mandibular anterior teeth Over-retained maxillary deciduous canines bilaterally and impacted maxillary canines bilaterally		
Alignment	2 mm of crowding in mandibular arch 4 mm of spacing in maxillary arch		
Dimension	**Skeletal**	**Dental**	**Soft Tissue**
Vertical		Altered gingival margins in maxillary anerior region due to presence of primary canines	
Anteroposterior		Retroclined maxillary and mandibular anterior teeth Obtuse interincisal angle	Retrusive upper and lower lips Obtuse nasolabial angle
Transverse		Mandibular midline 2 mm to the left of facial Primary maxillary canines in crossbite with corresponding teeth in the mandibular arch	

TREATMENT OBJECTIVES			
Pathology/Others	Extract over-retained maxillary deciduous canines bilaterally Exposure of impacted maxillary canines and bond gold chain for orthodontic eruption		
Alignment	Flare mandibular incisors to correct 2 mm of crowding in mandibular arch Close 4 mm of space to accommodate unerupted maxillary canines		
Dimension	**Skeletal**	**Dental**	**Soft Tissue**
Vertical		Intrude slightly lower incisors by leveling to improve OB	Assess gingival margins of permanent canines after completion of orthodontic treatment
Anteroposterior		Flare mandibular incisors to correct crowding and improve inclination	
Transverse		Move mandibular midline to the right to match facial midline	

OB, overbite.

Treatment Options

In the present case, the maxillary canines, although impacted, are placed favorably within the dentoalveolar region. The prognosis is very good. Orthodontic eruption could be carried out with the help of various methods such as elastomeric chain/thread, cantilevers, etc. With a cantilever approach, the amount of force and direction can be delivered precisely, making it a precision appliance for orthodontic directed eruption.

Eruption of the permanent canines was accomplished with cantilever mechanics.

TREATMENT SEQUENCE AND BIOMECHANICAL PLAN

Maxilla	Mandible
Extract over-retained maxillary deciduous canines bilaterally.	
Band molars, bond maxillary arch, level with .016-inch NiTi arch wires.	Band molars and bond mandibular arch, level with .016-inch NiTi arch wires.
Continue leveling with .016 × .022 inch NiTi arch wire.	Continue leveling with .016 × .022 inch NiTi arch wire.
Continue leveling up to a .017 × .025 inch SS arch wire, place push coils between maxillary first premolar and lateral incisors bilaterally to close up spaces between maxillary incisors and open up spaces for canines.	Continue leveling with .017 × .025 inch NiTi arch wire.
Exposure of impacted maxillary canines and bond gold chain for orthodontic eruption.	
Place .019 × .025 inch SS base arch wire, place cantilever from auxiliary slots on the molar brackets fabricated from .017 × .025 inch CNA. Direction of the vector should be occlusal with an approximate force magnitude of 25 g.	Continue leveling with .017 × .025 inch NiTi arch wire.
Place .016 inch NiTi piggyback arch wire and continue alignment of the canines into the arch.	Continue leveling with .019 × .025 inch NiTi arch wire.
Engage canines with leveling wire; continue leveling with .016 × .022 inch NiTi arch wire.	Continue leveling with .019 × .025 inch SS arch wire.
Continue leveling with .019 × .025 inch NiTi arch wire.	
.017 × .025 inch CNA with finishing bends.	.017 × .025 inch CNA with finishing bends.
Debond and deliver wrap around retainer.	Debond and bond lingual 3-3 retainer.
6-month recall appointment for retention check.	6-month recall appointment for retention check.

CNA, Connecticut new arch wire; *NiTi,* nickel titanium; *SS,* stainless steel.

■TREATMENT SEQUENCE

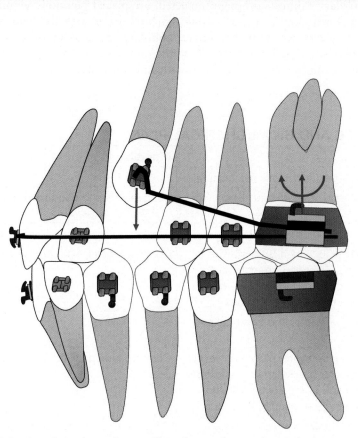

Figure 10-2-3 Cantilever from the maxillary first molar results in clockwise moment and intrusive force on the molar and extrusive force on the canine.

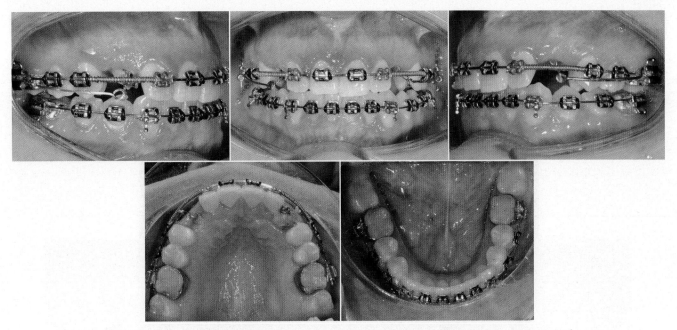

Figure 10-2-4 Intraoral photographs show cantilevers from maxillary molars. Direction of the eruptive force is in an occlusal direction.

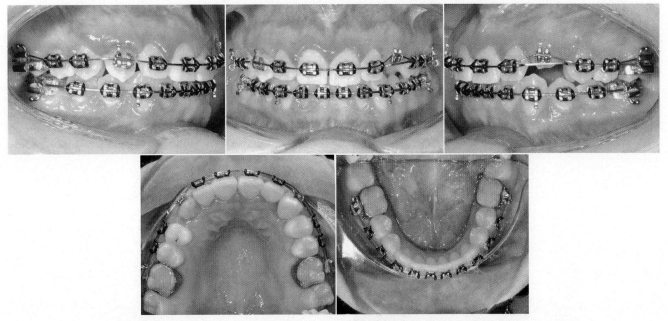

Figure 10-2-5 Intraoral photographs show .016 inch nickel titanium "piggyback" arch wire over the .019 × .025 inch stainless steel base arch wire for alignment of the maxillary canines.

■ FINAL RESULTS

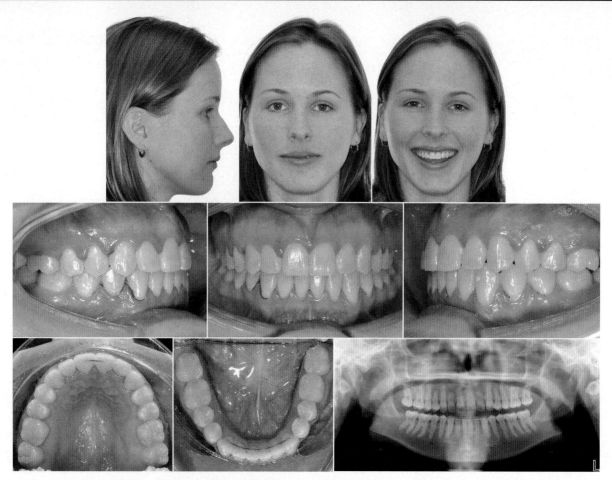

Figure 10-2-6 Posttreatment extraoral/intraoral photographs and panoramic radiograph.

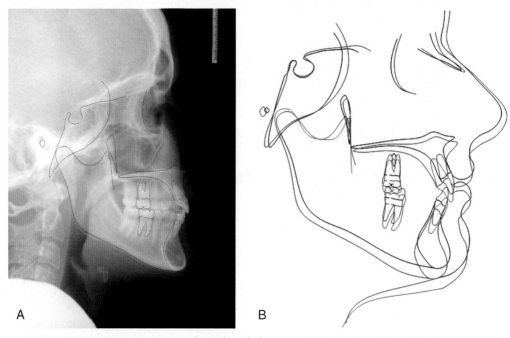

A

B

Figure 10-2-7 **A,** Posttreatment lateral cephalogram. **B,** Superimposition. *Black,* pretreatment; *red,* posttreatment.

What important considerations are needed when cantilevers are used to extrude maxillary canines?

Cantilevers can deliver precise directional forces, which make them a great tool for eruption of impacted canines. The line of force is defined by the wire in its preactivated state and the location where it will be tied. It is important to consider that this force has side effects on the other end of the wire (usually the molar). A moment that will tend to rotate and tip mesially the molar is generated. This moment can be considered most often a side effect. For this side effect to be counteracted, a couple of options are available: (1) place a transpalatal arch to splint the molars together; this would counteract mostly the rotational tendencies and minimize the tipping effects. (2) Place a large-dimension stiff arch wire from molar to molar bypassing the canines. This would act similarly to the transpalatal arch in minimizing the side effects.

Eruption of Maxillary Impacted Canines and Mandibular Second Premolar with Cantilever Mechanics

A 14-year-old postpubertal female patient was referred by her general dentist for treatment of impacted teeth in the maxillary arch. Medical and dental histories were noncontributory, and findings from a temporomandibular joint (TMJ) examination were normal with adequate range of jaw movements.

■ PRETREATMENT

Extraoral Analysis (Fig. 10-3-1)

Facial Form	Euryprosopic
Facial Symmetry	No gross asymmetries noticed
Chin Point	Coincidental with facial midline
Occlusal Plane	Normal
Facial Profile	Straight
Facial Height	Upper Facial Height/Lower Facial Height: Increased
	Lower Facial Height/Throat Depth: Normal
Lips	Competent, Upper: Normal; Lower: Normal
Nasolabial Angle	Normal
Mentolabial Sulcus	Normal

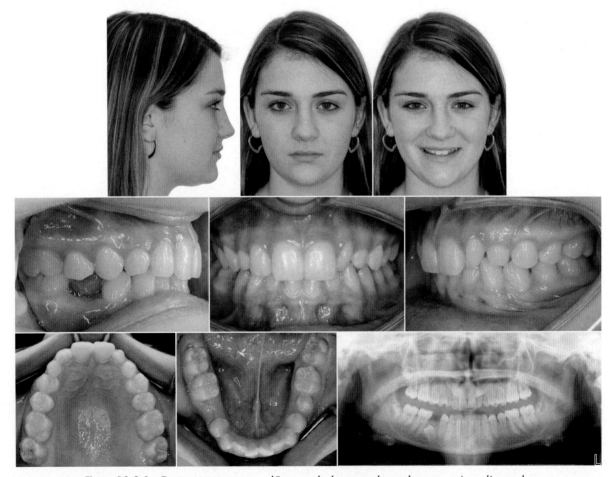

Figure 10-3-1   Pretreatment extraoral/intraoral photographs and panoramic radiograph.

Smile Analysis (Fig. 10-3-2)

Smile Arc	Consonant
Incisor Display	Rest: 3 mm
	Smile: 8 mm
Lateral Tooth Display	First premolar to first premolar
Buccal Corridor	Medium
Gingival Tissue	Margins: Canine margins are low (primary canines)
	Papilla: Present
Dentition	Tooth size and proportion: Maxillary left lateral incisor (peg shaped) and mandibular left second premolar are small mesiodistally
	Tooth shape: Abnormal for maxillary left lateral incisor and mandibular left second premolar
	Axial inclination: Normal
	Connector space and contact area: Normal between maxillary central incisors; abnormal between maxillary left central and lateral incisor (peg lateral)
Incisal Embrasure	Normal
Midlines	Maxillary and mandibular midline are coincidental with facial midline

Intraoral Analysis (see Fig. 10-3-2)

Teeth Present	7654C21/12C4567 (Impacted maxillary canines bilaterally and delayed eruption of mandibular right second premolar. Delayed formation of mandibular 8's and maxillary right 8. Maxillary left 8 formation not evidenced radiographically.)
	764321/1234567
Molar Relation	Class II end on relationship on the right
Canine Relation	Not Applicable
Overjet	2 mm
Overbite	4 mm
Maxillary Arch	U shaped, symmetric with crowding of 3 mm present
Mandibular Arch	U shaped with crowding of 4 mm and normal curve of Spee
Oral Hygiene	Fair

Functional Analysis

Swallowing	Normal adult pattern
Temporomandibular joint	Normal with normal range of jaw movements

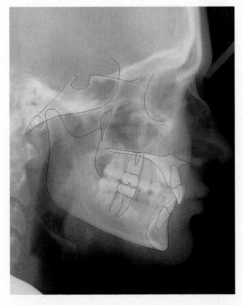

Parameter	Norm	Value
SNA (°)	82	75
SNB (°)	80	74
ANB (°)	2	1
FMA (°)	24	15
MP-SN (°)	32	28
U1-NA (mm/°)	4/22	4/20
L1-NA (mm/°)	4/25	1/20
IMPA (°)	95	96
U1-L1 (°)	130	140
OP-SN (°)	14	21
Upper Lip – E Plane (mm)	−4	−4
Lower Lip – E Plane (mm)	−2	−2
Nasolabial Angle (°)	103	106
Soft Tissue Convexity (°)	135	135

Figure 10-3-2 Pretreatment lateral cephalogram with tracing and cephalometric analysis.

Diagnosis and Case Summary

A 14-year-old postpubertal female patient had a straight soft tissue profile and dental Class II subdivision right malocclusion. She also exhibited a low mandibular plane angle, reduced lower facial height, over-retained deciduous maxillary canines, bilateral impacted maxillary canines, and delayed eruption of the mandibular right second premolar.

PROBLEM LIST			
Pathology/Others	Over-retained deciduous maxillary canines, bilaterally absent maxillary left third molar with delayed formation of the other third molars Impacted maxillary canines, bilaterally Delayed eruption of mandibular right second premolar Peg maxillary right lateral incisor		
Alignment	3 mm of crowding present in maxillary arch 4 mm of crowding present in mandibular arch		
Dimension	**Skeletal**	**Dental**	**Soft Tissue**
Anteroposterior		Class II end on molar relationship on the right	
Vertical	Reduced mandibular plane angle and lower facial height	Slightly increased overbite	
Transverse			

TREATMENT OBJECTIVES			
Pathology/Others	Extract over-retained deciduous maxillary canines, bilaterally Orthodontic eruption of impacted maxillary canines and mandibular right second premolar		
Alignment	Flare maxillary and mandibular incisors to align the incisors and relieve the crowding		
Dimension	**Skeletal**	**Dental**	**Soft Tissue**
Anteroposterior		Improve dental Class II end on relation by mesializing mandibular arch with help of Class II elastics	
Vertical		Reduce overbite	
Transverse			

Treatment Options

As evident from the pretreatment panoramic radiograph, crowns of the impacted maxillary canines have fully crossed the roots of the maxillary lateral incisors. A high probability that the crowns of the impacted canines are in close approximation with the roots of the maxillary central/lateral incisors is assumed. Therefore for the canines to be erupted into the arch, direction of the eruptive force should be in a distal direction during the first stages of orthodontic traction (to move the maxillary canines away from the roots of the maxillary central/lateral incisors). During the second stage, the direction of force should be occlusal to erupt the tooth into the dental arch. Finally, in the third stage, the crown should be brought into the arch labially.

Cantilever mechanics, which were applied to the eruption of the impacted teeth in this patient, create a one-couple system in which the clinician can apply a full array of force vectors in the desired direction.

TREATMENT SEQUENCE AND BIOMECHANICAL PLAN

Maxilla	Mandible
Surgical exposure and bonding of gold chain on the impacted maxillary canines.	Surgical exposure and bonding of gold chain on the mandibular right second premolar.
Band molars, bond maxillary arch, level the arch with .016, .016 × .022, and .019 × .025 inch NiTi arch wires. Place .016 × .022 inch SS arch wire and apply traction from lingual aspect of first molars to distalize the canines.	Band molars, bond maxillary arch, level the arch with .016, .016 × .022, and .019 × .025 inch NiTi arch wire.
Fabricate cantilever made from .017 × .025 inch CNA arch wire, place it in the auxiliary slot of the first molar bracket, tie the gold chain to the loop in the mesial end of the cantilever, and place 25 g of force directed occlusally.	Continue leveling with .019 × .025 inch SS arch wire.
Place lingual attachment on canine and bring it into the arch with elastomeric thread.	Fabricate cantilever made from .017 × .025 inch CNA, place it in the auxiliary slot of the right first molar bracket, tie the gold chain to the loop in the mesial end of the cantilever, place 25 g of force directed occlusally.
.018 inch CNA with finishing bends.	.016 × .022 inch CNA with finishing bends.
Debond and deliver wrap around retainer.	Debond and deliver a Hawley retainer.
6-month recall appointment for retention check. Refer patient for restoration of right peg lateral and gingivectomy/crown lengthening right canine.	6-month recall appointment for retention check.

CNA, Connecticut new arch wire; *NiTi,* nickel titanium; *SS,* stainless steel.

■TREATMENT SEQUENCE

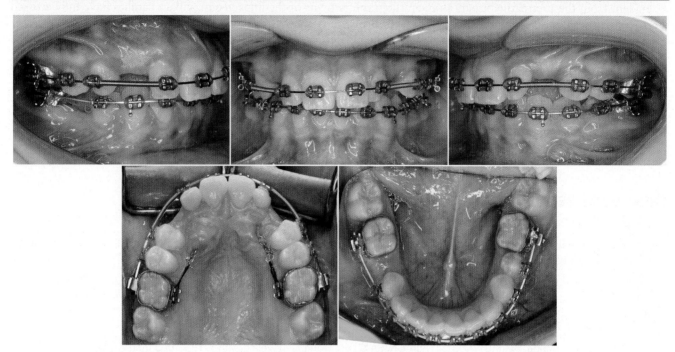

Figure 10-3-3   Intraoral photographs showing initial alignment of maxillary and mandibular arch. Distal force on the maxillary impacted canines by connecting the gold chain to the lingual aspect of the maxillary molars with an elastomeric chain.

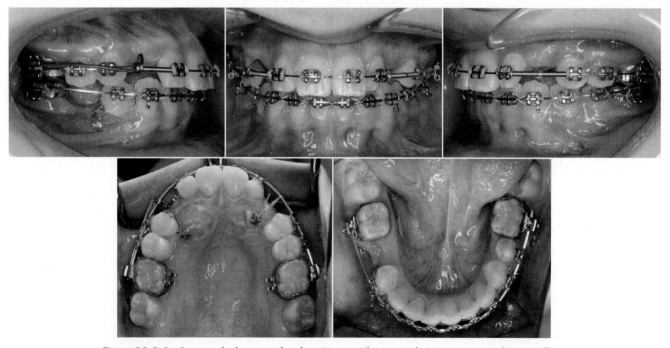

Figure 10-3-4   Intraoral photographs showing cantilever mechanics to erupt the maxillary right canine in an occlusal and distal direction.

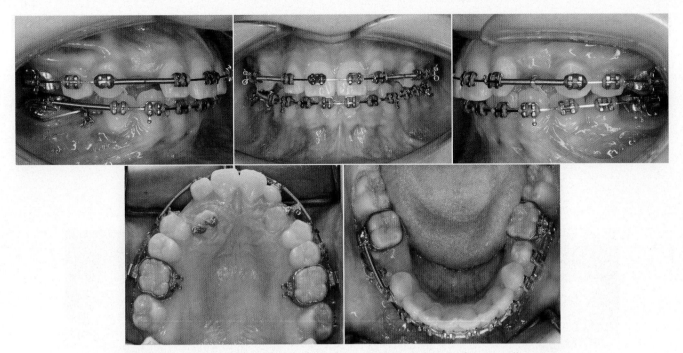

Figure 10-3-5 Intraoral photographs showing continued alignment of the maxillary canines and cantilever mechanics to erupt the right mandibular second premolar in an occlusal direction.

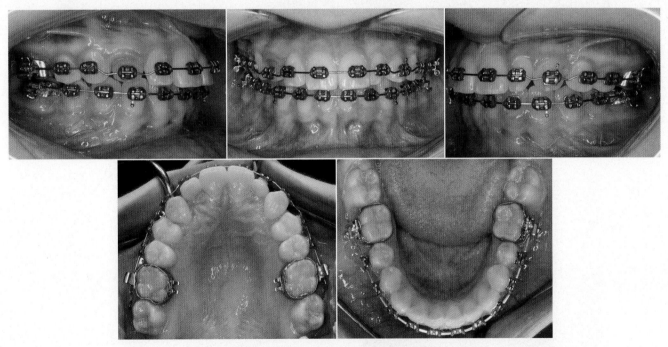

Figure 10-3-6 Finishing stage and settling of occlusion.

■ FINAL RESULTS

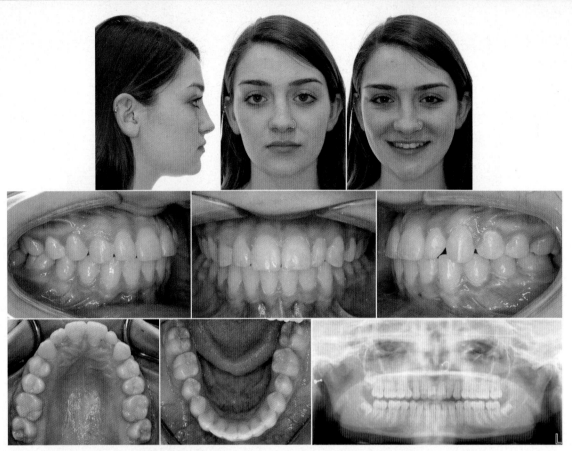

Figure 10-3-7 Posttreatment extraoral/intraoral photographs and panoramic radiograph. Patient was referred for composite buildup of maxillary right lateral incisors and gingivectomy/crown lengthening of maxillary right canine.

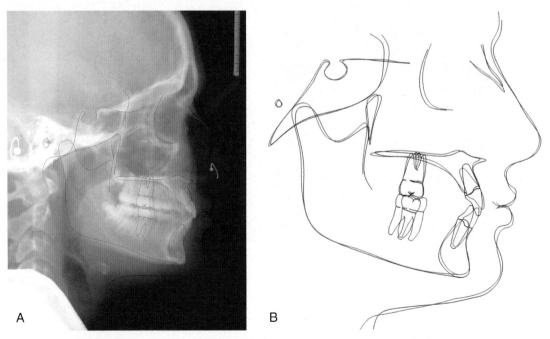

A   B

Figure 10-3-8   A, Posttreatment lateral cephalogram. **B,** Superimposition. *Black,* Pretreatment; *red,* posttreatment.

What options are available to extrude an unerupted premolar?

Cantilevers can also be applied to erupt unerupted/impacted premolars into the arch. The same principles apply as those considered for the eruption of impacted canines. The only difference is that when a cantilever is placed on a premolar, the activation distance is significantly reduced, especially if it is a second premolar as it is observed in this case. To increase the activation distance, the cantilever is engaged from the distal of the first molar.

An alternative to a cantilever for the eruption of unerupted/impacted premolars is the placement of a elastomeric thread from the base arch wire. The disadvantage of this approach is the quick deactivation of the force after placement due to the material properties of the elastomeric thread. On the other hand, cantilevers provide a more constant force level with a low load/deflection rate.

CASE 10-4
Use of Lip Bumper for Severely Impacted Mandibular Canines*

A 10-year-old prepubertal female patient was referred by her general dentist for assessment of impacted mandibular canines. Medical and dental histories were noncontributory, and findings from a temporomandibular joint (TMJ) examination were normal with adequate range of jaw movements.

■ PRETREATMENT

Extraoral Analysis (Fig. 10-4-1)

Facial Form	Mesoprosopic
Facial Symmetry	No gross asymmetries noticed
Chin Point	Coincidental with facial midline
Occlusal Plane	Normal
Facial Profile	Convex
Facial Height	Upper Facial Height/Lower Facial Height: Normal
	Lower Facial Height/Throat Depth: Reduced
Lips	Incompetent due to maxillary incisor protrusion, Upper: Protrusive; Lower: Protrusive
Nasolabial Angle	Normal
Mentolabial Sulcus	Deep

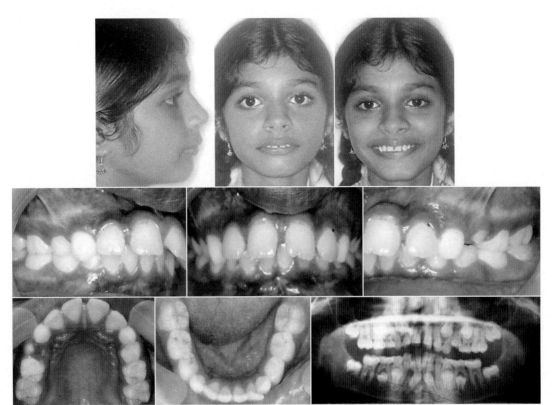

Figure 10-4-1 Pretreatment extraoral/intraoral photographs and panoramic radiograph.

*Portions of Case 10-4 from Agarwal S, Yadav S, Shah NV, Valiathan A, Uribe F, Nanda R. Correction of bilateral impacted mandibular canines with a lip bumper for anchorage reinforcement. *Am J Orthod Dentofacial Orthop.* 2013;143:393-403.

Smile Analysis (Fig. 10-4-2)

Smile Arc	Flat
Incisor Display	Rest: 3 mm
	Smile: 8 mm
Lateral Tooth Display	Maxillary: First premolar to first premolar
Buccal Corridor	Narrow
Gingival Tissue	Margins: Canine margins are more incisal compared with the lateral and central incisors
	Papilla: Present in all teeth
Dentition	Tooth size and proportion: Normal
	Tooth shape: Normal
	Axial inclination: Maxillary incisors are flared
	Connector space and contact area: Not present between maxillary central incisors and central incisors and lateral incisors due to diastemas
Incisal Embrasure	Unable to evaluate between maxillary central incisors due to diastema
Midlines	Lower dental midline is on with the facial midline. Maxillary dental midline is on with the facial midline on the mesial aspect of the right central incisor.

Intraoral Analysis (see Fig. 10-4-2)

Teeth Present	6E4C21/12CDE6 (Unerupted 7s developing normally)
	76EDC21/12CDE6
Molar Relation	Class II end on bilaterally
Canine Relation	N/A
Overjet	8 mm
Overbite	3 mm
Maxillary Arch	U shaped, symmetric with 5 mm of spacing (mixed dentition analysis)
Mandibular Arch	U shaped with impacted canines (labial to incisors) in the symphysis, 4 mm of spacing and deep curve of Spee
Oral Hygiene	Fair

Functional Analysis

Swallowing	Adult pattern
Temporomandibular joint	Normal with adequate range of jaw movements

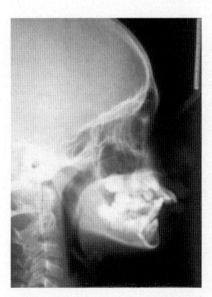

Parameter	Norm	Value
SNA (°)	82	78
SNB (°)	80	75
ANB (°)	2	3
FMA (°)	24	20
MP-SN (°)	32	29
U1-NA (mm/°)	4/22	12/59
L1-NA (mm/°)	4/25	4/27
IMPA (°)	95	101
U1-L1 (°)	130	100
OP-SN (°)	14	14
Upper Lip – E Plane (mm)	−4	1
Lower Lip – E Plane (mm)	−2	0
Nasolabial Angle (°)	103	97

Figure 10-4-2   Pretreatment lateral cephalogram and cephalometric analysis.

Diagnosis and Case Summary

A 10-year-old female patient had a mildly convex soft and hard tissue profile. She had a Class II Division 1 malocclusion with impacted mandibular canines in the symphysial region, significantly labially inclined maxillary incisors, and protrusive upper and lower lips. Vertically, she had a short facial height with a flat mandibular plane angle and deep overbite.

PROBLEM LIST

Pathology/Others	Impacted mandibular canines in the symphysial region labial to the mandibular incisors		
Alignment	5 mm of spacing in the maxillary arch and 4 mm of spacing in the mandibular arch		
Dimension	**Skeletal**	**Dental**	**Soft Tissue**
Anteroposterior	Mild convexity	Class II end on molar relation bilaterally OJ: 8 mm Labially inclined maxillary incisors Acute interincisal angle	Protrusive upper and lower lips
Transverse			
Vertical	Short lower facial height Flat mandibular plane angle	Deep OB Deep curve of Spee	Lip incompetence due to protrusion of maxillary incisors Gingival heights of the maxillary canines more incisal that adjacent anterior teeth

OB, overbite; *OJ*, overjet.

TREATMENT OBJECTIVES

Pathology/Others	Erupt impacted mandibular canines into the arch		
Alignment	Close maxillary and mandibular spacing		
Dimension	**Skeletal**	**Dental**	**Soft Tissue**
Anteroposterior		Retract maxillary anterior teeth to close the anterior spacing and correct the incisor inclination, reduce the overjet and improve interincisal angle Correct Class II end on molar relation into Class I	Improve the protrusive upper and lower lips by anterior tooth retraction
Transverse			
Vertical		Reduce OB by levelling the lower curve of Spee	Achieve lip competence Evaluate maxillary anterior gingival heights after completion of orthodontic treatment

OB, overbite.

Treatment Options

Three general treatment options are available for this patient:

1. Orthodontic correction of impacted mandibular canines.
2. Extraction of bilaterally impacted mandibular canines, while preserving the deciduous canines, to allow them to function in place of the permanent canines. Although there was no obvious external apical root resorption evident on the deciduous mandibular canines, these teeth would have to be left out during the fixed-appliance treatment phase to prevent any resorption of their roots. After the fixed-appliance phase, the vertical dimension of these teeth would need to be restored.
3. Extraction of deciduous canines and autotransplantation of the permanent mandibular canines was considered as another possible solution. The root formation of mandibular canines was two-thirds complete, making them ideal to be transplanted, but the procedure required extensive removal of bone from the thin midsymphyseal region of the mandible, which could jeopardize the adjacent teeth.

The patient chose option 1, which involved orthodontic correction of the impacted canines.

TREATMENT SEQUENCE AND BIOMECHANICAL PLAN

Maxilla	Mandible
Band first molars and bond incisors. Initiate leveling with .016 × .022 inch NiTi arch wire. Place elastomeric chain to close up the spacing between incisors.	Fit band on first molars and take a pick-up impression. Fabricate appliance for canine eruption into the arch (Fig. 10-4-4). Cement the appliance onto the first molars.
	Refer the patient to periodontist for surgical exposure of mandibular canines and to bond a gold chain on the crowns (closed eruption).
	Place 50 g of distal and occlusal force with the help of an elastomeric chain by connecting the elastomeric chain from the gold chain to the small steel hook soldered on to the distal legs of the lip bumper (Fig. 10-4-6).
Bond 5-5 and initiate leveling with .016 × .022, and .019 × .025 inch NiTi arch wires.	Bond 5-5 and initiate leveling with .016 × .022, and .019 × .025 inch NiTi arch wires.
Finish with .016 × .022 inch CNA.	Finish with .016 × .022 inch CNA.
Debond and bond lingual 3-3 retainer.	Debond and bond lingual 3-3 retainer.
6-month recall appointment for retention check.	6-month recall appointment for retention check.

CNA, Connecticut new arch wire; *NiTi,* nickel titanium.

■ TREATMENT SEQUENCE

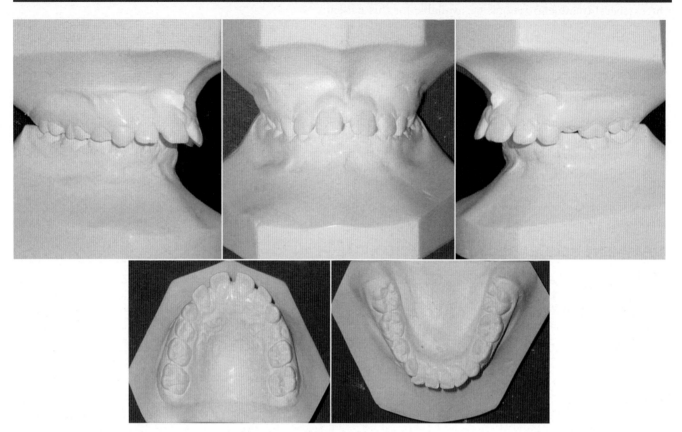

Figure 10-4-3　Pretreatment dental cast.

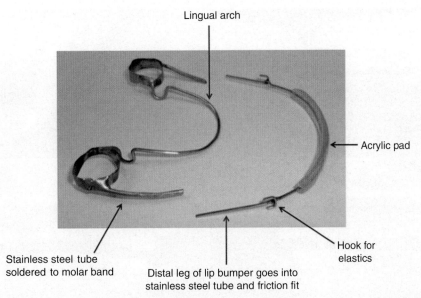

Lingual arch

Acrylic pad

Hook for elastics

Stainless steel tube soldered to molar band

Distal leg of lip bumper goes into stainless steel tube and friction fit

Figure 10-4-4 Appliance design: For anchorage to be reinforced, an assembly was fabricated in which both permanent first molars were connected with a .040-inch stainless steel (SS) lingual arch. On the buccal side of the molar bands, SS tubes with internal diameter of .030 inch were soldered. The length of the tube was adjusted so that the mesial end was at the mid buccal point of deciduous first molar. The SS tubes were curved according to their respective arch form segments. A lip bumper was fabricated from .021 × .027 inch SS ovoid arch wire by adding self-cured acrylic resin in the incisor region. In the distal legs of the lip bumper few bends were made which would friction lock it once the distal legs are drawn through the SS tubes. Small steel hooks were soldered onto the wire of the lip bumper just distal to the acrylic part for engaging the elastics. These hooks limited the distance that the leg of the lip bumper could go into the SS tube, thus keeping the acrylic pad 4 mm away from the mandibular incisor teeth and transfer the distal force from lip to the molars.

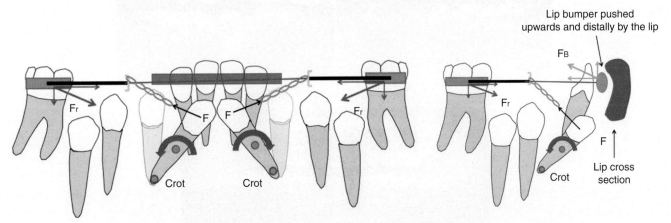

Lip bumper pushed upwards and distally by the lip

F_B

F_r

F

F_r

F F

F_r

Crot   Crot   Crot

Lip cross section

Figure 10-4-5 A distalizing and extrusive force (F) was applied by the elastomeric chain onto the canines from steel hooks soldered on the lip bumper. This force was expected to produce a controlled tipping of the canines around the center of rotation located at the root tip apex. A reactionary force (F_R) will be acting on the molar, which may result in mesial tipping of the molar. Because the acrylic pad of the lip bumper was at the middle of the crown of lower incisors, a distal force (F_B) was expected to be experienced by the molars to counteract the mesial reactionary force (F_R). B, Biomechanics; *Crot*, center of rotation; *F*, force applied by elastic power chain on the canines; *Fr*, reactionary force felt by molars due to F.

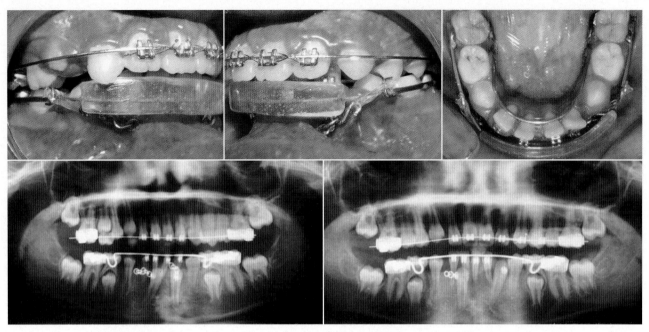

Figure 10-4-6 Lip bumper in place. Radiographs showing initial uprighting of impacted canines.

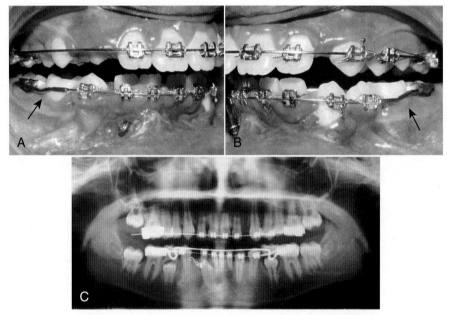

Figure 10-4-7 Left lower canine erupted into the oral cavity. Arrows in Figures **A** and **B** pointing toward the crimped steel tube to friction lock the .016-inch nickel titanium wire. **C,** Panoramic radiographs showing continued uprighting of the right lower canine.

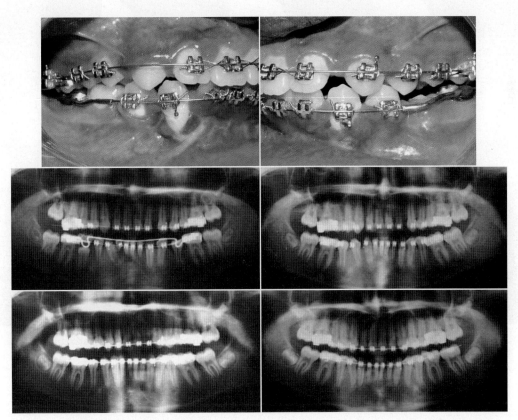

Figure 10-4-8 Right lower canine erupted into the oral cavity. Panoramic radiographs showing continued root correction of the right mandibular canine.

FINAL RESULTS

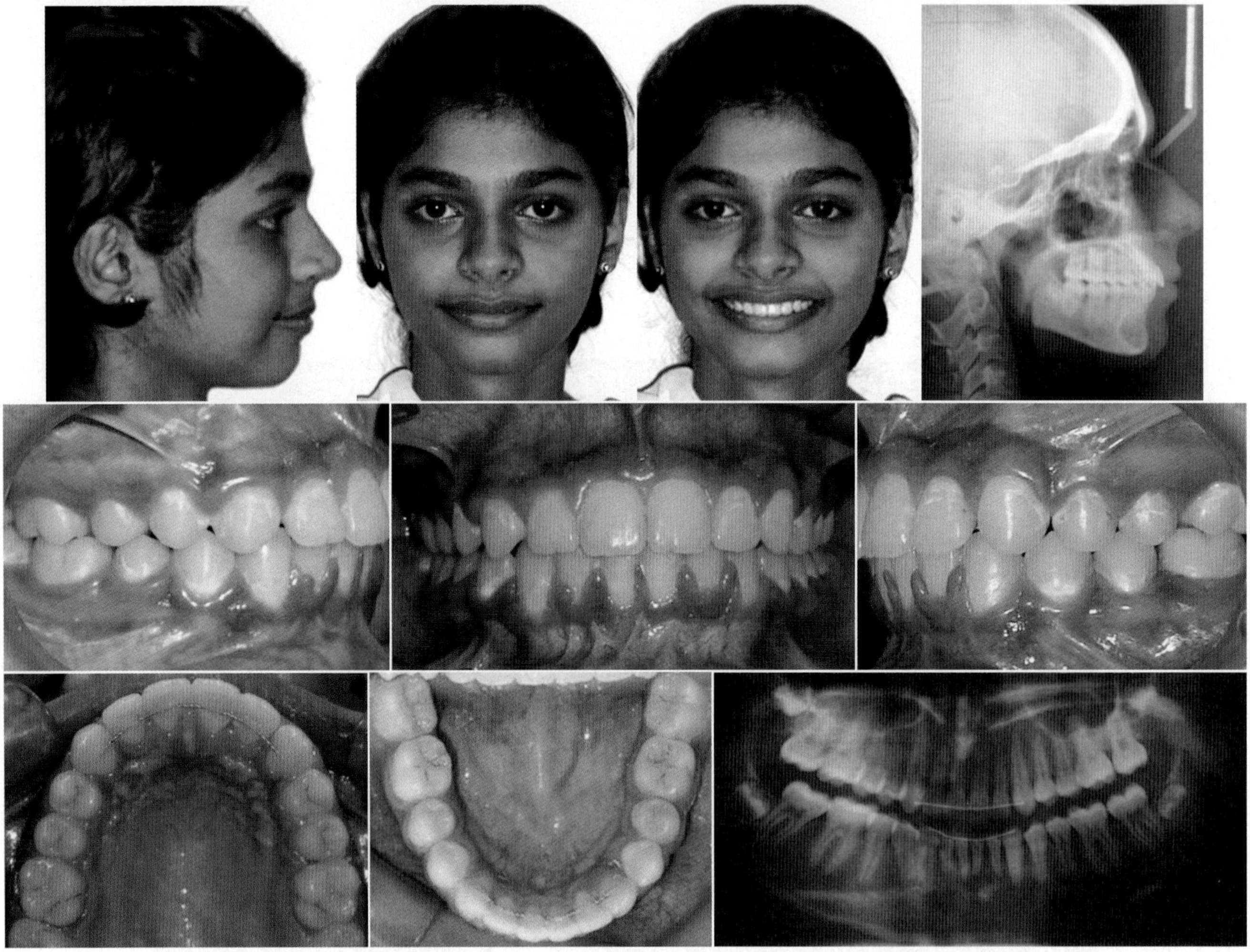

Figure 10-4-9   Postreatment extraoral/intraoral photographs and panoramic radiograph.

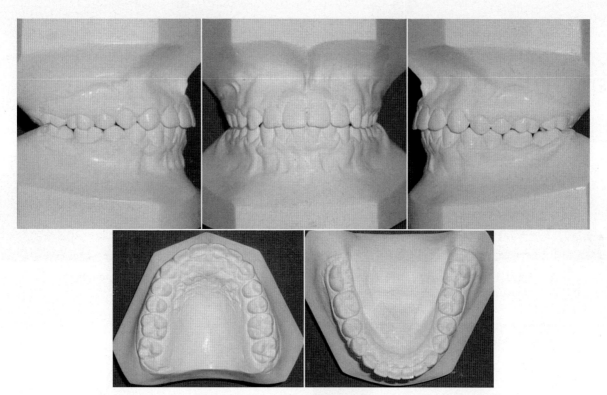

Figure 10-4-10   Posttreatment dental casts.

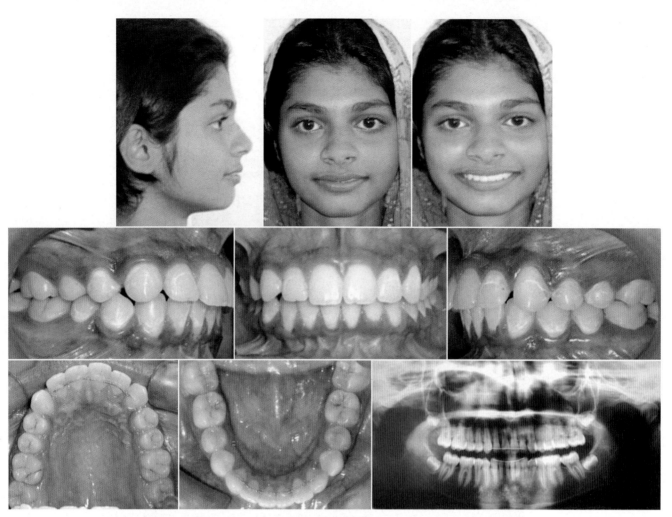

Figure 10-4-11   Two years' postretention extraoral/intraoral photographs and panoramic radiograph.

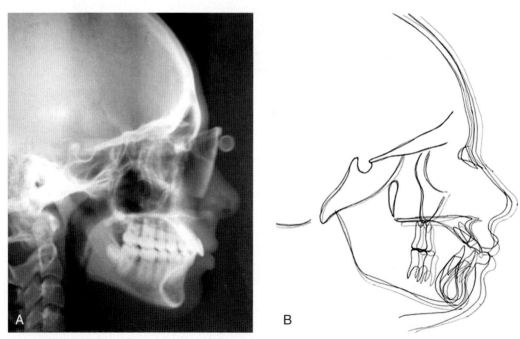

Figure 10-4-12   **A,** Posttreatment lateral cephalogram. **B,** Cephalometric superimposition. *Black,* pretreatment; *red,* posttreatment; *green,* postretention.

Why was it necessary to start the orthodontic treatment at an early stage instead of waiting until all the permanent teeth were erupted (permanent teeth could have served as anchors for forced eruption of the mandibular canines)?

Although none of the mandibular canines crossed the midline at the pretreatment stage (thus ectopic canines; not transmigrated), further eruption of ectopic canines always occurs in the direction of the crowns. Therefore intervention was indicated to reduce the odds of the ectopic canines crossing the mandibular midline and transmigrating to the opposite side, which would require more complex treatment at a later date.

CASE 11-1
Molar Uprighting of Severely Mesioangulated Mandibular Second Molars

A 13-year-old female patient was referred by her dentist for consultation regarding impacted mandibular second molars and crowding in upper and lower arches. Medical and dental histories were noncontributory, and findings from a temporomandibular joint (TMJ) examination were normal with adequate range of jaw movements.

■ PRETREATMENT

Extraoral Analysis (Fig. 11-1-1)

Facial Form	Mesoprosopic
Facial Symmetry	No gross asymmetries noticed
Chin Point	Coincidental with facial midline
Occlusal Plane	Normal
Facial Profile	Orthognathic
Facial Height	Upper Facial Height/Lower Facial Height: Normal
	Lower Facial Height/Throat Depth: Normal
Lips	Competent, Upper: Slight protrusion; Lower: Normal
Nasolabial Angle	Normal
Mentolabial Sulcus	Normal

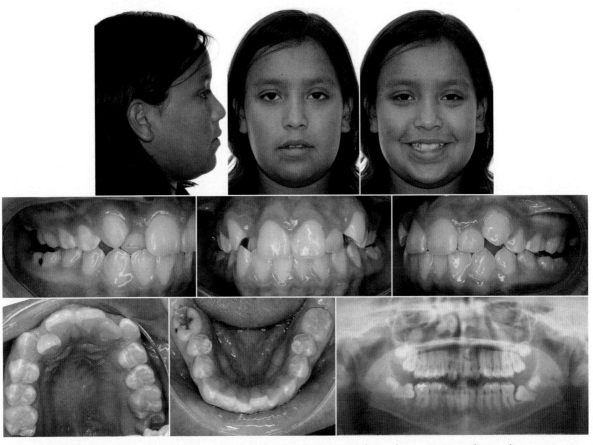

Figure 11-1-1   Pretreatment extraoral/intraoral photographs and panoramic radiograph.

Smile Analysis (Fig. 11-1-2)

Smile Arc	Consonant
Incisor Display	Rest: 3 mm
	Smile: 7 mm
Lateral Tooth Display	Maxillary first premolar to first premolar
Buccal Corridor	Slightly wide
Gingival Tissue	Margins: Irregular due to maxillary anterior crowding and lingual inclination of lateral incisors
	Papilla: Present in all teeth
Dentition	Tooth size and proportion: Normal
	Tooth shape: Normal
	Axial inclination: Normal
	Connector space and contact area: Closed contacts
Incisal Embrasure	Normal between central incisors
Midlines	Upper dental midline shifted to right of facial midline by 1 mm

Intraoral Analysis (see Fig. 11-1-2)

Teeth Present	7654321/1234567 (Impacted mandibular 7s and unerupted 8s)
	654321/123456
Molar Relation	End on Class II right
Canine Relation	End on Class II right
Overjet	2 mm
Overbite	2 mm
Maxillary Arch	U shaped, asymmetric with crowding
Mandibular Arch	U shaped, symmetric, normal curve of Spee and mandibular second molars in crossbite and first molars distally tipped and not in occlusion
Oral Hygiene	Fair

Functional Analysis

Swallowing	Adult pattern
Temporomandibular joint	Normal with adequate range of jaw movements

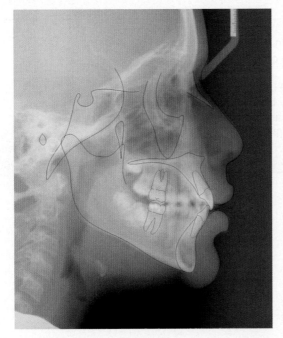

Parameter	Norm	Value
SNA (°)	82	80
SNB (°)	80	77
ANB (°)	2	3
FMA (°)	24	35
MP-SN (°)	32	43
U1-NA (mm/°)	4/22	5/21
L1-NA (mm/°)	4/25	8/28
IMPA (°)	95	89
U1-L1 (°)	130	125
OP-SN (°)	14	19
Upper Lip – E Plane (mm)	−4	0
Lower Lip – E Plane (mm)	−2	−1
Nasolabial Angle (°)	103	113
Soft Tissue Convexity (°)	135	137

Figure 11-1-2 Pretreatment lateral cephalogram with tracing and cephalometric analysis.

Diagnosis and Case Summary

A 13-year-old female patient had orthognathic soft and hard tissue profiles and a dental Class II subdivision right malocclusion. Her maxillary right lateral incisor was in crossbite; her mandibular first molars were in buccal crossbite, distally tipped and not in occlusion; and she had mesioangular impaction of mandibular second molars.

PROBLEM LIST				
Pathology/Others	Possibility of root resorption of the distal root of the mandibular first molars			
Alignment	Mesioangular impaction of mandibular second molars bilaterally 6 mm of crowding present in maxillary arch and 2 mm of crowding present in mandibular arch			
Dimension	**Skeletal**	**Dental**		**Soft Tissue**
Transverse		Maxillary midline shifted to right side by 1 mm Mandibular first molars in buccal crossbite		

Anteroposterior		End on Class II molar and canine relation on
		  the right side
		Maxillary right lateral incisor in crossbite
		Decreased interincisal angle
		Mandibular incisors labial to the apical base
		Distally tipped mandibular first molars
				Slightly protrusive upper
				  and lower lips

Vertical	Increased FMA	Mandibular first molars not in occlusion		Uneven gingival margins in
				  anterior maxilla due to
				  crowding and lingual
				  position of the lateral
				  incisors

FMA, Frankfort-mandibular plane angle.

TREATMENT OBJECTIVES				
Pathology/Others	Evaluate root integrity of first mandibular molars after disimpaction of second molars			
Alignment	Upright/disimpact mandibular second molar and align into the arch Create space to relieve the crowding in maxillary and mandibular arch by flaring the anterior teeth			
Dimension	**Skeletal**	**Dental**		**Soft Tissue**
Transverse		Correct the dental buccal crossbite by arch wire coordination		

Anteroposterior		Correct inclination of distally tipped mandibular
		  first molars
		Correct the lingual crossbite of maxillary right
		  lateral incisor by bringing it into the arch
		Correct the molar and canine relationship into
		  Class I on the right side		

Vertical				Align and level anterior teeth and reassess gingival levels

Treatment Options

The patient could be treated with four first premolar extractions which would facilitate the disimpaction of mandibular second molar or as a nonextraction case with disimpaction of mandibular second molar. Extraction of the mandibular second molars possesses great risk of injury to the mandibular first molars. Advantages of an extraction treatment option would be correction of the labially placed lower incisors, alignment of the maxillary arch, and availability of increased amount of space (due to some anchorage loss) for disimpaction/eruption of the impacted mandibular second molars. Contraindications for the extraction approach are increasing the nasolabial angle and the extraction of sound mandibular premolars with the uncertainty of the diagnosis related to the aberrant positioning of the mandibular first molars. Specifically, the vertical position of the mandibular first molars suggested primary failure of eruption, which would not respond to an orthodontic force. Therefore if these teeth would be unresponsive to extrusion mechanics, extraction of these teeth instead of mandibular premolars would be the approach in conjunction with the extraction of maxillary premolars.

A nonextraction plan was selected by the patient with reassessment after uprighting the mandibular second molars and initial response to orthodontic forces of the mandibular first molars.

TREATMENT SEQUENCE AND BIOMECHANICAL PLAN

Maxilla	Mandible
Band molars and bond maxillary arch.	Band molars and bond mandibular arch.
Level with .016, .018, and .016 × .022 inch NiTi arch wires.	Level with .016, .018, and .016 × .022 inch NiTi arch wires.
Leveling with .017 × .025 inch NiTi arch wire.	Refer patient to periodontist for exposure of second molars and bond molar tubes, .016 × .022 inch SS first molar to first molar base arch wire. Place sectional .016 inch NiTi arch wire between auxiliary slot of mandibular first molars and second molars for tipping second molars distally.
Leveling with .019 × .025 inch NiTi arch wire.	Cantilever with .017 × .025 inch CNA placed from mandibular second molars to further upright the second molars.
Continue with .019 × .025 inch NiTi arch wire.	Engage mandibular second molars into the base arch wire and start alignment with .016 × .022 inch NiTi arch wire.
Arch wire coordination and finishing with .016 × .022 inch CNA.	Arch wire coordination and finishing with .016 × .022 inch CNA.
Debond and deliver wraparound retainer.	Debond and bond a lingual 3-3 retainer.
6-month recall appointment for retention check.	6-month recall appointment for retention check.

CNA, Connecticut new arch wire; *NiTi,* nickel titanium; *SS,* stainless steel.

TREATMENT SEQUENCE

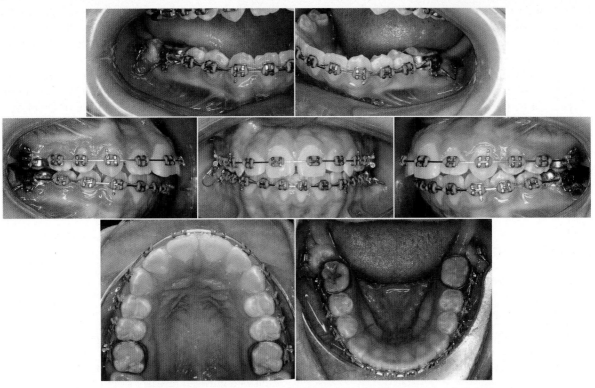

Figure 11-1-3 Compressed nickel titanium wire between mandibular first and second molars for distal tipping of mandibular second molars and also desired tipping of first molars.

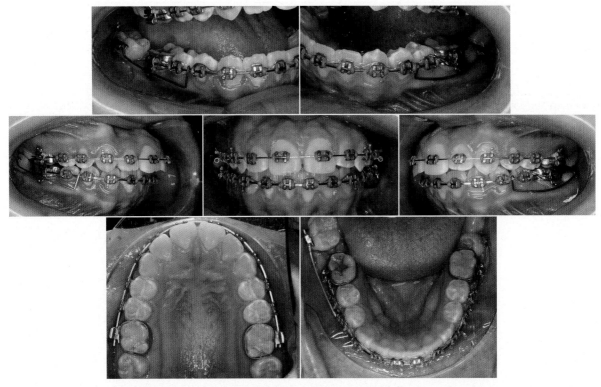

Figure 11-1-4 Cantilever to further upright the mandibular second molars.

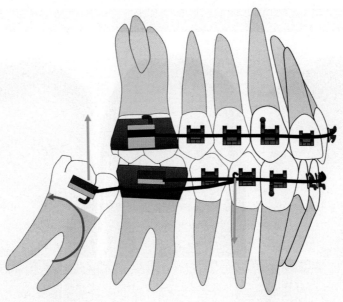

Figure 11-1-5 Cantilever results in the counterclockwise moment and extrusive force on the mandibular second molars and intrusive force on the anterior segment.

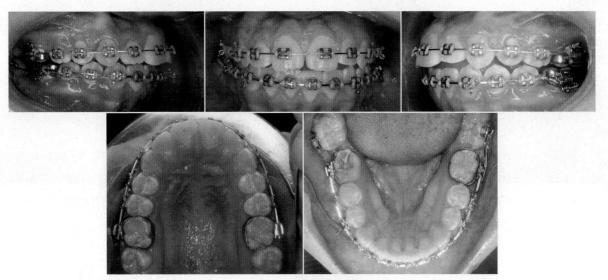

Figure 11-1-6 Mandibular second molars engaged into the base arch wire for further alignment.

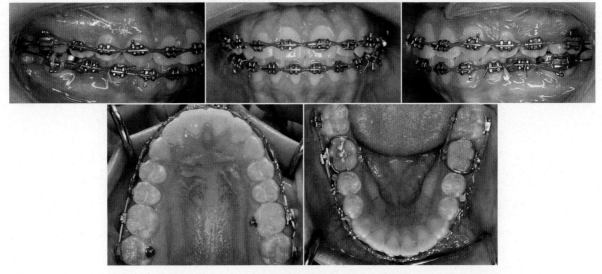

Figure 11-1-7 Finishing and arch wire coordination.

■ FINAL RESULTS

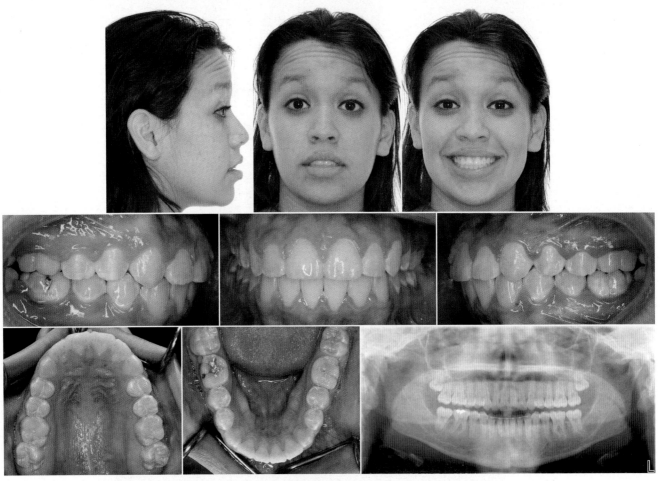

Figure 11-1-8   Posttreatment extraoral/intraoral photographs and panoramic radiograph.

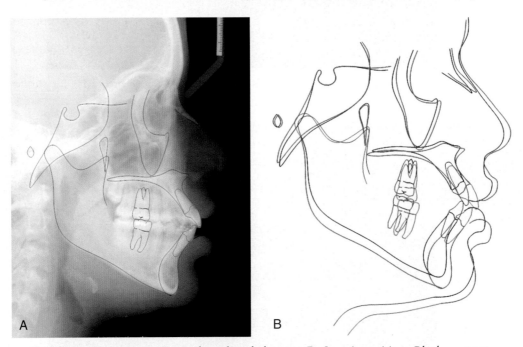

Figure 11-1-9   **A,** Posttreatment lateral cephalogram. **B,** Superimposition. *Black*, pretreatment; *red*, posttreatment.

Why was a cantilever used to upright the mandibular second molars?
The one-couple system or cantilever applies a couple and force at one end of the system and a single force at the other end. For uprighting a molar, the moment and force can be used consistently to tip back the molar and simultaneously erupt this tooth. It is important to also evaluate the single force being generated at the other end. For molar uprighting, the anterior force is intrusive, which may be a negative side effect in an open bite tendency. If that is the case, the magnitude of the force should be minimized, and anterior seating elastics may be worn at the same time to prevent any bite-opening effect.

Section 5

Multidisciplinary Treatment

CASE 12-1
Restoration of a Mutilated Dentition with Preprosthetic TADs to Intrude the Mandibular Dentition*

A 46-year-old male patient presented with a chief complaint of, "I want a nicer smile and to be able to eat." Medical history revealed penicillin allergy, and the patient reported clenching when lifting heavy things (plumber by profession). He possibly chews with his anterior teeth and first noticed wear on the anterior teeth about 8 to 10 years ago. Findings from a temporomandibular joint (TMJ) examination were normal with adequate range of jaw movements.

■ PRETREATMENT

Extraoral Analysis (Fig. 12-1-1)

Facial Form	Mesoprosopic
Facial Symmetry	No gross asymmetries noticed
Chin Point	Coincidental with facial midline
Occlusal Plane	Flat; supraerupted mandibular canines and first premolars and maxillary first molars and left first premolar
Facial Profile	Straight
Facial Height	Upper Facial Height/Lower Facial Height: Normal
	Lower Facial Height/Throat Depth: Normal
Lips	Competent, Upper: Retrusive, Lower: Retrusive. Obtuse cervicomental angle.
Nasolabial Angle	Normal
Mentolabial Sulcus	Normal

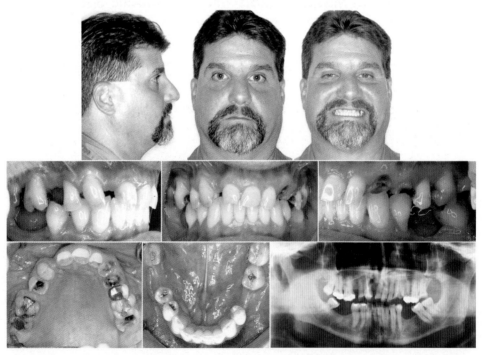

Figure 12-1-1   Pretreatment extraoral/intraoral photographs and panoramic radiograph.

---

*Portions of Case 12-1 from Bidra AS, Uribe F. Preprosthetic orthodontic intervention for management of a partially edentulous patient with generalized wear and malocclusion. *J Esthet Restor Dent.* 2012;24:88-100.

Smile Analysis (Fig. 12-1-2)

Smile Arc	Reverse (incisor wear)
Incisor Display	Rest: 0 mm
	Smile: 4 mm
Lateral Tooth Display	Second premolar to second premolar
Buccal Corridor	Normal
Gingival Tissue	Margins: Right canine margin is high. Significant recession on maxillary first molars, left mandibular first premolar, and right second premolar.
	Papilla: Present
Dentition	Tooth size and proportion: Heavily worn dentition with reduced occlusogingival height
	Tooth shape: Abnormal due to tooth wear
	Axial inclination: Maxillary central incisors tipped to the right
	Connector space and contact area: Contact at tip of the papilla in the maxillary incisors
	Incisal Embrasure: Open between maxillary central incisors due to wear of right incisor
Midlines	Upper shifted to the right by 2 mm as compared to facial midline with axial inclination of incisors inclined to the right

Intraoral Analysis (see Fig. 12-1-2)

Teeth Present	876 431/1234567
	854321/123478
Molar Relation	Could not be established
Canine Relation	Right side Class I and left side could not be established
Overjet	3 mm
Overbite	4 mm
Maxillary Arch	U shaped, symmetric with multiple missing teeth and grossly broken restorations
Mandibular Arch	U shaped with multiple missing in the posterior segment and deep curve of Spee
Oral Hygiene	Fair

Functional Analysis

Swallowing	Normal
Temporomandibular joint	Normal with adequate range of jaw movements
Vertical dimension of occlusion	Reduced, with increased freeway space

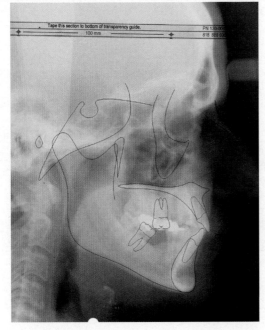

Parameter	Norm	Value
SNA (°)	82	77
SNB (°)	80	77
ANB (°)	2	0
FMA (°)	24	22
MP-SN (°)	32	29
U1-NA (mm/°)	4/22	7/33
L1-NA (mm/°)	4/25	2/23
IMPA (°)	95	95
U1-L1 (°)	130	123
OP-SN (°)	14	7.5
Upper Lip – E Plane (mm)	−4	−6
Lower Lip – E Plane (mm)	−2	−7
Nasolabial Angle (°)	103	107
Soft Tissue Convexity (°)	135	135

Figure 12-1-2 Pretreatment lateral cephalogram with tracing and cephalometric analysis.

Diagnosis and Case Summary

A 46-year-old male patient presented with a straight soft and hard tissue profile and a dental Class I malocclusion, multiple missing teeth, broken restorations, and severe attrition on remaining teeth. He had a reduced incisor display at rest and a smile with reduced vertical dimension of occlusion, increased freeway space, and deep curve of Spee.

PROBLEM LIST

Pathology/Others	Missing teeth: #4, 7, 11, 12, 16, 19, 20, 30, 31
	Severe attrition present: #5, 6, 8, 9, 10, 15
	Large restorations present: #2, 3, 13 ,14
	Root canal treatment: #6, 11, 12
	Broken restorations: #5, 11, 12, 15
	Mesially inclined: #17, 18, 32
	Gingival recession: #2, 3, 13, 14, 12, 29
	Oral hygiene: Fair
Alignment	Spacing in maxillary and mandibular arch due to multiple missing teeth
	Significantly rotated #29

Dimension	Skeletal	Dental	Soft Tissue/Function
Vertical	Reduced FMA and reduced vertical dimension of occlusion	OB: 4 mm Deep curve of Spee Reduced amount of maxillary incisor show upon smiling and at rest Supraerupted mandibular canines and first premolars and maxillary first molars and left second premolar	Increased freeway space
Anteroposterior			
Transverse		Maxillary dental midline is shifted to the right by 2 mm with axial inclination of the incisors	

FMA, Frankfort-mandibular plane angle; *OB,* overbite.

TREATMENT OBJECTIVES

Pathology/Others	Extraction of teeth #1, 2, 12, 15, 17, 32
	RCT: Redo RCT on teeth #6 and 11
	Crown lengthening procedure: #11, 13
	Post and core: #6, 11, 13
	Crown: #9, 10, 11, 13, 14
	Fixed partial denture: #3-5, 6-8, and 18-21
	Implant: #30
Alignment	

Dimension	Skeletal	Dental	Soft Tissue/Function
Vertical		Reduce overbite and curve of Spee by intrusion of mandibular anterior teeth (intrude 21-28 by 2 mm)	
Anteroposterior		Bodily move #3 mesially by 4 mm Bodily move #13 and 14 mesially by 4 mm Upright #31 by mesial root correction	
Transverse		Shift maxillary dental midline to the left by opening space for pontic in #7	

RCT, root canal treatment.

Treatment Options

In the present case, we have three options. The first one is extraction of all the maxillary teeth and replacement of maxillary teeth with implant-supported denture and replacement of missing mandibular teeth with implants or fixed partial dentures. The second option is full-mouth rehabilitation with the help of crowns and fixed partial dentures. The third option is to perform a preprosthetic orthodontic treatment, an extraction of hopeless teeth, and an increase in the vertical dimension of occlusion complemented by the restoration of the occlusion with implants/crowns/fixed partial dentures. Although this option would extend the total treatment time significantly, it would allow optimal placement of remaining teeth for the best possible aesthetic, functional, and long-term results before extensive restorative work is undertaken. The patient elected the third option.

TREATMENT SEQUENCE AND BIOMECHANICAL PLAN

Maxilla	Mandible
	Band molars and bond mandibular incisors, sectional leveling with .016, .018, and .016 × .022 inch NiTi arch wire.
	Sectional leveling of mandibular incisor with .016 × .022 inch SS wire segment and cantilever made out of .017 × .025 inch CNA from molar tubes on the mandibular right third molar and left second molar. Intrusive force of 40 g.
	Place TADs distal to mandibular first premolars.
Band molars and bond maxillary arch, leveling with .016, .018, and .016 × .022 inch NiTi arch wire. Use #2 to protract #3. Open space for pontic of #7 correcting maxillary midline. Close up space of tooth #12 by protracting teeth #13 and 14 and distalizing #11.	Fabricate a stiff extension arm with .040 inch SS wire mesially to the labial side of premolars and canines and intrude premolars and canines by connecting teeth with cantilever arm using elastomeric chain. Intrusive force of 40 g.
.016 × .022 inch CNA with finishing bends.	Level lower arch once intrusion of premolars is accomplished and place continuous .016 × .022 inch CNA with finishing bends.
Debond. Start restorative phase. Perform root canal treatments, post and cores, crown lengthening procedures, implant and tooth preparation for restorations. Place temporary restorations with increased vertical dimension of occlusion by 2 mm for 6 months.	Debond. Place temporary restoration on the mandibular left posterior segment with increased vertical dimension of occlusion by 2 mm.
Place final restorations.	Place final restorations.
Tooth #5 broke unfavorably below the gingival margin during orthodontic treatment and was deemed unrestorable. Porcelain fused to a metal bridge from #3 to #6 was fabricated. Tooth #13 had an unfavorable tooth fracture after orthodontic appliance removal and was replaced with the help of an implant.	

CNA, Connecticut new arch wire; NiTi, nickel titanium; SS, stainless steel; TAD, temporary anchorage device.

▪ TREATMENT SEQUENCE

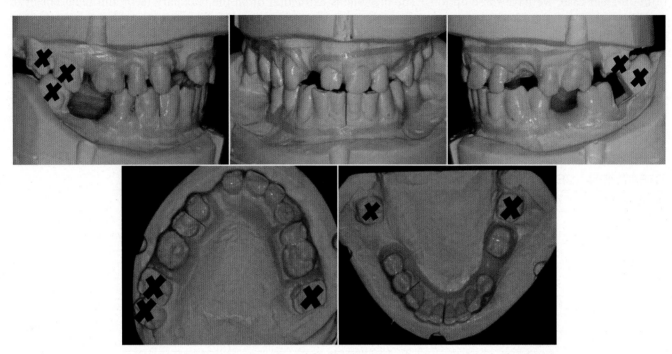

Figure 12-1-3 Diagnostic wax-up models demonstrating the proposed orthodontic movements and teeth to be extracted.

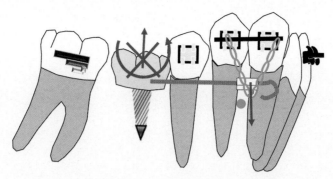

Figure 12-1-4   A mesial extension arm from the temporary anchorage device (TAD), when connected to premolars and canines with an elastomeric chain, will produce a one-couple system, with pure intrusive force on premolars and canines and extrusive force with counterclockwise moment on TAD, which will be negated as the TAD is anchored to the bone.

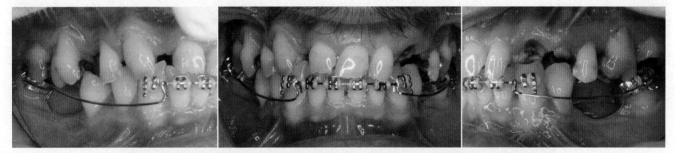

Figure 12-1-5   Cantilevers used to intrude the mandibular incisors from the mandibular molars before the extraction of teeth numbers 17 and 32.

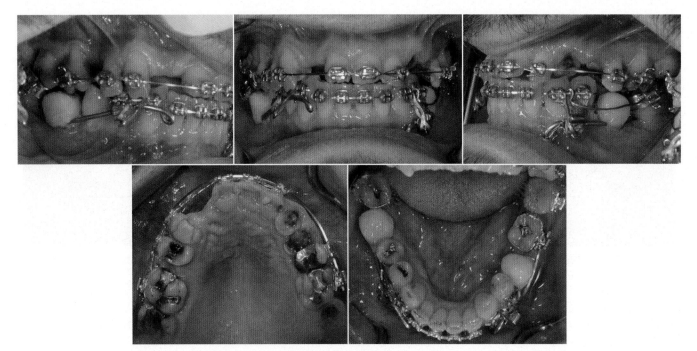

Figure 12-1-6 Mesial extension arm from temporary anchorage devices to intrude premolar and canines in mandibular arch using elastomeric chain.

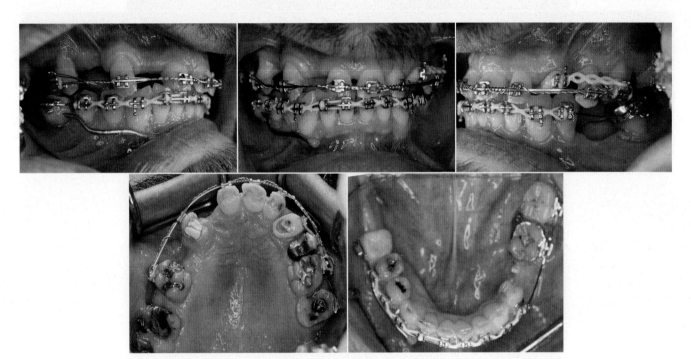

Figure 12-1-7   Intrusion of mandibular arch complete, finishing of both maxillary and mandibular arches.

■ FINAL RESULTS

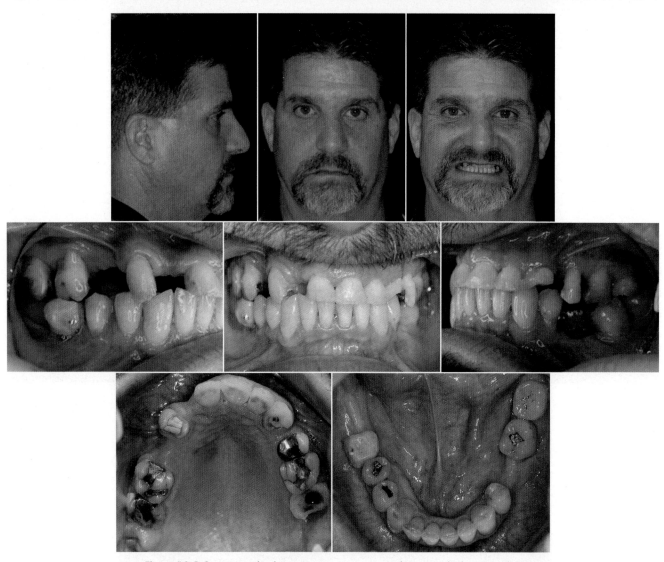

Figure 12-1-8   Postorthodontic treatment extraoral/intraoral photographs.

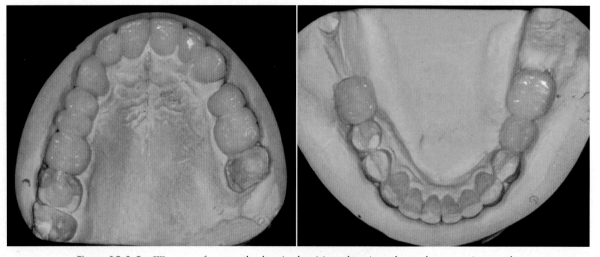

Figure 12-1-9   Wax-up of postorthodontic dentition showing planned restorative work.

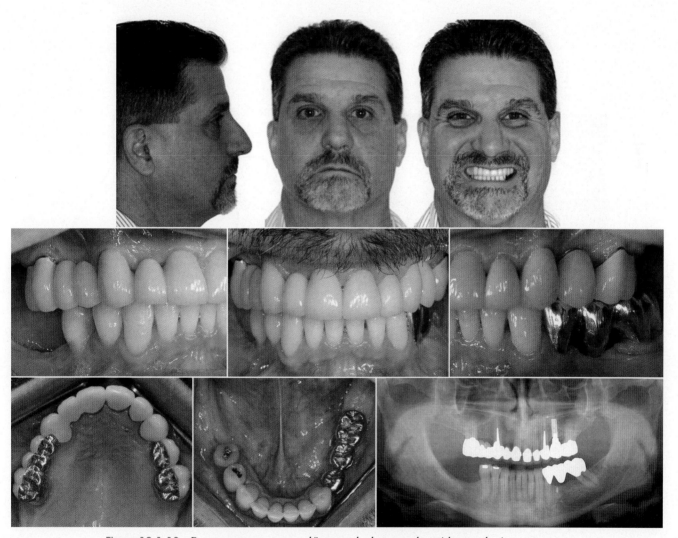

Figure 12-1-10 Posttreatment extraoral/intraoral photographs with prosthetic reconstruction and panoramic radiograph. Patient declined implant on #30 due to financial reasons.

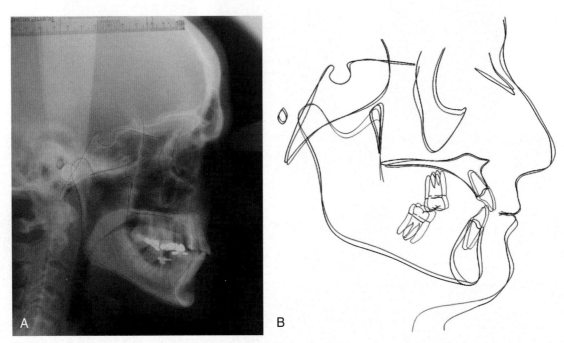

Figure 12-1-11 **A,** Posttreatment lateral cephalogram. **B,** Superimposition. *Black,* pretreatment; *red,* posttreatment.

Why were the mini-implants placed in the mandibular alveolar ridge instead of the labial aspect of the alveolar bone?

Mini-implants placed in the alveolar ridge serve a similar purpose to endosseous implants that can be used for anteroposterior movement of the adjacent teeth. Also, these mini-implants can be used for intrusion of the adjacent teeth and to intrude teeth at a distance by means of extension wires as shown in this patient. One of the advantages of the placement on the ridge is that with the use of extension arms for anterior intrusion, the moment generated is counteracted by the length the mini-implant instead of the width, as is the case when mini-implants are placed in the labial aspect of the alveolar bone. This favors the stability of the mini-implants in the long term when this type of force system is applied.

CASE 13-1
Unilateral Canine Impaction with Maxillary Canine Substitution

A 14-year-old postpubertal female patient presented with a chief complaint of irregular teeth present in the front region of the upper and lower jaws. Medical and dental histories were noncontributory, and findings from a temporomandibular joint (TMJ) examination were normal with adequate range of jaw movements.

■ PRETREATMENT

Extraoral Analysis (Fig. 13-1-1)

Facial Form	Mesoprosopic
Facial Symmetry	No gross asymmetry noticed
Chin Point	Coincidental with facial midline
Occlusal Plane	Normal
Facial Profile	Convex due to prognathic maxilla and retrognathic mandible
Facial Height	Upper Facial Height/Lower Facial Height: Normal
	Lower Facial Height/Throat Depth: Normal
Lips	Competent, Upper: Protrusive; Lower: Protrusive
Nasolabial Angle	Obtuse
Mentolabial Sulcus	Normal

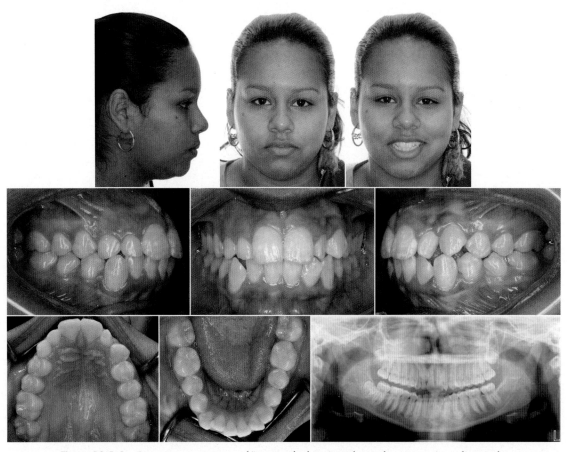

Figure 13-1-1   Pretreatment extraoral/intraoral photographs and panoramic radiograph.

Smile Analysis (Fig. 13-1-2)

Smile Arc	Consonant
Incisor Display	Rest: 3 mm
	Smile: 8 mm
Lateral Tooth Display	Right canine to left first premolar
Buccal Corridor	Small
Gingival Tissue	Margins: Maxillary right canine and lateral margins are more coronal (primary teeth)
	Maxillary left lateral margin is also more coronal than central incisors
	Papilla: Present
Dentition	Tooth size and proportion: Maxillary left lateral incisor is peg shaped
	Tooth shape: Normal
	Axial inclination: Maxillary teeth inclined normal and mandibular incisors are proclined
	Connector space and contact area: Large connector between central incisor with apically displaced papilla; low contact (at the interproximal papilla) between maxillary left lateral incisor and canine
Incisal Embrasure	Minimal between central incisors; large (between maxillary left lateral incisor and canine due to morphology)
Midlines	Upper and lower dental midlines are coincidental with facial midline

Intraoral Analysis (see Fig. 13-1-2)

Teeth Present	7654CB1/1234567
	7654321/1234567 Unerupted 8s except for congenitally missing mandibular left third molar
Molar Relation	Class I bilaterally
Canine Relation	Class II left side, not applicable on right side
Overjet	2 mm
Overbite	2 mm
Maxillary Arch	U shaped, symmetric, with over-retained deciduous maxillary right canine and lateral incisor, impacted right canine and congenitally missing maxillary right lateral incisor
Mandibular Arch	U shaped with crowding of 6 mm and normal curve of Spee
Oral Hygiene	Fair

Functional Analysis

Swallowing	Normal adult pattern
Temporomandibular joint	Normal with normal range of jaw movements

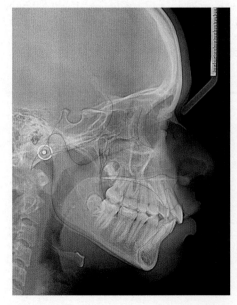

Parameter	Norm	Value
SNA (°)	82	84
SNB (°)	80	78.5
ANB (°)	2	5.5
FMA (°)	24	24.5
MP-SN (°)	32	35.5
U1-NA (mm/°)	4/22	5.5/25
L1-NA (mm/°)	4/25	9/35
IMPA (°)	95	101
U1-L1 (°)	130	113
OP-SN (°)	14	18
Upper Lip – E Plane (mm)	−4	0.4
Lower Lip – E Plane (mm)	−2	2
Nasolabial Angle (°)	103	104
Soft Tissue Convexity (°)	135	127

Figure 13-1-2 Pretreatment lateral cephalogram with tracing and cephalometric analysis.

Diagnosis and Case Summary

A 14-year-old postpubertal female had a convex soft tissue profile mainly due to a prognathic maxilla and retrognathic mandible. She had a Class I malocclusion with an impacted maxillary right canine, over-retained maxillary right deciduous canine and lateral incisor, a congenitally missing right maxillary right lateral incisor, and a left peg lateral incisor.

PROBLEM LIST			
Pathology/Others	Congenitally missing maxillary right lateral incisor and mandibular left third molar Impacted maxillary right canine Over-retained deciduous maxillary right lateral incisor and canine Peg-shaped maxillary left lateral incisor Radiopaque structure related to apex of mandibular left first premolar compatible with condensing osteitis		
Alignment	6 mm crowding in mandibular arch		
Dimension	**Skeletal**	**Dental**	**Soft Tissue**
Anteroposterior	Convex profile due to prognathic maxilla and retrognathic mandible	Class II end on canine relation on left side; proclined maxillary and mandibular anterior teeth Acute interincisal angle	Protrusive upper and lower lips
Vertical		Impacted maxillary right canine	
Transverse			

TREATMENT OBJECTIVES			
Pathology/Others	Monitor radiopaque structure associated to the mandibular left first premolar Extract over-retained deciduous maxillary right lateral incisor and canine Extract mandibular first premolars bilaterally and permanent maxillary left lateral incisor Exposure and bond gold chain to impacted maxillary right canine (closed eruption) Contour maxillary canines into maxillary lateral incisors		
Alignment	Extract first premolars in the mandibular arch to relieve crowding		
Dimension	**Skeletal**	**Dental**	**Soft Tissue**
Anteroposterior		Maintain Class I molar relationship and achieve Class I "canine" relationship with maxillary first premolars Retract maxillary and mandibular incisors to correct the proclination of incisors	Retract upper and lower lips to correct the protrusion of lips
Vertical		Orthodontic traction to erupt impacted right maxillary canine	
Transverse			

Treatment Options

An extraction approach was necessary in this patient because of the protrusive maxillary and mandibular lips. Because the maxillary right lateral incisor is congenitally missing and the left lateral incisor is peg shaped, the first option could be to extract the maxillary left peg-shaped lateral incisor and mandibular first premolars. The maxillary lateral incisors would be substituted for maxillary canines finishing in a Class I molar and "canine" relationship.

The second option could be to extract all the first premolars for profile improvement, build up the maxillary left lateral incisor, and restore the missing right lateral incisor with a prosthetic implant. Because the patient was still growing and did not want to wait long to receive an implant, she chose the first option.

TREATMENT SEQUENCE AND BIOMECHANICAL PLAN

Maxilla	Mandible
Extract over-retained deciduous maxillary right lateral incisor and canine and permanent maxillary left lateral incisor.	Extract mandibular first premolars bilaterally.
Band molars, bond maxillary arch, level using .016 inch NiTi arch wire.	Band molars and bond mandibular arch. Level using .016 inch NiTi arch wire.
Continue leveling with .016 × .022 inch NiTi arch wire.	Continue leveling with .016 × .022 inch NiTi arch wire.
Continue leveling with .017 × .025 inch NiTi arch wire.	Continue leveling with .017 × .025 inch NiTi arch wire.
Place .017 × .025 inch SS base arch wire. Exposure and bond gold chain to impacted maxillary right canine.	Continue leveling with .017 × .025 inch NiTi arch wire.
	Continue leveling with .019 × .025 inch NiTi arch wire.
Bond lingual button on the lingual surface of right maxillary canine, place .016 inch NiTi piggyback arch wire gingival to the lingual button to move the canine in a labial direction.	Continue leveling with .019 × .025 inch NiTi arch wire.
Place a .018 × .025 inch SS arch wire with arch wire hooks distal to the laterals. Extend .017 × .025 inch NiTi intrusion arch from the auxiliary slots of the molar tubes as an overlay to the main arch wire. Place elastomeric chain from first molar hooks to the arch wire hooks to retract the anterior teeth and close the spaces.	Place .018 × .025 inch SS arch wire with arch wire hooks distal to the lateral incisors. Place elastomeric chain from first molar hook to the arch wire hook to retract the anterior teeth and close the spaces.
.017 × .025 inch CNA with finishing bends. Reshape maxillary canines into maxillary lateral incisors.	.017 × .025 inch CNA with finishing bends.
Debond and deliver wrap around retainer.	Debond and deliver Hawley retainer.

CNA, Connecticut new arch wire; *NiTi*, nickel titanium; *SS*, stainless steel.

■ TREATMENT SEQUENCE

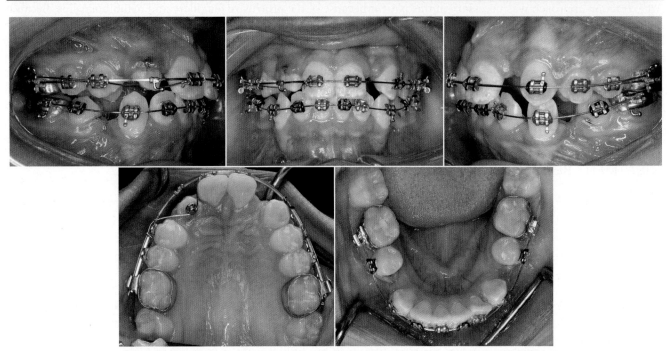

Figure 13-1-3 Piggyback nickel titanium arch wire placed gingival to the lingual button bonded on the lingual surface of the maxillary right canine to move the canine labially and incisally.

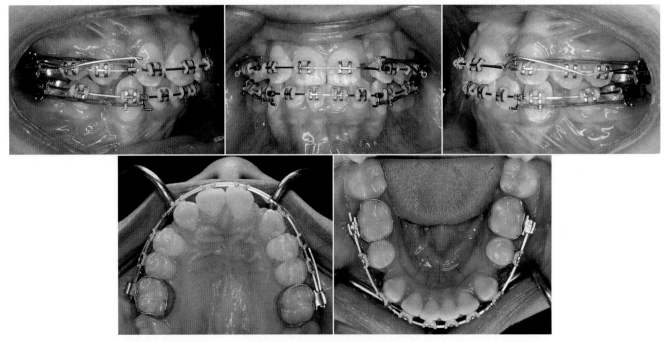

Figure 13-1-4 En masse retraction of the maxillary and mandibular anterior to close extraction spaces. The intrusion arch in the maxillary arch helps to maintain maxillary anchorage by means of the distal tip moments on the maxillary first molars.

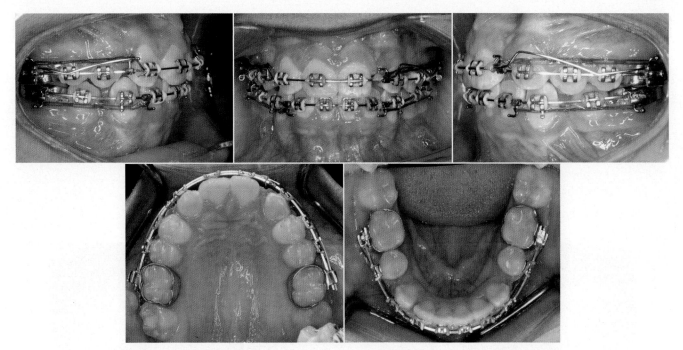

Figure 13-1-5 Continuation of en masse retraction of the maxillary and mandibular anterior to close the extraction spaces.

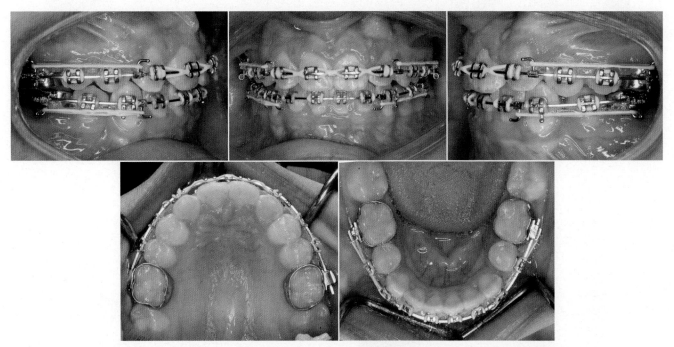

Figure 13-1-6 En masse retraction of maxillary and mandibular anterior to close extraction spaces completed.

■ FINAL RESULTS

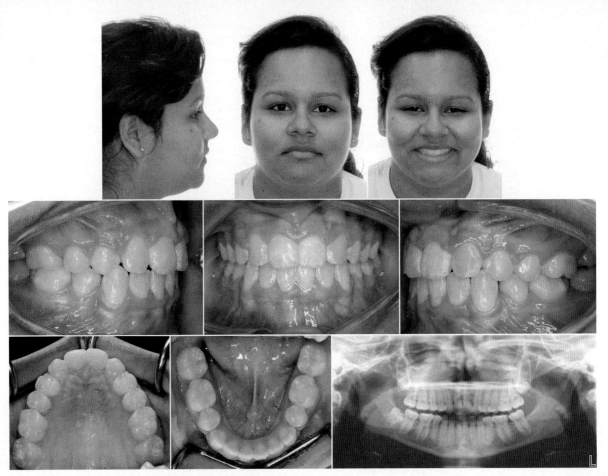

Figure 13-1-7 Posttreatment extraoral/intraoral photographs and panoramic radiograph. Note the canine substitution for the congenitally missing maxillary lateral incisor and extracted peg lateral.

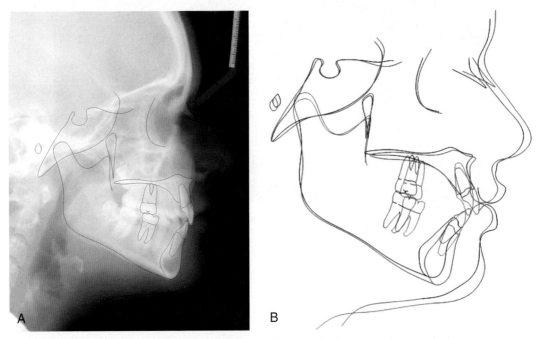

Figure 13-1-8 **A,** Posttreatment lateral cephalogram. **B,** Superimposition. *Black,* pretreatment; *red,* posttreatment.

Why is a base arch wire placed while the right maxillary canine is being brought into the arch?

The base arch wire counteracts the side effects that may be observed when a continuous arch wire is deflected. In this patient the maxillary arch already had a nice form. For this form to be maintained and for the side effects of the adjacent teeth to the canine minimized, a piggyback nickel titanium (NiTi) sectional arch wire is added to move the canine labially and incisally. A lingual button is also added to increase the range of activation of the NiTi wire.

CASE 13-2
Multidisciplinary Approach of Multiple Missing Teeth with Bone Grafts and Endosseous Implants

A 34-year-old female patient was referred by her restorative dentist for consultation regarding opening up spaces for missing maxillary lateral incisors. Medical and dental histories were noncontributory, and findings from a temporomandibular joint (TMJ) examination were normal with adequate range of jaw movements.

■ PRETREATMENT

Extraoral Analysis (Fig. 13-2-1)

Facial Form	Leptoprosopic
Facial Symmetry	No gross asymmetry noticed
Chin Point	Coincidental with facial midline
Occlusal Plane	Normal
Facial Profile	Straight
Facial Height	Upper Facial Height/Lower Facial Height: Normal
	Lower Facial Height/Throat Depth: Long lower facial height
Lips	Competent, Upper: Normal; Lower: Normal
Nasolabial Angle	Normal
Mentolabial Sulcus	Normal

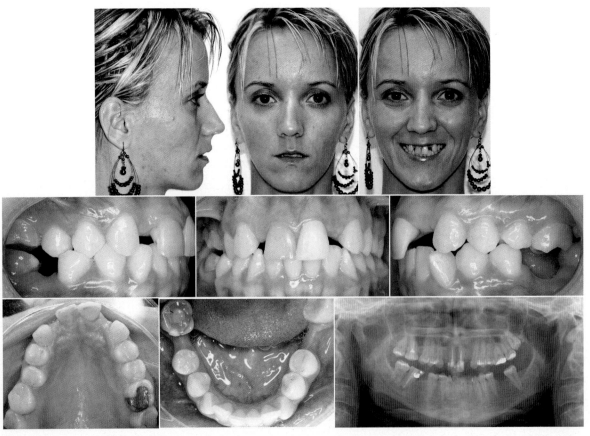

Figure 13-2-1   Pretreatment extraoral/intraoral photographs and panoramic radiograph.

Smile Analysis (Fig. 13-2-2)

Smile Arc	Consonant
Incisor Display	Rest: 2 mm
	Smile: 10 mm
Lateral Tooth Display	Maxillary second premolar to second premolar
Buccal Corridor	Medium
Gingival Tissue	Margins: Irregular between central incisors
	Papilla: Present in all teeth
Dentition	Tooth size and proportions: Normal
	Tooth shape: Normal
	Axial inclination: Normal, except maxillary central incisors, which are tipped to the right
	Connector space and contact area: Closed contacts
Incisal Embrasure	Normal
Midlines	Upper dental midline shifted to right of facial midline by 2 mm
Other	Discoloration of maxillary right central incisor

Intraoral Analysis (see Fig. 13-2-2)

Teeth Present	875431/1345678 Congenitally missing maxillary lateral incisors and mandibular left third molar
	8754321/123457
Molar Relation	Not applicable
Canine Relation	Class I bilaterally
Overjet	2 mm
Overbite	3 mm
Maxillary Arch	Asymmetric with spacing
Mandibular Arch	U shaped with normal curve of Spee
Oral Hygiene	Fair
Other	Atrophic alveolar ridge with respect to missing maxillary lateral incisors
	Multiple posterior restoration
	Occlusal attrition with respect to lower second molar
	Root canal therapy on lower right second molar with associated periapical lesion and a cervical restoration as a result of a tooth perforation
	Root canal therapy on maxillary central incisors and right second molar

Functional Analysis

Swallowing	Tongue thrust present
Temporomandibular joint	Normal with adequate range of jaw movements

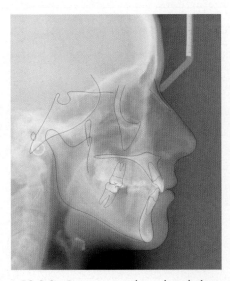

Parameter	Norm	Value
SNA (°)	82	80
SNB (°)	80	77
ANB (°)	2	3
FMA (°)	24	28
MP-SN (°)	32	37
U1-NA (mm/°)	4/22	3/20
L1-NA (mm/°)	4/25	4/28
IMPA (°)	95	88
U1-L1 (°)	130	133
OP-SN (°)	14	15
Upper Lip – E Plane (mm)	−4	−4.6
Lower Lip – E Plane (mm)	−2	−1.7
Nasolabial Angle (°)	103	122
Soft Tissue Convexity (°)	135	127

Figure 13-2-2   Pretreatment lateral cephalogram with tracing and cephalometric analysis.

Diagnosis and Case Summary

A 34-year-old female patient presented with skeletal and dental Class I malocclusion with straight soft and hard tissue profiles, as well as multiple missing permanent teeth including congenitally absent maxillary lateral incisors.

PROBLEM LIST			
Pathology/Other	Heavily restored maxillary central incisor and extensive amalgam restoration on maxillary left first molar		
	Missing maxillary right first molar, lateral incisors bilaterally, mandibular left third molar, and first molars; previous root canal treatment of maxillary centrals, right second molar and right mandibular second molar		
	Periapical lesion associated to root canal treatment of right mandibular second molar and mesial perforation at the level of the cementoenamel junction		
	Occlusal attrition on the mandibular second molars		
	Atrophic ridge in edentulous sites		
Alignment	Insufficient space for restoration of missing maxillary lateral incisors		
	Rotated mandibular canines		
Dimension	**Skeletal**	**Dental**	**Soft Tissue**
Transverse		Maxillary midline shifted to the right side by 2 mm	
		Mandibular right second premolar in crossbite	
		Mandibular left second molar significantly tipped lingually	
Anteroposterior			
Vertical			

TREATMENT OBJECTIVES			
Pathology/Other	Restoration of missing teeth with prosthetic implants, extraction of right mandibular second molar		
Alignment	Create space for restoration of missing maxillary lateral incisors and align mandibular arch		
	Space appropriation for edentulous sites of the first mandibular molars		
Dimension	**Skeletal**	**Dental**	**Soft Tissue**
Transverse		Correct the maxillary midline and correct the crossbite with respect to mandibular right second premolar	
Anteroposterior		Protract mandibular right third molar into the second molar site	
Vertical			

Treatment Options

In the maxillary arch, spaces present as a result of congenitally missing lateral incisors and can be treated by either opening up these edentulous sites for restoration with implants or closing up the spaces through protraction of the maxillary posterior dentition and substituting canines for the lateral incisors. In an adult patient with canines Class I relation, protraction of the entire maxillary dentition to close the edentulous lateral incisor spaces is a difficult, time-consuming procedure.

In the mandibular arch, the mandibular right second molar had a questionable prognosis due to cervical perforation on the mesial side and had to be extracted. The right third molar can be substituted for the right second molar, and both missing first molars could be restored with prosthetic implants. Although full space closure of the mandibular edentulous spaces could be performed by means of temporary anchorage devices (TADs), length of treatment and unopposed maxillary terminal molars precluded this option. The patient opted for space appropriation for implant placement on the missing maxillary lateral incisors and mandibular first molars.

TREATMENT SEQUENCE AND BIOMECHANICAL PLAN

Maxilla	Mandible
Diagnostic wax-up (Fig. 13-2-3).	Diagnostic wax-up (Fig. 13-2-3).
Bond maxillary arch.	Bond mandibular arch bypassing right first molar.
Level with .016, .018, and .016 × .022 inch NiTi arch wire (Fig. 13-2-4).	Level with .016, .018, and .016 × .022 inch NiTi arch wire.
.020 inch SS arch wire.	.017 × .022 inch SS arch wire, protract right second and third molars while retracting right first and second premolars to correct right canine rotation (Fig. 13-2-5).
Space appropriation for lateral incisors.	Extract mandibular right second molar.
Perform autogenous bone graft for missing lateral incisors and place implants (Fig. 13-2-9).	Place implant for missing first molars with simultaneous allograft and guided bone regeneration. Use mandibular right implant to protract right third molar (Fig. 13-2-8).
Debond and deliver wrap around retainer.	Debond and bond lingual 3-3 fixed retainer.
Restoration with crowns (Fig. 13-2-12).	Restoration with crowns (Fig. 13-2-12).
6-month recall appointment for retention check.	6-month recall appointment for retention check.

NiTi, nickel titanium; *SS,* stainless steel.

■ TREATMENT SEQUENCE

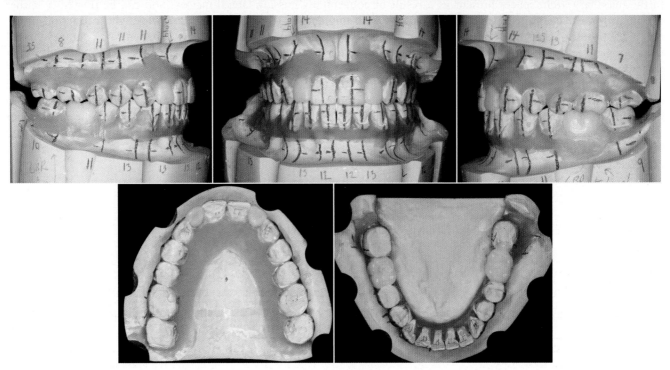

Figure 13-2-3   Diagnostic wax-up.

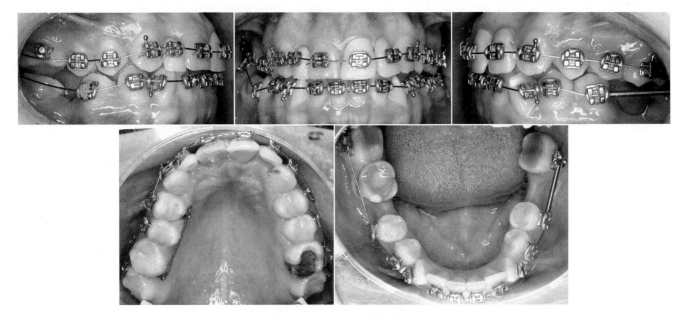

Figure 13-2-4   Initial leveling.

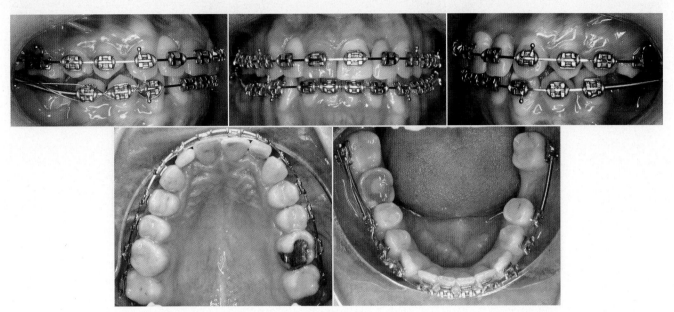

Figure 13-2-5 Continuation of leveling and protraction of mandibular right molars.

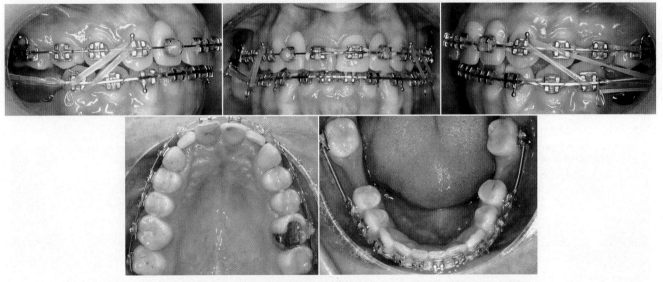

Figure 13-2-6 Continuation of leveling and extraction of right mandibular second molar.

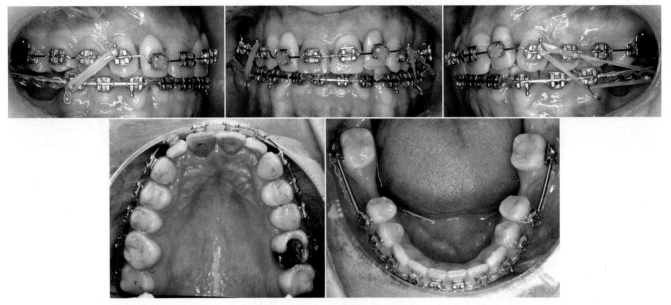

Figure 13-2-7   Finishing details.

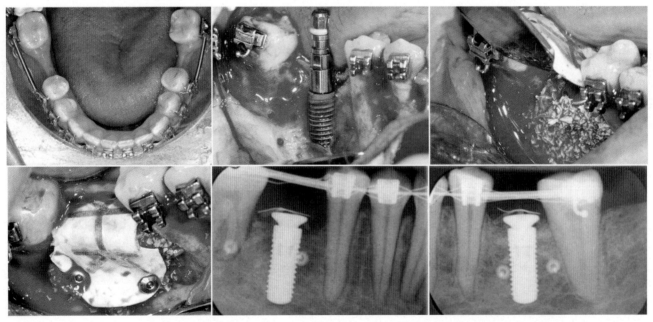

Figure 13-2-8   Placement of prosthetic implants with allograft and guided bone regeneration for missing mandibular first molars bilaterally.

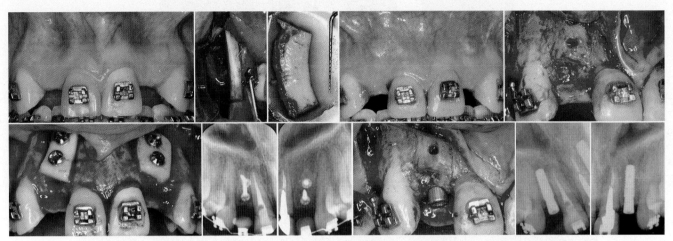

Figure 13-2-9 Placement of autogenous block bone graft to increase the thickness of the alveolar bone in the region of missing maxillary lateral incisors and placement of prosthetic implants (5 months later).

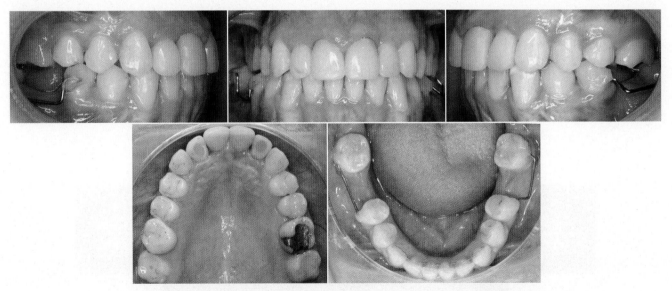

Figure 13-2-10 Posttreatment intraoral photographs before the final implant-supported restorations.

■ FINAL RESULTS

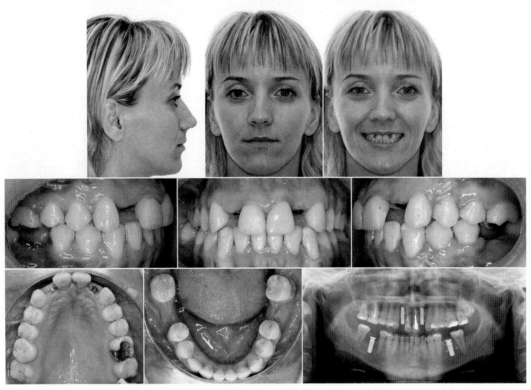

Figure 13-2-11 Posttreatment extraoral/intraoral photographs and panoramic radiograph.

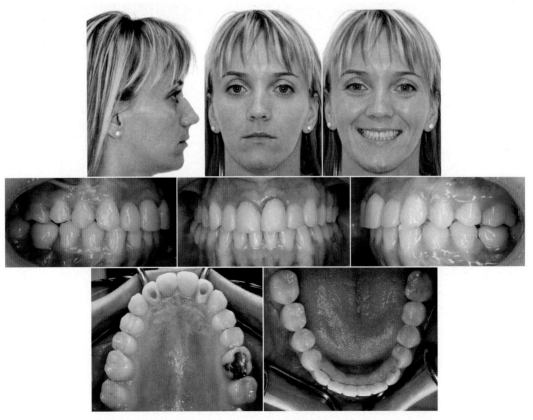

Figure 13-2-12 Posttreatment extraoral/intraoral photographs with restorations.

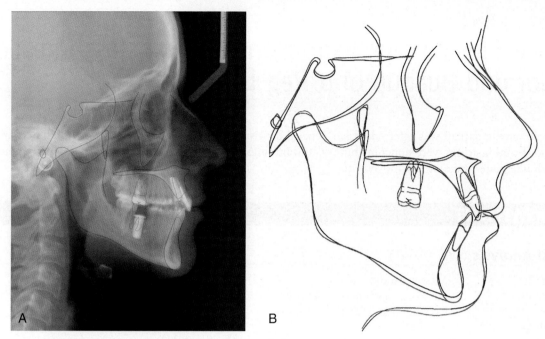

Figure 13-2-13   A, Posttreatment lateral cephalogram. **B,** Superimposition. *Black,* Pretreatment; *red,* posttreatment.

Why was a wax-up depicting the treatment objective performed for this patient?
In patients receiving multiple implants after orthodontic treatment, it is mandatory to fabricate a wax-up depicting the orthodontic tooth movements and the implants to be placed at the end of treatment. The lines on the wax-up serve as reference for the required tooth movements based on the specific objectives of the plan. These reference lines also help to define the mechanics plan to be delivered.

CASE 14-1

Space Closure after Extraction of a Hopeless Maxillary Molar and Buildup of a Peg Lateral

A 13-year-old female patient was referred by her general dentist for assessment of an impacted mandibular premolar. Medical and dental histories were noncontributory, and findings from a temporomandibular (TMJ) examination were normal with adequate range of jaw movements.

■ PRETREATMENT

Extraoral Analysis (Fig. 14-1-1)

Facial Form	Mesoprosopic
Facial Symmetry	No gross asymmetries noticed
Chin Point	Coincidental with facial midline
Occlusal Plane	Normal
Facial Profile	Convex
Facial Height	Upper Facial Height/Lower Facial Height: Normal
	Lower Facial Height/Throat Depth: Normal
Lips	Competent, Upper: Protrusive, Lower: Protrusive
Nasolabial Angle	Normal
Mentolabial Sulcus	Deep

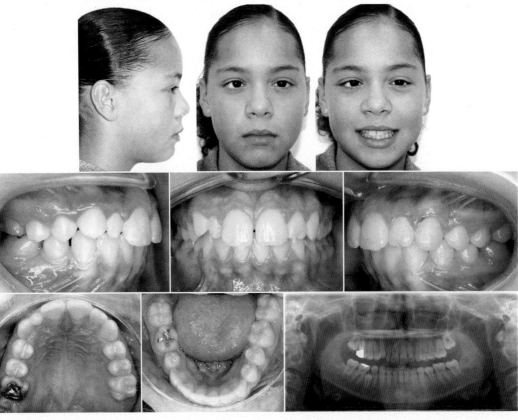

Figure 14-1-1   Pretreatment extraoral/intraoral photographs and panoramic radiograph.

Smile Analysis (Fig. 14-1-2)

Smile Arc	Flat
Incisor Display	Rest: 2 mm
	Smile: 6 mm (asymmetric)
Lateral Tooth Display	Maxillary: Canine to canine
Buccal Corridor	Narrow
Gingival Tissue	Margins: Irregular on the right side due to peg lateral incisor and erupting canine
	Papilla: Present
Dentition	Tooth size and proportion: Peg-shaped right maxillary lateral incisor
	Tooth shape: Normal except for the right maxillary lateral incisor
	Root canal therapy and extensive restoration on maxillary right first molar
	Axial inclination: Normal
	Connector space and contact area: Not present between maxillary central incisors due to diastema
Incisal Embrasure	Unable to evaluate between maxillary central incisors due to diastema
Midlines	Lower dental midline 1 mm right of the facial midline

Intraoral Analysis (see Fig. 14-1-2)

Teeth Present	7654321/123456 Unerupted maxillary left 7, impacted mandibular right 5 and delayed development of 8s
	764321/1234567
Molar Relation	Class I bilaterally
Canine Relation	Class I bilaterally
Overjet	3 mm
Overbite	3 mm
Maxillary Arch	Symmetric with spacing
Mandibular Arch	U-shaped with impacted right second premolar and normal curve of Spee
Oral Hygiene	Fair

Functional Analysis

Swallowing	Adult pattern
Temporomandibular joint	Normal with adequate range of jaw movements

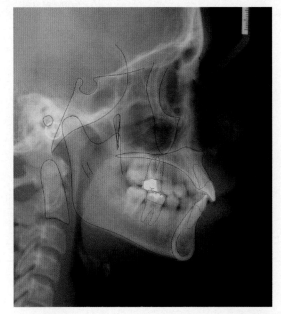

Parameter	Norm	Value
SNA (°)	82	77
SNB (°)	80	74
ANB (°)	2	3
FMA (°)	24	23
MP-SN (°)	32	38
U1-NA (mm/°)	4/22	5/27
L1-NA (mm/°)	4/25	5/28
IMPA (°)	95	95
U1-L1 (°)	130	121
OP-SN (°)	14	20
Upper Lip – E Plane (mm)	−4	2.9
Lower Lip – E Plane (mm)	−2	2.3
Nasolabial Angle (°)	103	113

Figure 14-1-2 Pretreatment lateral cephalogram with tracing and cephalometric analysis.

Diagnosis and Case Summary

A 13-year-old female patient had a skeletal and dental Class I malocclusion with a convex soft tissue profile, impacted right mandibular second premolar, and peg-shaped right lateral incisor.

PROBLEM LIST			
Pathology/Other	Root canal treatment of maxillary right first molar and defective restoration Peg maxillary right lateral incisor Delayed development of 8s		
Alignment	Maxillary crowding of 2.5 mm due to peg-shaped lateral incisor Mandibular crowding of 8 mm due to impacted mandibular right second premolar		
Dimension	**Skeletal**	**Dental**	**Soft Tissue**
Anteroposterior		Class II canine relation on right side 3-mm overjet	Convex profile
Transverse		Mandibular midline 1 mm to the right of the facial midline	
Vertical		50% overbite	Coronal gingival margin of the maxillary right lateral incisor in relation to the contralateral

TREATMENT OBJECTIVES			
Pathology/Others	Reevaluate/extract maxillary right first molar Restore right maxillary lateral incisor to proper dimension Monitor development of 8s		
Alignment	Create space for restoration of peg-shaped maxillary right lateral incisor Create space for eruption of mandibular right second premolar		
Dimension	**Skeletal**	**Dental**	**Soft Tissue**
Anteroposterior		Correct Class II canine on the right side and reduce overjet	
Transverse		Coordinate mandibular to maxillary midline	
Vertical		Reduce overbite by leveling arches	Match gingival margin of maxillary right lateral incisor to contralateral

Treatment Options

In the maxillary arch, the peg-shaped lateral incisor could be extracted and the right side buccal segment protracted mesially to achieve canine substitution. Alternatively, space appropriation for the proper dimension of the lateral incisor could be obtained by distalization of the right-side buccal segment. Because the right-side first molar was grossly decayed with a defective restoration and a root canal treatment, the extraction of this tooth would be recommended. The extraction would result in 10 mm of space used to retract the right buccal segment by 4 mm into Class I relation. The rest of the space would be closed by protracting the right second molar in place of the first molar.

In the mandibular arch, the right-side second premolar was impacted, resulting in a Class II canine relationship. A push coil mechanism could be used to protract the canine mesially and simultaneously create space for the impacted second premolar.

Another option could be to perform extraction of the peg-shaped lateral incisor in the maxilla, perform canine substitution, extract the impacted second premolar, and finish the case in Class I molar and canine relationship. The disadvantage of this option is that it will result in uneven gingival margins due to canine substitution on one side, especially between the right canine (lateral) and right first premolar (canine).

Patient elected to extract the maxillary right molar, build up the right lateral incisor and bring the mandibular right second premolar into the arch.

TREATMENT SEQUENCE AND BIOMECHANICAL PLAN

Maxilla	Mandible
Band molars and bond maxillary arch.	Band molars and bond mandibular arch.
Leveling with .016, .018, and .016 × .022 inch NiTi arch wires.	Leveling with .016, .018, and .016 × .022 inch NiTi arch wires.
.019 × .025 inch NiTi arch wire and send for extraction of maxillary right first molar.	.019 × .025 inch NiTi arch wire with push coil to create space for impacted right second premolar.
.017 × .025 inch SS arch wire with Class V geometry and elastomeric chain for protraction of right second molar (Fig. 14-1-6).	
Maintain the space distal to right lateral incisor open with dead coil and finish with .016 × .022 inch CNA (Fig. 14-1-7).	Finish with .016 × .022 inch CNA.
Debond and deliver wrap around retainer. Refer for restoration of right peg lateral.	Debond and deliver lower Hawley retainer.
6-month recall appointment for retention check. Monitor eruption of right third molar in future retention checks.	6-month recall appointment for retention check.

CNA, Connecticut new arch wire; *NiTi,* nickel titanium; *SS,* stainless steel.

■ TREATMENT SEQUENCE

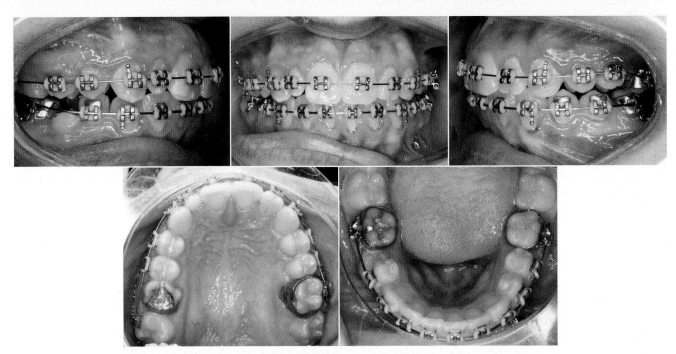

Figure 14-1-3   Initial leveling.

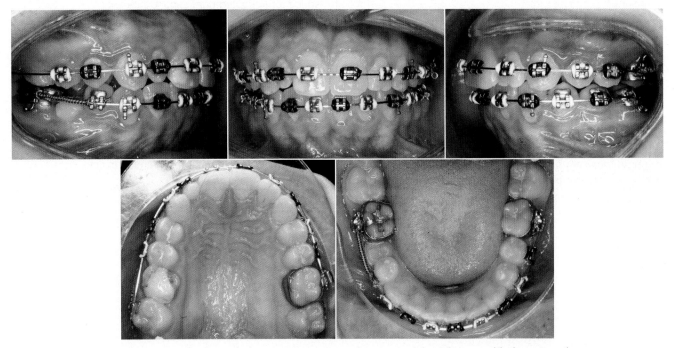

Figure 14-1-4   Push coil for creating space for impacted right mandibular second premolar.

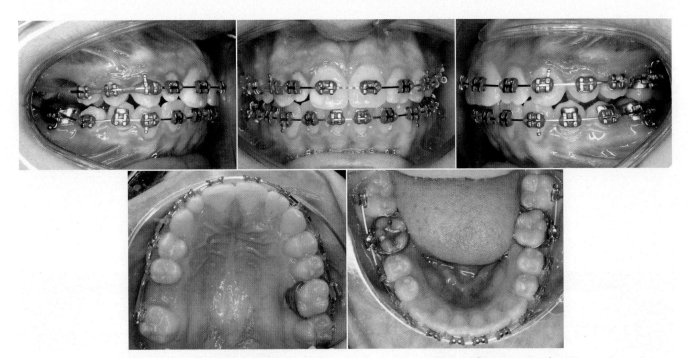

Figure 14-1-5 Extraction of the maxillary right first molar and space closure using Class V geometry.

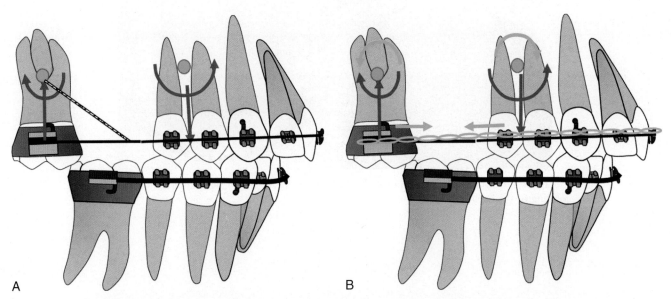

A   B

Figure 14-1-6 **A,** Class V geometry results in a bigger moment on the segment closer to the asymmetric V bend. In this case, the V bend was placed closer to the anterior segment, resulting in a counterclockwise moment and an extrusive force on the anterior segment and a clockwise moment and an intrusive force on the right maxillary second molar. The counterclockwise moment on the anterior segment will reinforce the anterior anchorage during protracting of the maxillary second molar. **B,** Green arrows represent the forces delivered by the elastomeric chain during space closure and the resultant moments on the estimated center of resistance of the molar and anterior anchorage segment.

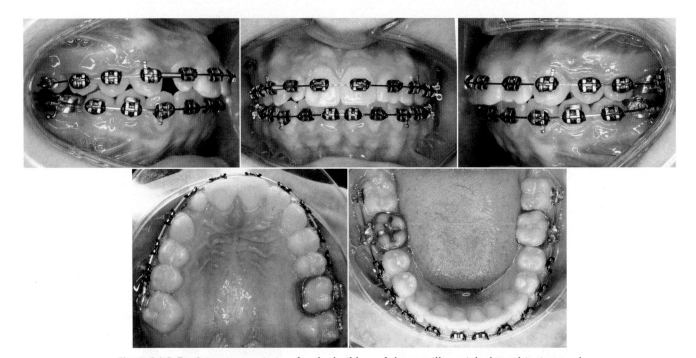

Figure 14-1-7 Space appropiation for the buildup of the maxillary right lateral incisor and settling of the occlusion.

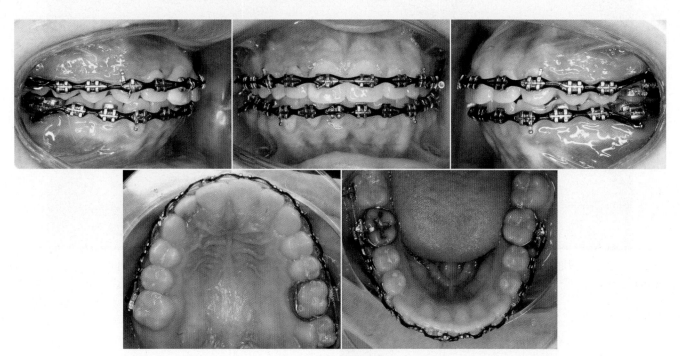

Figure 14-1-8 Finishing and detailing after temporary buildup of the maxillary right lateral incisor.

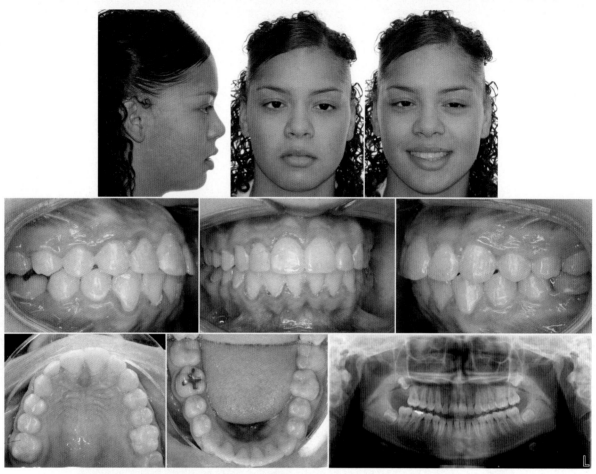

Figure 14-1-9 Posttreatment extraoral/intraoral photographs and panoramic radiograph with final buildup of the maxillary right lateral incisor.

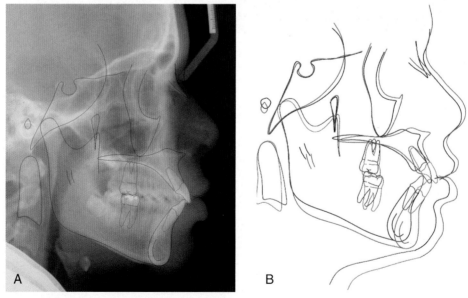

Figure 14-1-10 **A,** Posttreatment lateral cephalogram with tracing. **B,** Superimposition. *Black,* pretreatment; *red,* posttreatment.

Why wasn't a mini-implant used to protract the maxillary right second molar?
Anchorage requirements for molar protraction in the maxilla are not as high as in the mandible. Also, on the basis of the treatment objectives, space closure of the extracted maxillary right first molar required some anchorage loss of the teeth anterior to the molar. The patient also could use Class III elastics to facilitate space closure if anterior anchorage was required.

Mini-Implant–Supported Space Closure of Missing Left First Molar and Extracted Maxillary Premolars

A 26-year-old female patient was referred by her general dentist for assessment of crowding present in the maxillary anterior region and the possibility of closure of edentulous spaces present due to extraction of mandibular molars. Medical and dental histories were noncontributory, and findings from a temporomandibular joint (TMJ) examination were normal with adequate range of jaw movements.

■ PRETREATMENT

Extraoral Analysis (Fig. 14-2-1)

Facial Form	Mesoprosopic
Facial Symmetry	No gross asymmetries noticed
Chin Point	Coincidental with facial midline
Occlusal Plane	Normal
Facial Profile	Convex due to prognathic maxilla
Facial Height	Upper Facial Height/Lower Facial Height: Normal
	Lower Facial Height/Throat Depth: Normal
Lips	Competent, Upper: Protrusive, Lower: Normal
Nasolabial Angle	Obtuse
Mentolabial Sulcus	Normal

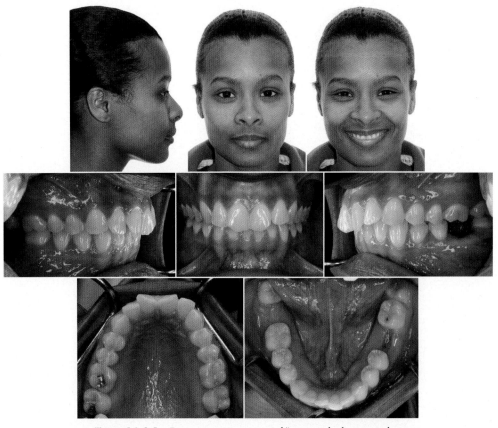

Figure 14-2-1   Pretreatment extraoral/intraoral photographs.

Smile Analysis (Fig. 14-2-2)

Smile Arc	Consonant
Incisor Display	Rest: 2 mm
	Smile: 8 mm
Lateral Tooth Display	Maxillary molar to molar
Buccal Corridor	Narrow
Gingival Tissue	Margins: Irregular; reverse architecture between maxillary centrals and incisors
	Papilla: Present in all teeth
Dentition	Tooth size and proportion: Normal
	Tooth shape: Triangular shaped maxillary central incisors
	Connector space and contact area: Closed contacts
Incisal Embrasure	Not present due to incisor wear on mesial aspect on maxillary central incisors
Midlines	Mandibular dental midline shifted to the left by 3 mm with respect to the facial midline

Intraoral Analysis (see Fig. 14-2-2)

Teeth Present	7654321/1234567
	8654321/1234578
Molar Relation	Class II end on right side, left side N/A
Canine Relation	Class I on right side and Class II on the left side
Overjet	4 mm
Overbite	4 mm
Maxillary Arch	U shaped with crowding
Mandibular Arch	U shaped with missing molars and normal curve of Spee
Oral Hygiene	Fair
	Alveolar ridges: Adequate ridge width of mandibular edentulous sites; slight reduced ridge height on the right side
	Gingival biotype: Thin gingival biotype on labial of the lower incisors

Functional Analysis

Swallowing	Adult pattern
Temporomandibular joint	Normal with adequate range of jaw movements

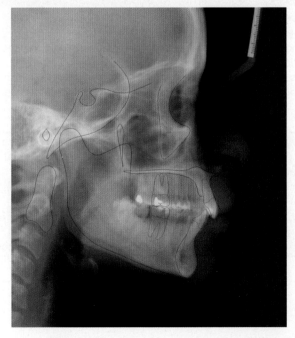

Parameter	Norm	Value
SNA (°)	82	90
SNB (°)	80	82
ANB (°)	2	8
FMA (°)	24	25
MP-SN (°)	32	32
U1-NA (mm/°)	4/22	0/8
L1-NA (mm/°)	4/25	6/28
IMPA (°)	95	95
U1-L1 (°)	130	134
OP-SN (°)	14	16
Upper Lip – E Plane (mm)	−4	0
Lower Lip – E Plane (mm)	−2	−1
Nasolabial Angle (°)	103	117
Soft Tissue Convexity (°)	135	128

Figure 14-2-2 Pretreatment lateral cephalogram with tracing and cephalometric analysis.

Diagnosis and Case Summary

A 26-year-old female patient with skeletal and dental Class II malocclusion with convex soft tissue profile mainly due to a prognathic maxilla. Maxillary anterior teeth are retroclined and mandibular incisors are slightly proclined and labially placed. The mandibular right second molar and left first molar are missing in the mandible.

PROBLEM LIST			
Pathology/Others	Missing mandibular right second molar and left first molar Incisal wear in the mesial aspect of the maxillary central incisors Thin gingival biotype on labial of the mandibular incisors		
Alignment	2 mm of crowding present in maxillary arch and 3 mm of crowding present mesial to molars in mandibular arch 20 mm of space due to missing mandibular left first molar and right second molar		
Dimension	**Skeletal**	**Dental**	**Soft Tissue**
Anteroposterior	Class II denture base due to prognathic maxilla	Class II canine relation on the left side Class II end on molar relation on right side OJ: 4 mm Retroclined maxillary incisors Slightly proclined and labially positioned mandibular incisors	Protrusive upper lip Obtuse nasolabial angle
Transverse		Mandibular midline shifted to the left side by 3 mm	
Vertical		OB: 4 mm	Reverse architecture in gingival heights between maxillary central and lateral incisors

OB, overbite; *OJ*, overjet.

TREATMENT OBJECTIVES			
Pathology/Others	Restore mesial aspect of maxillary central incisors with composite restorations Monitor for recession in the mandibular anterior segment		
Alignment	Relieve the crowding in maxillary and mandibular arches using the extraction spaces in the maxilla and the right mandibular molar edentulous site Close spaces due to missing molars by protracting the lower left second molar and third molar into the space of the first molar and the mandibular right third molar into the space of the second molar		
Dimension	**Skeletal**	**Dental**	**Soft Tissue**
Anteroposterior		Retract maxillary anterior teeth to correct overjet and Class II canine relationship	Retraction of maxillary incisors to correct protrusion of upper lip
Transverse		Shift the mandibular midline to the right side by 3 mm using the mandibular right second molar space	
Vertical		Reduce OB by leveling maxillary and mandibular arches	Evaluate gingival margins of maxillary anterior teeth for possible periodontal esthetic contouring

OB, overbite.

Treatment Options

For the Class II canine relationship to be corrected on the left side, either upper premolars could be extracted and space could be closed by retracting the maxillary anterior teeth or the entire left mandibular buccal segment could be protracted mesially. For space due to a missing mandibular left first molar to be closed up, the mandibular left second and third molars could be protracted mesially with the help of temporary anchorage devices (TADs). This space closure will not correct the Class II canine occlusion unless a space for an implant is developed after the protraction of the left mandibular second and third molars. This option would increase the proclination of the mandibular incisors, would not allow for reducing maxillary lip protrusion, and increase treatment costs.

Therefore a maxillary premolar extraction plan is recommended in conjunction with closure of the extraction space of the right second mandibular molar, which could be managed with Group B space closure by protracting the mandibular right third molar mesially and retracting the right mandibular buccal segment distally simultaneously with the retraction of the maxillary right canine. A TAD would protract the left mandibular second and third molar. This treatment option was selected by the patient.

TREATMENT SEQUENCE AND BIOMECHANICAL PLAN

Maxilla	Mandible
Band molars and bond maxillary arch.	Band molars and bond mandibular arch.
Leveling with .016, .018, .016 × .022, and .019 × .025 inch NiTi arch wires.	Leveling with .016, .018, .016 × .022, and .019 × .025 inch NiTi arch wires.
.019 × .025 inch SS wire, TADs between first molars and second premolars, and start en-masse space closure with 200 g NiTi coil spring (Fig. 14-2-5).	.019 × .025 inch SS arch wire, TAD between left first and second premolars, and start protraction of left lower second and third molar with 200 g NiTi coil spring (Fig. 14-2-6).
Continue en-masse space closure.	Group B space closure on mandibular right side to close up space of the missing second molar with elastomeric chain.
.016 × .022 inch CNA with finishing bends, finish Class II molar and Class I canine relationship bilaterally.	.016 × .022 inch CNA with finishing bends.
Debond and deliver wrap around retainer.	Debond and deliver Hawley retainer.
6-month recall appointment for retention check.	6-month recall appointment for retention check.

CNA, Connecticut new arch wire; *NiTi,* nickel titanium; *SS,* stainless steel; *TAD,* temporary anchorage device.

■ TREATMENT SEQUENCE

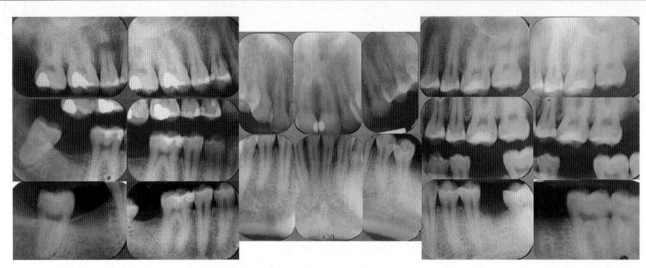

Figure 14-2-3   Pretreatment full mouth series.

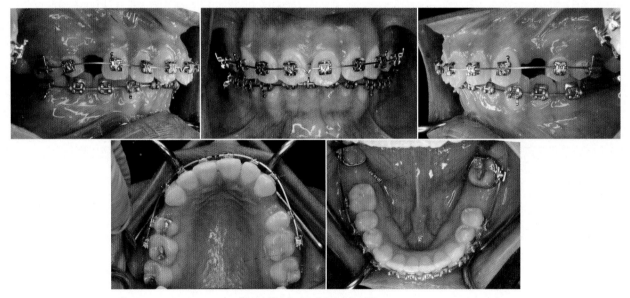

Figure 14-2-4   Initial leveling.

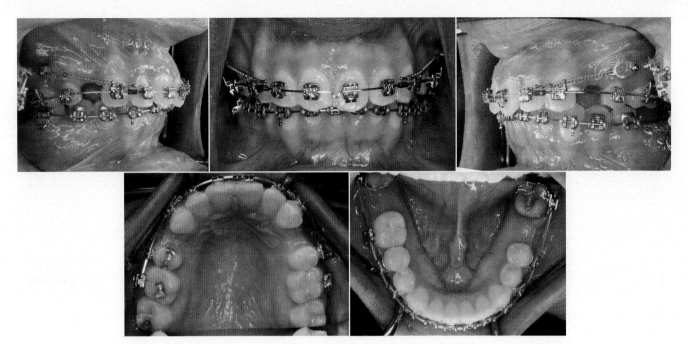

Figure 14-2-5 Temporary anchorage device supported maxillary anterior en-masse retraction.

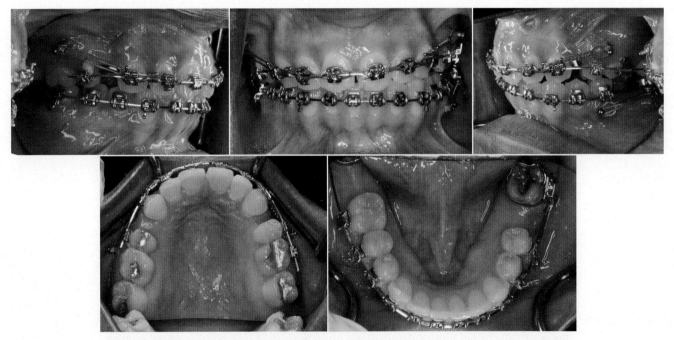

Figure 14-2-6 Temporary anchorage device supported mesial protraction of the mandibular left second molar.

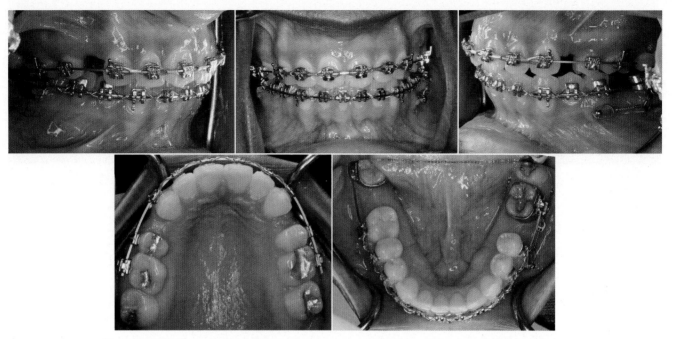

Figure 14-2-7 Temporary anchorage device supported mesial protraction of the mandibular left second molar almost complete.

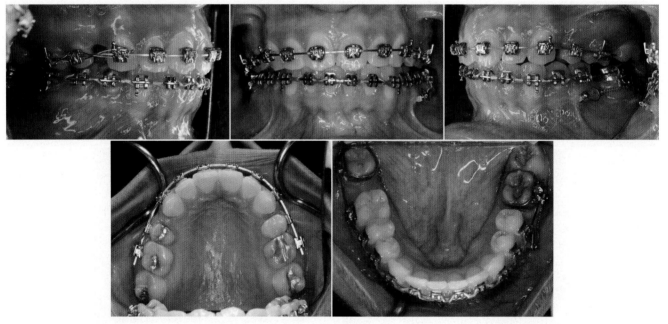

Figure 14-2-8 Group B space closure on the mandibular right side results in mesial protraction of the mandibular right third molar and distal retraction of the right mandibular buccal segment.

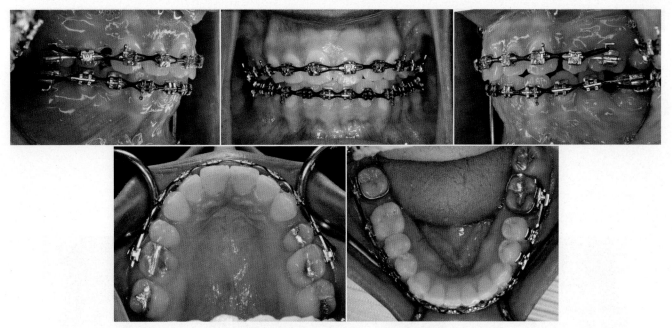

Figure 14-2-9   Finishing.

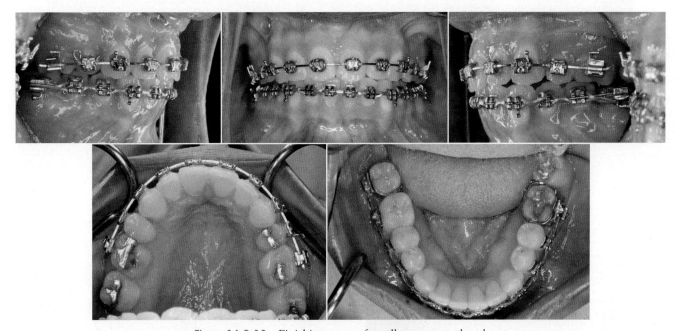

Figure 14-2-10   Finishing stage after all spaces are closed.

■ FINAL RESULTS

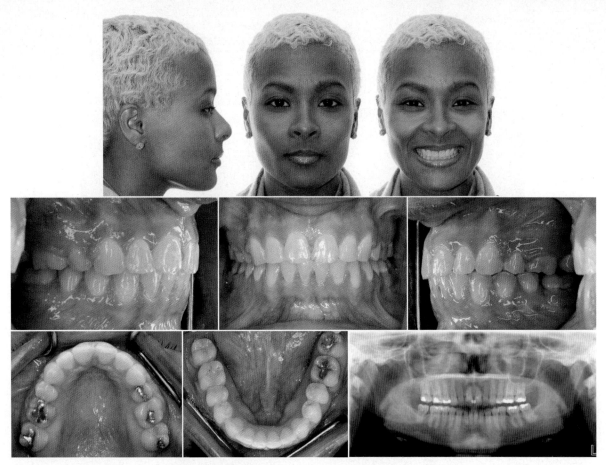

Figure 14-2-11   Posttreatment extraoral/intraoral photographs and panoramic radiograph.

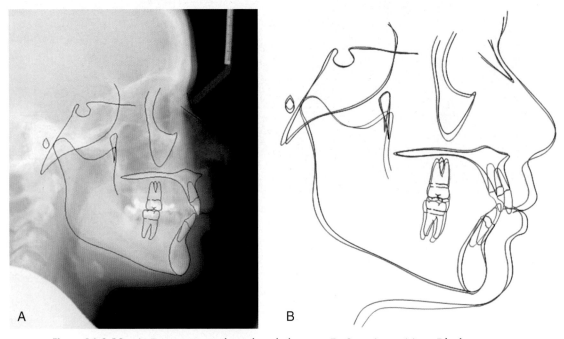

Figure 14-2-12   **A,** Posttreatment lateral cephalogram. **B,** Superimposition. *Black,* pretreatment; *red,* posttreatment.

Why was a mini-implant placed on the left mandibular region?
Perfect anchorage was required in the maxilla to retract the left canine, which was obtained with a mini-implant placed mesial to the canine. Full protraction without any anchorage loss was also necessary on the left mandibular second and third molar. For this objective to be achieved, a mini-implant was also required in that quadrant.

Mandibular Second Molar Protraction into a First Molar Space with a Fixed Functional Appliance*

A 14-year-old male patient presented with chief complaint related to the appearance of his maxillary canines. Medical history was noncontributory. Dental history revealed extraction of the right mandibular first molar 3 years prior due to caries. Findings from a temporomandibular joint (TMJ) examination were normal with adequate range of jaw movements.

■ PRETREATMENT

Extraoral Analysis (Fig. 14-3-1)

Facial Form	Euryprosopic
Facial Symmetry	No gross asymmetries noticed
Chin Point	Coincidental with facial midline
Occlusal Plane	Normal
Facial Profile	Straight
Facial Height	Upper Facial Height/Lower Facial Height: Normal
	Lower Facial Height/Throat Depth: Normal
Lips	Competent, Upper: Normal; Lower: Normal
Nasolabial Angle	Normal
Mentolabial Sulcus	Deep

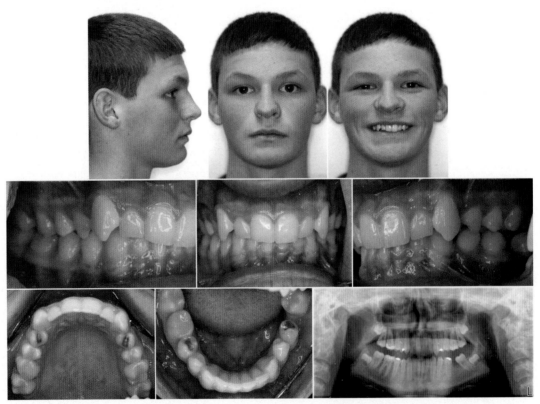

Figure 14-3-1 Pretreatment extraoral/intraoral photographs and panoramic radiograph.

*Portions of Case 14-3 from Davoody AR, Feldman J, Uribe FA, Nanda R. Mandibular molar protraction with the Twin Force Bite Corrector in a Class II patient. *J Clin Orthod.* 2011;45:223-228.

Smile Analysis (Fig. 14-3-2)

Smile Arc	Flat
Incisor Display	Rest: 3 mm
	Smile: 8 mm
Lateral Tooth Display	Maxillary first premolar to first premolar
Buccal Corridor	Narrow
Gingival Tissue	Margins: Irregular; maxillary central and lateral incisor margins are more incisal in relation to the canines
	Papilla: Present in all teeth
Dentition	Tooth size and proportion: Long height of maxillary canines
	Tooth shape: Small occlusogingival height of maxillary lateral incisors; sharp incisal tip of maxillary canines
	Connector space and contact area: Closed contacts
Incisal Embrasure	Large incisal embrasure between maxillary incisors and canines due to the morphology of the canine's incisal edge
Midlines	Maxillary and mandibular dental midline are on with the facial midline

Intraoral Analysis (see Fig. 14-3-2)

Teeth Present	7654321/1234567
	7654321/123457 (Unerupted 8s)
Molar Relation	Class II end on right side, left side not applicable
Canine Relation	Class II end on bilaterally
Overjet	3 mm
Overbite	5 mm
Maxillary Arch	U shaped with labially placed canines and reverse curve of Spee
Mandibular Arch	U shaped with spacing in the left buccal segment from the missing left first molar, mesially inclined left second molar and normal curve of Spee
Oral Hygiene	Fair
Alveolar Ridges	Reduced ridge width of mandibular edentulous site
Gingival Biotype	Thin gingival biotype on labial of lower incisors

Functional Analysis

Swallowing	Normal adult pattern
Temporomandibular joint	Normal with adequate range of jaw movements

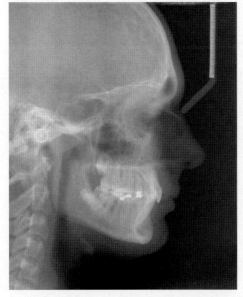

Parameter	Norm	Value
SNA (°)	82	82
SNB (°)	80	81
ANB (°)	2	1
FMA (°)	24	20
MP-SN (°)	32	23
U1-NA (mm/°)	4/22	4/18
L1-NA (mm/°)	4/25	2/28
IMPA (°)	95	95
U1-L1 (°)	130	135
OP-SN (°)	14	15
Upper Lip – E Plane (mm)	−4	−4
Lower Lip – E Plane (mm)	−2	−2
Nasolabial Angle (°)	103	105

Figure 14-3-2   Pretreatment lateral cephalogram and cephalometric analysis.

Diagnosis and Case Summary

A 14-year-old male patient had orthognathic soft and hard tissue profiles; a vertically, flat mandibular plane angle and deep overbite; and Class II malocclusion with retroclined maxillary incisors and missing left mandibular first molar.

PROBLEM LIST			
Pathology/Others	Missing mandibular left first molar Mesially inclined left mandibular second molar Reduced ridge width of the edentulous site Sharp incisal tip on maxillary canines Thin biotype on the labial aspect of the mandibular incisors		
Alignment	Spacing in mandibular left buccal segment due to missing first molar		
Dimension	**Skeletal**	**Dental**	**Soft Tissue**
Anteroposterior		Class II end on canine relation bilaterally Class II end on molar relation on the right side Retroclined maxillary incisors	Deep mentolabial fold
Transverse		Maxillary canines labially placed	
Vertical	Reduced mandibular plane angle	OB: 5 mm Reverse maxillary curve of Spee	Gingival margins of the maxillary central and lateral incisors are more incisal in relation to the canines

OB, overbite.

TREATMENT OBJECTIVES			
Pathology/Others	Close edentulous mandibular left first molar space by protracting the mandibular left second molar mesially Monitor eruption of mandibular left third molar and labial gingival margins of mandibular anterior segment Contour incisal edge of maxillary canines		
Alignment			
Dimension	**Skeletal**	**Dental**	**Soft Tissue**
Anteroposterior		Correct Class II molar and canine relationship with help of Class II corrector appliance Improve maxillary incisor inclination	Reduce mentolabial fold
Transverse		Match maxillary canine width to mandibular canine width	
Vertical		Reduce OB and eliminate reverse curve of Spee by leveling the maxillary arch	Extrude maxillary canines to match the gingival margins and contour incisal edges

OB, overbite.

Treatment Options

The following four treatment alternatives were considered.

The first alternative involved a nonextraction approach through protraction of the mandibular left second molar and simultaneous correction of the Class II occlusion with a fixed functional appliance. The disadvantage of this option is the extended total treatment time.

The second nonextraction option entailed opening the mandibular left first molar space for a prosthodontic restoration. The advantage of this option could be shorter duration of total treatment time as compared with the first option, but this option would be more expensive when the restoration is included in the cost.

The third option involved the extraction of the maxillary first premolars to correct the canine relationship and protraction of the mandibular left second molar to close up the edentulous space. Less amount of mandibular left second molar protraction is required with this option with the potential of reducing treatment duration.

The fourth alternative included the extraction of the maxillary first premolars for the correction of the canine relationship and opening of the mandibular left first molar space for prosthodontic restoration.

The patient chose to close orthodontically the mandibular left first molar space without maxillary extractions. For the occlusal objectives to be achieved, molar protraction requires no anterior anchorage loss, thereby two options are available. The first option is to draw anchorage from a temporary anchorage device (TAD); the second option is to use a fixed functional appliance such as the Twin Force Bite Corrector (Ortho Organizers, a subsidiary of Henry Schein, Carlsbad, California) or Forsus (3M Unitek, Orthodontic Products, Monrovia, California) for anchorage, which not only reinforces the anterior anchorage during molar protraction into the edentulous site, but also corrects the Class II occlusion.

A fixed functional appliance option without TADs was selected to protract the left mandibular second molar.

TREATMENT SEQUENCE AND BIOMECHANICAL PLAN

Maxilla	Mandible
Band molars and bond maxillary arch.	Band molars and bond mandibular arch.
Leveling with .016, .018, .016 × .022, and .019 × .025 inch NiTi arch wires.	Leveling with .016, .018, .016 × .022, and .019 × .025 inch NiTi arch wires.
.019 × .025 inch SS wire with cinch back behind the first molars. Place .032 inch CNA transpalatal arch and insert Twin Force Bite Corrector.	.019 × .025 inch SS with cinch back and attach Twin Force Bite Corrector.
	Place elastomeric chain from the right first molar to left second molar to protract the left second molar mesially.
.016 × .022 inch CNA with finishing bends, finish Class I molar, and Class I canine relationship bilaterally.	.016 × .022 inch CNA with finishing bends.
Debond and deliver wrap around retainer.	Debond and deliver Hawley retainer. Place fixed labial-bonded retainer between mandibular left second premolar and second molar.
6-month recall appointment for retention check.	6-month recall appointment for retention check.

CNA, Connecticut new arch wire; *NiTi,* nickel titanium; *SS,* stainless steel.

■ TREATMENT SEQUENCE

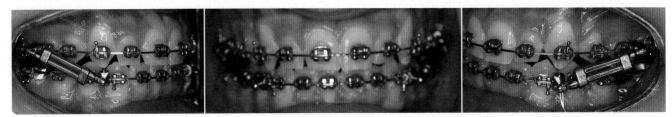

Figure 14-3-3   Intraoral photographs after Twin Force Bite Corrector delivery.

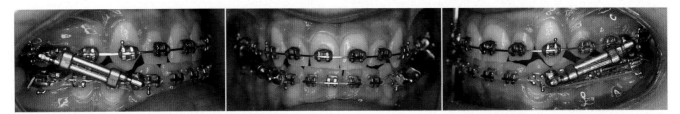

Figure 14-3-4   Intraoral photographs after the start of molar protraction.

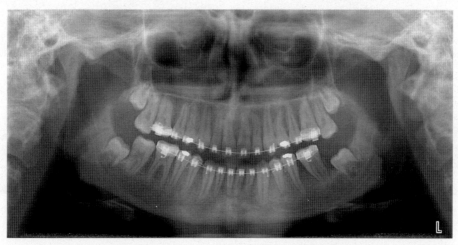

Figure 14-3-5   Progress panoramic radiograph.

▪ FINAL RESULTS

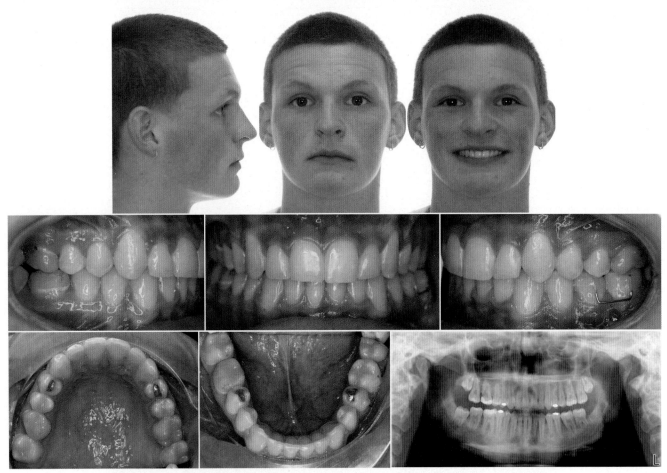

Figure 14-3-6 Posttreatment extraoral/intraoral photographs and panoramic radiograph. Note the full eruption of the left mandibular third molar into the second molar space.

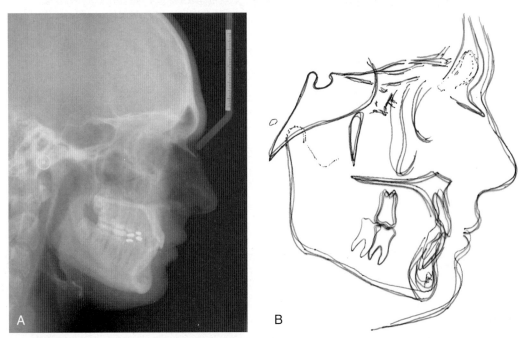

Figure 14-3-7 **A,** Posttreatment lateral cephalogram. **B,** Superimposition. *Blue,* Pretreatment; *red,* posttreatment.

How do interarch Class II correctors reinforce maxillary posterior and mandibular anterior anchorage?

Most fixed functional appliances deliver an anterior force to the mandibular anterior dentition that also results in a clockwise moment. This anterior force and moment counteracts the retraction force and moment from the intraarch mechanics to protract the mandibular left molar. In addition, the force system corrects that Class II molar occlusion by distalizing the maxillary dentition, mesializing the mandibular dentition, and steepening the occlusal plane.

Section 6

Strategies to Expedite Orthodontic Treatment

CASE 15-1
Corticotomy-Assisted and TAD-Supported Mandibular Molar Protraction with TAD-Based Intrusion of Maxillary Molars*

A 58-year-old female patient was referred by her prosthodontist for assessment of orthodontic protraction of the mandibular second molars into bilateral atrophied edentulous spaces of the first molar sites. Medical history revealed the patient had controlled diabetes, and dental history was noncontributory. Findings from a temporomandibular joint (TMJ) examination were normal with adequate range of jaw movements.

■ PRETREATMENT

Extraoral Analysis (Fig. 15-1-1)

Facial Form	Mesoprosopic
Facial Symmetry	No gross asymmetries noticed
Chin Point	Coincidental with facial midline
Occlusal Plane	Flat
Facial Profile	Straight
Facial Height	Upper Facial Height/Lower Facial Height: Normal
	Lower Facial Height/Throat Depth: Normal
Lips	Competent, Upper: Retrusive; Lower: Retrusive
Nasolabial Angle	Obtuse
Mentolabial Sulcus	Normal

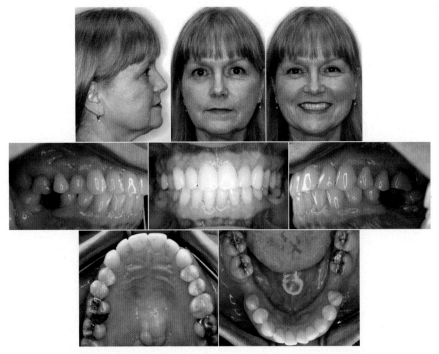

Figure 15-1-1 Pretreatment extraoral/intraoral photographs.

*Portions of Case 15-1 from Uribe F, Janakiraman N, Fattal AN, Schincaglia GP, Nanda R. Corticotomy-assisted molar protraction with the aid of temporary anchorage device. *Angle Orthod.* 2013;83:1083-1092.

Smile Analysis (Fig. 15-1-2)

Smile Arc	Consonant
Incisor Display	Rest: 0 mm
	Smile: 8 mm
Lateral Tooth Display	Maxillary molar to molar
Buccal Corridor	Narrow
Gingival Tissue	Margins: Normal relationship
	Papilla: Present in all teeth
	Periodontium: Mild attachment loss in maxillary and mandibular molars
Dentition	Tooth size and proportion: Normal
	Tooth shape: Normal
	Axial inclination: Maxillary teeth inclined labially
	Connector space and contact area: Closed contacts
Incisal Embrasure	Normal
Midlines	Maxillary: Coincidental with facial midline
	Mandibular: 1 mm to the right

Intraoral Analysis (see Fig. 15-1-2)

Teeth Present	87654321/12345678
	8754321/1234578
Molar Relation	N/A
Canine Relation	Class I bilaterally
Overjet	1 mm
Overbite	2 mm
Maxillary Arch	U shaped and symmetric
Mandibular Arch	U shaped with missing first molars and normal curve of Spee
Oral Hygiene	Fair
	Alveolar ridges: Atrophic ridge with reduced width and height of mandibular edentulous sites
	Gingival biotype: Thin gingival biotype with slight gingival recession on labial of lower incisors
Dentition	Heavily restored posterior dentition

Functional Analysis

Swallowing	Adult pattern
Temporomandibular joint	Normal with adequate range of jaw movements

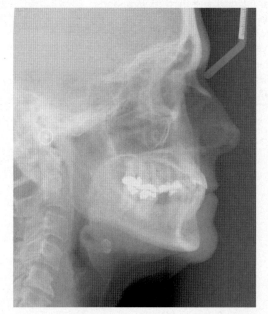

Parameter	Norm	Value
SNA (°)	82	78
SNB (°)	80	80
ANB (°)	2	−2
FMA (°)	24	22
MP-SN (°)	32	30
U1-NA (mm/°)	4/22	7/43
L1-NA (mm/°)	4/25	4/28
IMPA (°)	95	96
U1-L1 (°)	130	130
OP-SN (°)	14	5
Upper Lip – E Plane (mm)	−4	−5
Lower Lip – E Plane (mm)	−2	−6
Nasolabial Angle (°)	103	110

Figure 15-1-2 Pretreatment lateral cephalogram and cephalometric analysis.

Diagnosis and Case Summary

A 58-year-old female patient had a straight skeletal and soft tissue profile. She had a Class I malocclusion with labially inclined maxillary anterior teeth, retrusive upper and lower lips, and obtuse nasolabial angle. Mandibular first molars were missing, and edentulous ridges were atrophic with supraerupted maxillary first molars.

PROBLEM LIST			
Pathology/Others	Atrophic edentulous ridges in the region of the mandibular first molars Mild recession on labial aspect of mandibular incisors Heavily restored posterior dentition Slight periodontal attachment loss on maxillary and mandibular molars		
Alignment	Mild anterior mandibular crowding		
Dimension	**Skeletal**	**Dental**	**Soft Tissue**
Anteroposterior	Straight hard tissue profile	Proclined maxillary incisors Mandibular first and second molars mesially inclined	Retrusive upper and lower lips Straight soft tissue profile Obtuse nasolabial angle
Transverse		Mandibular midline 1 mm to the right of facial midline	
Vertical		Maxillary first molars are extruded into the edentulous space of the missing mandibular first molars Reduced incisor display at rest Flat occlusal plane	

TREATMENT OBJECTIVES			
Pathology/Others	Periodontal monitoring and maintenance every 4 months by periodontist Monitor recession in the labial aspect of mandibular incisors		
Alignment	Relieve mandibular anterior crowding		
Dimension	**Skeletal**	**Dental**	**Soft Tissue**
Anteroposterior		Maintain maxillary and mandibular incisor inclination Upright the mandibular second and third molars, and close the edentulous space by protracting the second and third molars into the extraction space with the help of miniscrews	
Transverse		Improve mandibular midline to match facial midline	
Vertical		Intrude the maxillary first molars to level the maxillary arch with help of miniscrews	

Treatment Options

In the present case, three options were available to restore the mandibular dental arch.

1. Intrusion of maxillary first molars with the aid of miniscrews, followed by restoration of missing mandibular first molars with endosseous implant supported prosthesis after orthodontic space appropriation.

2. Space closure of the edentulous mandibular first molar space by protraction of the mandibular second and third molars aided by miniscrew anchorage. In addition, miniscrews were to intrude both first maxillary molars to the level occlusal plane. The advantage of this option is the reduced cost compared with restorations with prosthetic implants. The disadvantage of this option is that because the ridges are atrophic, molar protraction can be time consuming and periodontal damage around the second and the third molars can occur.

3. Corticotomy-assisted second molar protraction as a possibility to reduce the treatment time with this procedure in addition to miniscrew-supported maxillary first molar intrusion. Additional bone grafting could also contribute to a wider ridge width and possible better posttreatment periodontal health of the protracted molars.

The patient chose the third option.

TREATMENT SEQUENCE AND BIOMECHANICAL PLAN

Maxilla	Mandible
Band first molars, place TPA made from .032-inch round SS wire. Place miniscrews on the palatal side between second premolar and first molar. Apply 100 g of intrusive force by connecting the first molars with the miniscrews through an elastomeric chain.	Corticotomy around the second and third molars, as well as in the edentulous space of the first molars. Demineralized freeze-dried bone allograft in the corticotomy area, an edentulous site.
	Band second molars and bond third molars. Segmental wire connecting first and second molars with .019 × .025 SS wire. Place .032-inch lingual arch. Place miniscrews distal to the second premolars and apply 150 g of mesial force by connecting second molars with the miniscrews through NiTi closed coil springs.
Bond maxillary arch and initiate leveling with .016, .018, .016 × .022, and .019 × .025 inch NiTi arch wires.	Place a power arm from the auxiliary slot of the second molar bracket and continue the protraction force.
.019 × .025 inch SS arch wire.	Bond mandibular arch and initiate leveling with .016, .018, .016 × .022, and .019 × .025 inch NiTi arch wires. .019 × .025 inch SS arch wire.
.016 × .022 inch CNA with finishing bends.	.016 × .022 inch CNA with finishing bends.
Debond and bond lingual 3-3 retainer.	Debond and bond lingual 3-3 retainer. Segmental wire bonded labially on the second and third molars and second premolar to prevent space from reopening.
6-month recall appointment for retention check.	6-month recall appointment for retention check.

CNA, Connecticut new arch wire; *NiTi,* nickel titanium; *SS,* stainless steel; *TPA,* transpalatal arch.

■ TREATMENT SEQUENCE

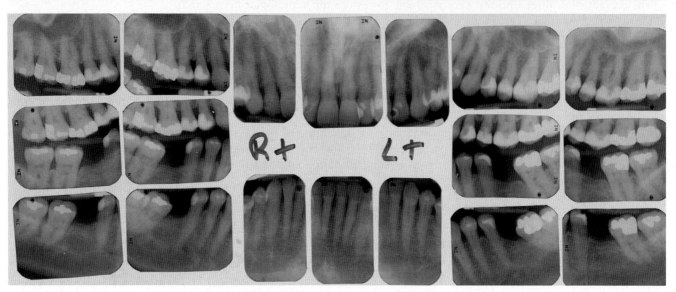

Figure 15-1-3   Pretreatment full-mouth series.

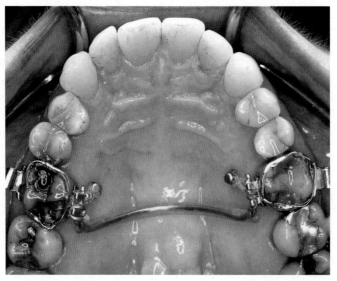

Figure 15-1-4   Miniscrews for intrusion of maxillary first molars.

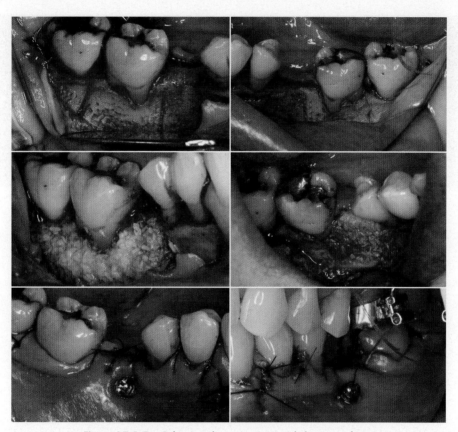

Figure 15-1-5 Selective decortication with bone grafting.

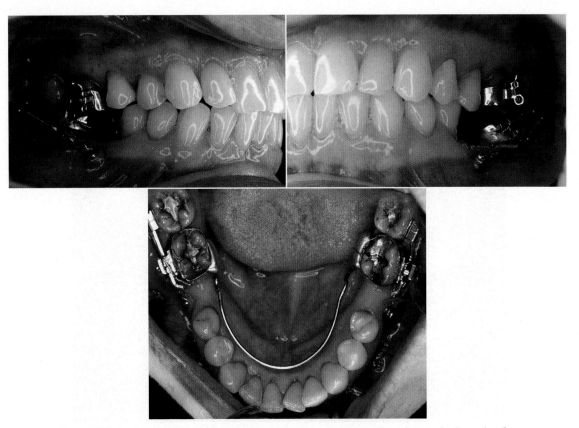

Figure 15-1-6 Molar protraction from miniscrews to a lingual arch attached to the first molars. A .019 × .025 stainless steel segment connects the first and second molars.

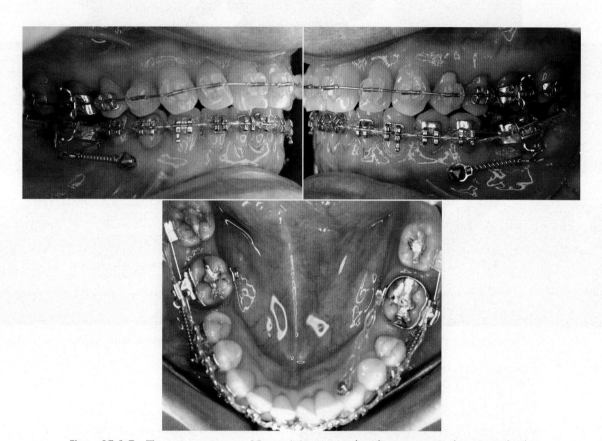

Figure 15-1-7   Treatment progress. Note miniscrews replaced more anteriorly to completely close the edentulous space.

■ FINAL RESULTS

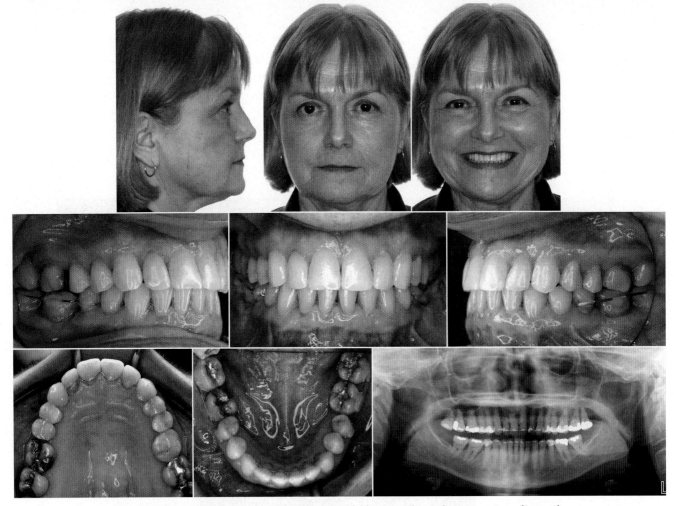

Figure 15-1-8   Posttreatment extraoral/intraoral photographs and panoramic radiograph.

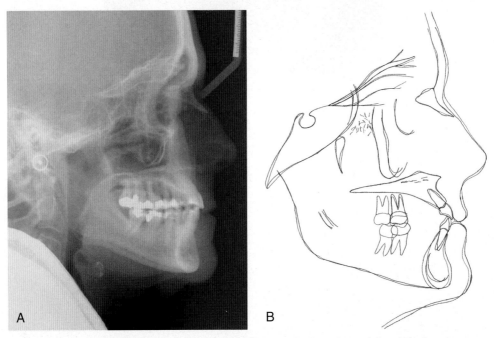

Figure 15-1-9   **A,** Posttreatment lateral cephalogram. **B,** Superimposition. *Black*, pretreatment; *red*, posttreatment.

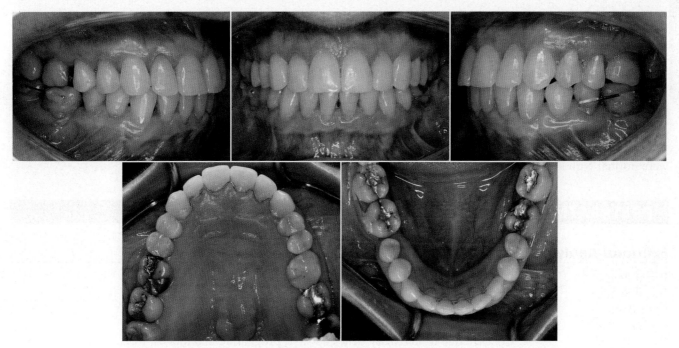

Figure 15-1-10   One-year postretention intraoral photographs.

?

Why was a corticotomy performed on the second molars?

Molar protraction into an edentulous space is one of the most time-consuming procedures in orthodontics. To reduce the duration of this procedure, a periodontally accelerated osteogenic orthodontic (PAOO) technique was used. Incidentally, the treatment duration was still prolonged even after this procedure. The total treatment time for this patient was 41 months.

CASE 16-1
Virtual Three-Dimensional Plan and Surgery-First Approach in Orthognathic Surgery

A 17-year-old female patient presented with a chief complaint that her lower teeth were in front of the upper teeth. Medical and dental histories were noncontributory, and findings from a temporomandibular joint (TMJ) examination were normal with adequate range of jaw movements.

▪ PRETREATMENT

Extraoral Analysis (Fig. 16-1-1)

Facial Form	Leptoprosopic
Facial Symmetry	Tip of the nose deviated to right side of the face
Chin Point	Shifted to the left side by 2 mm
Occlusal Plane	Normal
Facial Profile	Concave due to maxillary deficiency and prognathic mandible
Facial Height	Upper Facial Height/Lower Facial Height: Normal
	Lower Facial Height/Throat Depth: Normal
Lips	Competent, Upper: Retrusive; Lower: Normal
Nasolabial Angle	Obtuse
Mentolabial Sulcus	Normal
Malar Prominences	Deficient

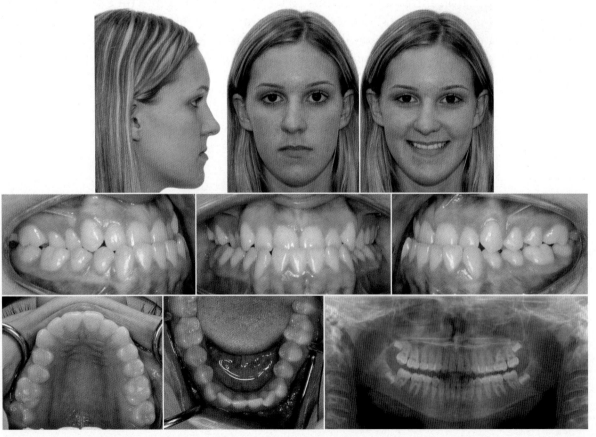

Figure 16-1-1   Pretreatment extraoral/intraoral photographs and panoramic radiograph.

Smile Analysis (Fig. 16-1-2)

Smile Arc	Consonant
Incisor Display	Rest: 2 mm
	Smile: 8 mm
Lateral Tooth Display	Second premolar to second premolar
Buccal Corridor	Large (especially on the right side)
Gingival Tissue	Margins: Adequate height relationships
	Papilla: Present
Dentition	Tooth size and proportion: Normal
	Tooth shape: Normal
	Axial inclination: Maxillary teeth inclined labially; mandibular incisors slightly upright
	Connector space and contact area: Present
Incisal Embrasure	Normal
Midlines	Lower midline shifted left side by 2 mm as compared with facial midline

Intraoral Analysis (see Fig. 16-1-2)

Teeth Present	7654321/1234567 (Unerupted 8s)
	7654321/1234567
Molar Relation	Class III bilaterally
Canine Relation	Class III bilaterally
Overjet	−3 mm
Overbite	3 mm
Maxillary Arch	U shaped, asymmetric with constricted right first and second premolars, anterior crossbite
Mandibular Arch	U shaped with crowding of 5 mm and flat curve of Spee
Oral Hygiene	Fair

Functional Analysis

Swallowing	Normal adult pattern
Temporomandibular joint	Normal with adequate range of jaw movements

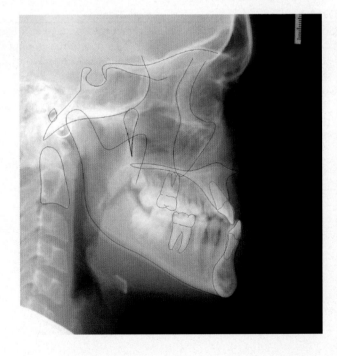

Parameter	Norm	Value
SNA (°)	82	82
SNB (°)	80	89
ANB (°)	2	−7
FMA (°)	24	24
MP-SN (°)	32	30
U1-NA (mm/°)	4/22	6/35
L1-NA (mm/°)	4/25	2/19
IMPA (°)	95	82
U1-L1 (°)	130	131
OP-SN (°)	14	11
Upper Lip – E Plane (mm)	−4	−8
Lower Lip – E Plane (mm)	−2	−3
Nasolabial Angle (°)	103	106
Soft Tissue Convexity (°)	135	136
N-A (HP) (mm)	−2	−2
N-B (HP) (mm)	−6.5	7

Figure 16-1-2 Pretreatment lateral cephalogram with tracing and cephalometric analysis.

Diagnosis and Case Summary

A 17-year-old female patient presented with concave soft hard and soft tissue profiles due to a combination of maxillary deficiency and mandibular prognathism. She had a dental Class III relationship with a mild to moderate mandibular asymmetry, negative overjet, flared maxillary incisors, retroclined mandibular incisors, and maxillary right first and second premolars in crossbite.

PROBLEM LIST			
Pathology/Others	Long mandibular condyle stalk on the right		
Alignment	5 mm of crowding present in mandibular arch		
Dimension	**Skeletal**	**Dental**	**Soft Tissue**
Anteroposterior	Concave profile due to maxillary deficiency and mandibular prognathism	OJ: –3 mm Slight proclination of maxillary incisors are retroclined lower incisors	Concave soft tissue profile Retrusive upper lip
Transverse	Chin point deviated to the left by 2 mm	Maxillary right first and second premolars in crossbite Mandibular midline shifted to the left side by 2 mm	Wider buccal corridor on the right than the left side
Vertical			Slightly reduced maxillary incisor display at rest and smile

OJ, overjet.

TREATMENT OBJECTIVES			
Pathology/Others			
Alignment	Relieve the mandibular crowding by flaring the incisors		
Dimension	**Skeletal**	**Dental**	**Soft Tissue**
Anteroposterior	Advance the maxilla approximately 4 mm Set back the mandible slightly	Correct the reverse overjet Correct the maxillary and mandibular incisor inclination	Correct the concave soft tissue profile and retrusive upper lip by surgical correction of the skeletal discrepancy
Transverse	Correct the chin point deviation to the facial midline by skeletal correction	Correct the maxillary right first and second premolar lingual crossbite Shift the mandibular midline 2 mm to the right	Reduce the size of the buccal corridor by expanding maxillary right premolars
Vertical			Improve incisor display with maxillary advancement

Treatment Options

Orthognathic surgery is indicated for the correction of skeletal facial concavity, paranasal deficiency, and Class III malocclusion with mandibular asymmetry.

Two surgical approaches were available, the first option being a conventional orthognathic surgery approach in which the teeth are aligned and leveled into an ideal relationship with their respective basal arches, followed by surgical correction. This treatment approach usually takes approximately 2 to 3 years to complete.

The second option is the surgery-first approach in which there is no presurgical orthodontic phase. The patient is banded and bonded a few weeks before the surgery, and the dental correction is done after the surgical procedure. Because both maxillary and mandibular arches are reasonably well aligned at the pretreatment stage and no occlusion interferences were noted when the models were articulated in ideal intercuspation, the surgery-first approach was indicated. Some of the advantages of this approach are reduced total treatment time, elimination of the unaesthetic period of decompensation of the dental arches, and addressing the patient chief complaint early in treatment. This patient was treated with a surgery-first approach.

TREATMENT SEQUENCE AND BIOMECHANICAL PLAN

Maxilla	Mandible
Band molars, bond both arches, impressions and CBCT for virtual 3D planning of the surgical movements and fabrication of the surgical splints.	
Place .016 × .022 inch NiTi arch wire with surgical hooks crimped to arch wire the day before surgery.	Place .016 × .022 inch NiTi arch wire with surgical hooks crimped to arch wire the day before surgery.
Orthognathic surgery.	Orthognathic surgery.
Two weeks from the day of surgery, remove the stent and check for appliance breakages, remove the surgical wires, replace all the debonded brackets, place .016 × .022 inch NiTi arch wires, and ligate securely. Wear intermaxillary elastics to seat the occlusion.	Two weeks from the day of surgery, remove the stent and check for appliance breakages, remove the surgical wires, replace all the debonded brackets, place .016 × .022 inch NiTi arch wires, and ligate securely. Wear intermaxillary elastics to seat the occlusion.
Continue leveling with .017 × .025 inch NiTi arch wire.	Continue leveling with .017 × .025 inch NiTi arch wire.
Continue leveling with .019 × .025 inch NiTi arch wire.	Continue leveling with .019 × .025 inch NiTi arch wire.
.016 × .022 inch CNA with finishing bends.	.016 × .022 inch CNA with finishing bends.
Debond and deliver wrap around retainer.	Debond and bond lingual 3-3 retainer.
6-month recall appointment for retention check.	6-month recall appointment for retention check.

CBCT, Cone beam computed tomography; *CNA,* connecticut new arch wire; *NiTi,* nickel titanium; *3D,* three-dimensional.

■ TREATMENT SEQUENCE

Surgical Plan: Preoperative Situation

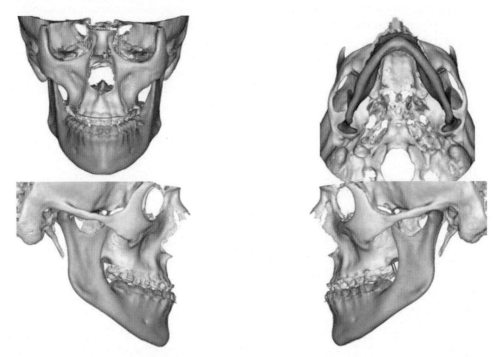

Surgical Plan: Intermediate Position (Maxilla Movement First)

4-mm advancement, yaw correction with CW rotation about midline. Uncut mandible rotated open slightly for splint design.

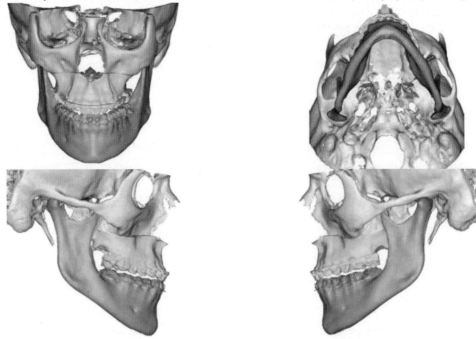

Figure 16-1-3 Virtual three-dimensional surgical planning. *CCW,* counterclockwise; *CT,* computed tomography; *CW,* clockwise; *SNA,* sella-nasion–A point angle; *SNB,* sella-nasion–B point angle.

Surgical Plan: Final Position

Mandible moved into final occlusion with maxilla (3-mm setback, 3 mm to the right, 2-mm impaction, CCW rotation about the midline).

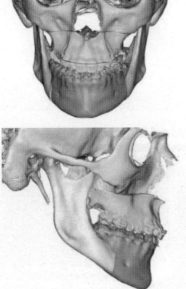
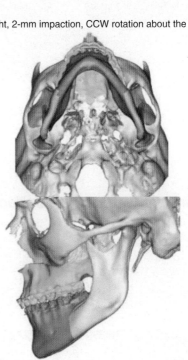

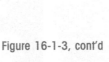

Figure 16-1-3, cont'd

Surgical Plan: Maxilla Movement

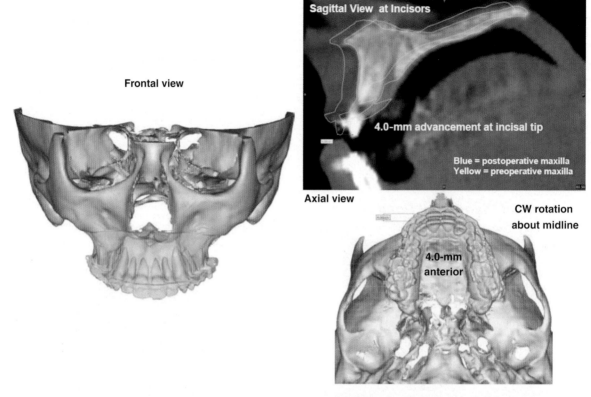

Surgical Plan: Maxilla Impaction/Disimpaction Measurements

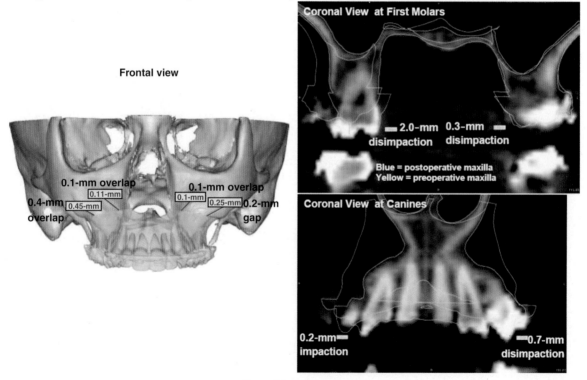

Figure 16-1-3, cont'd

Surgical Plan: Proximal Segment Measurements

Left Buccal View

Right Buccal View

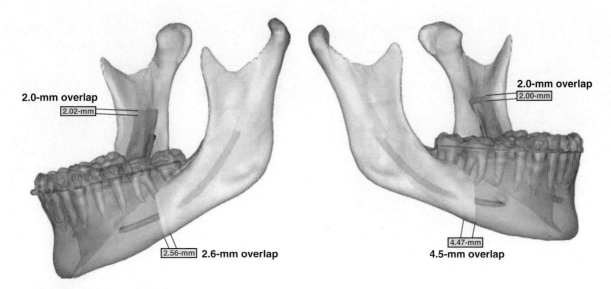

2.0-mm overlap
2.02-mm

2.0-mm overlap
2.00-mm

2.56-mm 2.6-mm overlap

4.47-mm
4.5-mm overlap

Surgical Plan: Mandible Movement

Frontal View

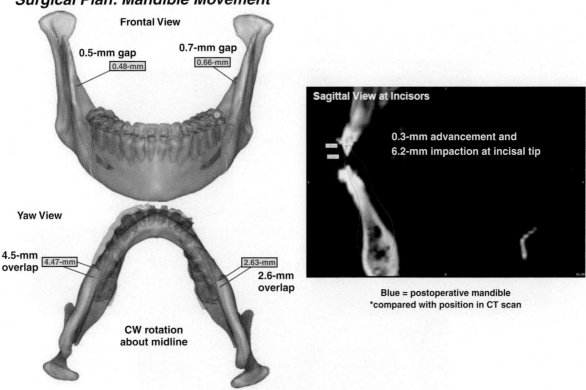

0.5-mm gap
0.48-mm

0.7-mm gap
0.66-mm

Sagittal View at Incisors

0.3-mm advancement and
6.2-mm impaction at incisal tip

Yaw View

4.5-mm
overlap
4.47-mm

2.63-mm
2.6-mm
overlap

CW rotation
about midline

Blue = postoperative mandible
*compared with position in CT scan

Figure 16-1-3, cont'd

Surgical Plan: Basic Lateral Cephalometry

Preoperative: SNA = 81.6°; SNB = 85.8°; ANB = 4.2°;
Postoperative: SNA = 85.6°; SNB = 84.2°; ANB = 1.4°;

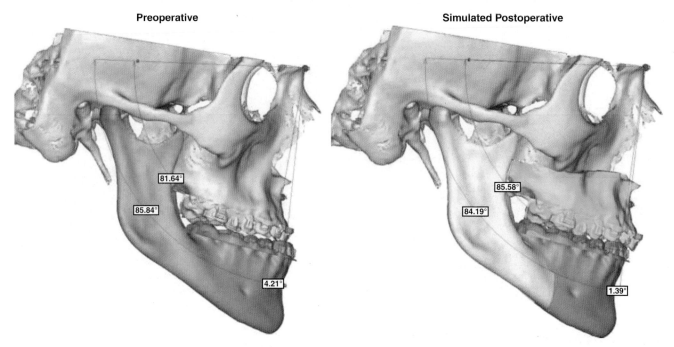

Figure 16-1-3, cont'd

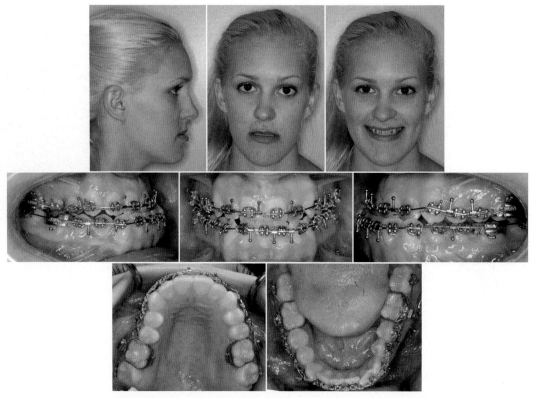

Figure 16-1-4   A .016 × .022 inch nickel titanium surgical arch wire with crimped surgical hooks placed the day before surgery.

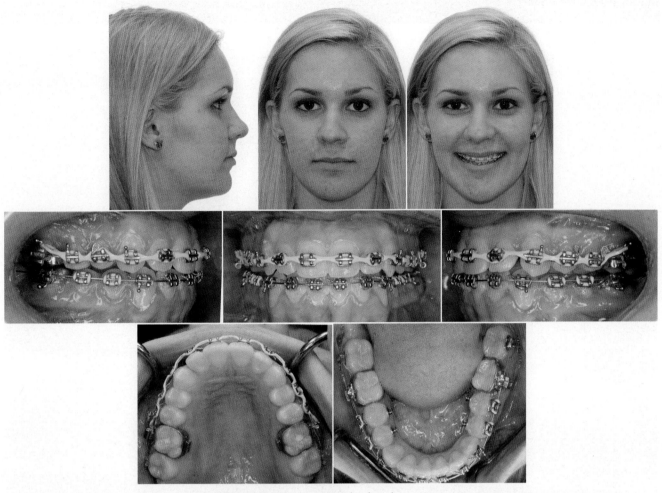

Figure 16-1-5   One month after the surgery.

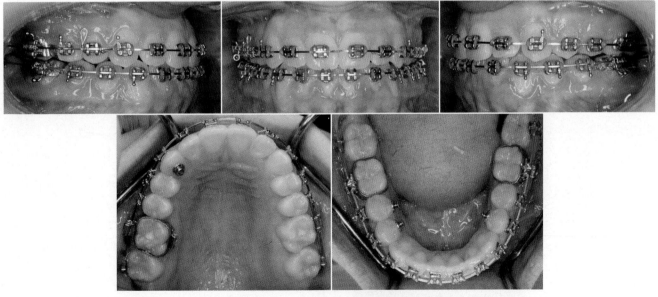

Figure 16-1-6   Finishing and settling of the occlusion.

■ FINAL RESULTS

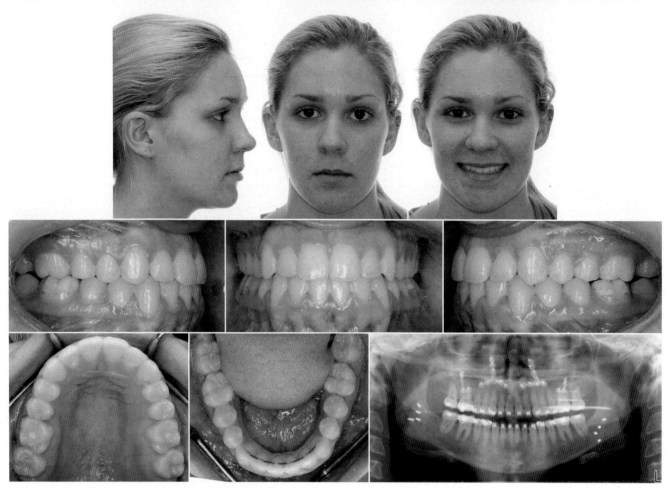

Figure 16-1-7   Posttreatment extraoral/intraoral photographs and panoramic radiograph. Treatment duration was 10 months.

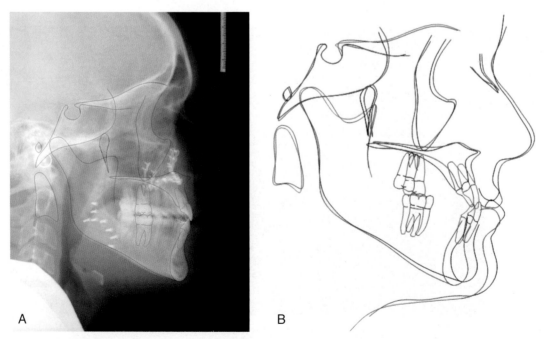

Figure 16-1-8   **A,** Posttreatment lateral cephalogram. **B,** Superimposition. *Black,* pretreatment; *red,* posttreatment.

Why was a three-dimensional (3D) virtual digital orthognathic surgery plan used?
Contemporary orthognathic surgery is relying more heavily on virtual 3D plans instead of model surgery for treatment planning and surgical guide fabrication. A definite indication for this approach is patients with asymmetries. Visualization of asymmetries in 3D allows one to evaluate the complexity of the deformity better than the classic multiple two dimensional (2D)–imaging approach. It also provides a template for the complex 3D surgical movements for which surgical guides can be fabricated with CAD/CAM (computer-aided design/computer-aided manufacturing) technology.

Why was the surgery-first approach used in this patient?
The surgery-first approach was used in this patient because many of the characteristics that indicate this approach were present. Some of these indications present in this patient were minimum to moderate crowding in the maxilla and mandible, adequate anteroposterior position of the maxillary incisor, and minimal transverse discrepancy of the arches when related in the ideal postsurgical occlusion.

CASE 17-1
Targeted Mechanics for Impacted Canines

A 14-year-old postpubertal female patient presented with a chief complaint of spacing present in the anterior region of the maxilla. Medical and dental histories were noncontributory, and findings from a temporomandibular joint examination were normal with adequate range of jaw movements.

▪ PRETREATMENT

Extraoral Analysis (Fig. 17-1-1)

Facial Form	Mesoprosopic
Facial Symmetry	No gross asymmetries noticed
Chin Point	Coincidental with facial midline
Occlusal Plane	Normal
Facial Profile	Normal for ethnicity
Facial Height	Upper Facial Height/Lower Facial Height: Normal
	Lower Facial Height/Throat Depth: Reduced due to increased throat depth
Lips	Competent, Upper: Slightly protrusive, Lower: Protrusive
Nasolabial Angle	Acute
Mentolabial Sulcus	Deep

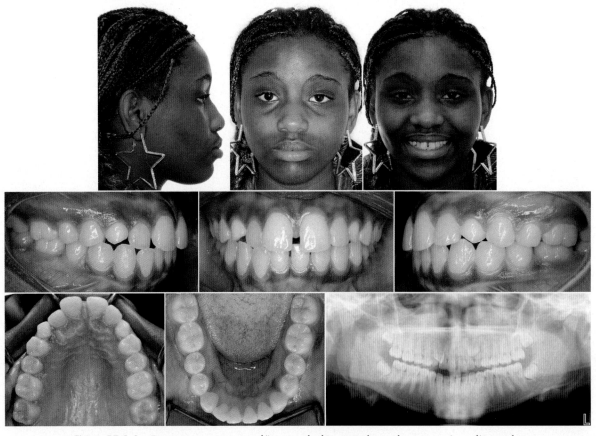

Figure 17-1-1 Pretreatment extraoral/intraoral photographs and panoramic radiograph.

Smile Analysis (Fig. 17-1-2)

Smile Arc	Consonant
Incisor Display	Rest: 3 mm
	Smile: 9 mm
Lateral Tooth Display	Second premolar to second premolar
Buccal Corridor	Narrow
Gingival Tissue	Margins: Primary canine margins are low (more incisal)
	Papilla: Present
	Thick labial frenum
Dentition	Tooth size and proportion: Normal
	Tooth shape: Normal
	Axial inclination: Normal
	Connector space and contact area: No contact between maxillary centrals
Incisal Embrasure	No contact between central incisors, thus not able to evaluate
Midlines	Mandibular midline shifted to the right by 1 mm
	Upper dental midline is coincidental with the facial midline

Intraoral Analysis (see Fig. 17-1-2)

Teeth Present	7654321/124567
	7654321/1234567 (Unerupted 8s)
Molar Relation	Class I bilaterally
Canine Relation	N/A
Overjet	2 mm
Overbite	2 mm
Maxillary Arch	U shaped, symmetric with impacted left canine and over-retained deciduous canines and midline diastema of 3 mm; ectopic eruption of maxillary right canine
Mandibular Arch	U shaped, normal curve of Spee
Oral Hygiene	Fair

Functional Analysis

Swallowing	Normal adult pattern
Temporomandibular joint	Normal with adequate range of jaw movements

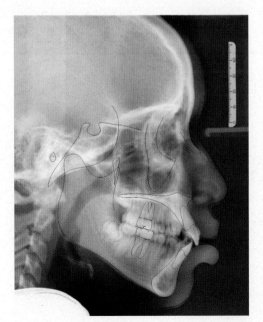

Parameter	Norm	Value
SNA (°)	85	85
SNB (°)	81	82
ANB (°)	4	3
FMA (°)	28	30
MP-SN (°)	38	38
U1-NA (mm/°)	7/22	6/21
L1-NA (mm/°)	9/33	7/32
IMPA (°)	98	92
U1-L1 (°)	119	122
OP-SN (°)	16	20
Upper Lip – E Plane (mm)	0	1.9
Lower Lip – E Plane (mm)	4	8.7
Nasolabial Angle (°)	90	81

Figure 17-1-2 Pretreatment lateral cephalogram with tracing and cephalometric analysis.

Diagnosis and Case Summary

A 14-year-old postpubertal female had orthognathic soft and hard tissue profiles and a dental Class I malocclusion, an impacted left maxillary canine, over-retained deciduous maxillary canines, and a maxillary midline diastema of 3 mm.

PROBLEM LIST			
Pathology/Others	Over-retained maxillary deciduous canines		
Alignment	Impacted maxillary left canine; ectopic eruption maxillary right canine Maxillary midline diastema of 3 mm 1 mm of spacing present in mandibular arch		
Dimension	**Skeletal**	**Dental**	**Soft Tissue**
Anteroposterior			Slightly protrusive lips
Transverse		Palatally placed maxillary right canine Mandibular midline shifted 1 mm to the right	
Vertical	Increased Frankfort-mandibular plane angle		

TREATMENT OBJECTIVES			
Pathology/Others	Extraction of retained maxillary deciduous canines		
Alignment	Orthodontic traction for eruption of the impacted maxillary left canine and the ectopic maxillary right canine Retract the maxillary and mandibular anterior teeth to close the spaces present in the arches		
Dimension	**Skeletal**	**Dental**	**Soft Tissue**
Anteroposterior			
Transverse		Align the palatally placed maxillary right canine Align mandibular midline to facial midline	
Vertical			Assess gingival heights of erupted maxillary canines after orthodontic treatment

Treatment Options

The patient's profile is in accordance with her ethnic pattern, so a nonextraction treatment strategy would be appropriate in the present case. In the maxillary arch, the left impacted canine is in a favorable position for eruption. Cantilevers from first molars could be used for eruption of the canines with orthodontic traction. In the mandibular arch, minor spacing could be closed using a fully banded appliance and elastic chain.

Because the pretreatment posterior occlusion was Class I with good interdigitation, an alternative method of gaining anchorage could be ideal so as to minimally disturb the relationship of posterior teeth. Temporary anchorage devices (TADs) could be a suitable alternative. First premolars could be stabilized by connecting them to TADs and leaving posterior occlusion undisturbed. A targeted mechanics approach was used for this patient to erupt the canines into the arch while maintaining the adequate posterior occlusion.

TREATMENT SEQUENCE AND BIOMECHANICAL PLAN

Maxilla	Mandible
Refer the patient to the periodontist for extraction of over-retained maxillary deciduous canines and a closed eruption approach of the maxillary left canine for orthodontic traction.	
Band molars, bond maxillary 4-4 with lingual brackets, place a TPA, and cantilever made out of .017 × .022 inch CNA from the molar tubes on the first molars for orthodontic eruption of the maxillary canines. Deliver a vertical eruption force of 25 g. Vector of the force is labial and occlusal on the canines.	Bond first premolar to first premolar, .016 inch NiTi arch wire.
Place TADs interdentally between first and second premolar in all the quadrants. Stabilize the first premolars with TADs using a sectional .019 × .025 inch SS wire. Bond labially first premolar to first premolar. Start aligning the canines with .016 and .016 × .022 inch NiTi arch wires.	Continue leveling with .016 × .022 inch NiTi arch wire.
Continue leveling with .019 × .025 inch NiTi arch wire.	Continue leveling with .017 × .025 inch NiTi arch wire.
Bond all remnant teeth and finish the occlusion with .016 × .022 inch CNA arch wire.	Bond all remnant teeth and finish the occlusion with .016 × .022 inch CNA arch wire.
Debond and deliver wrap around retainer.	Debond and bond lingual 3-3 retainer.
6-month recall appointment for retention check.	6-month recall appointment for retention check.

CNA, Connecticut new arch wire; *NiTi,* nickel titanium; *SS,* stainless steel; *TAD,* temporary anchorage device; *TPA,* transpalatal arch.

▪TREATMENT SEQUENCE

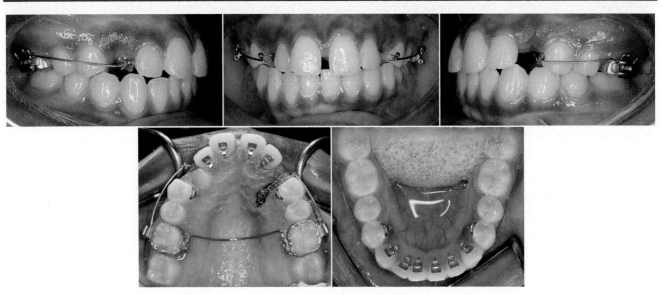

Figure 17-1-3 Cantilevers for force eruption of maxillary impacted canines.

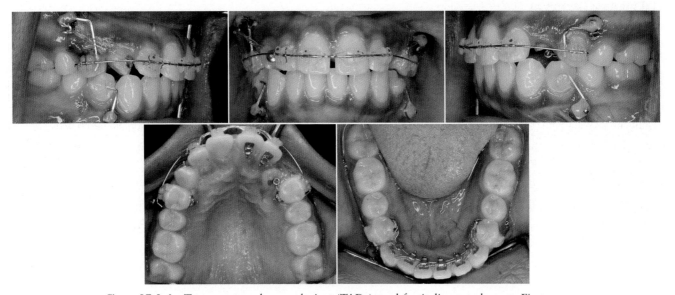

Figure 17-1-4 Temporary anchorage devices (TADs) used for indirect anchorage. First premolars are connected to TADs with the help of a sectional stainless steel wire. Alignment of the maxillary canines using a directional force from the TAD-supported sectional wire connected to the maxillary first premolars.

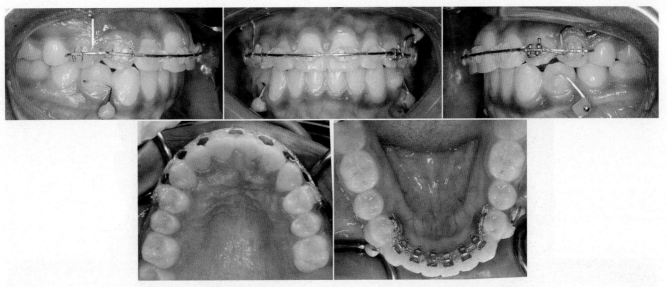

Figure 17-1-5   Continuation of alignment of the maxillary canines with a .016 × .022 inch nickel titanium arch wire.

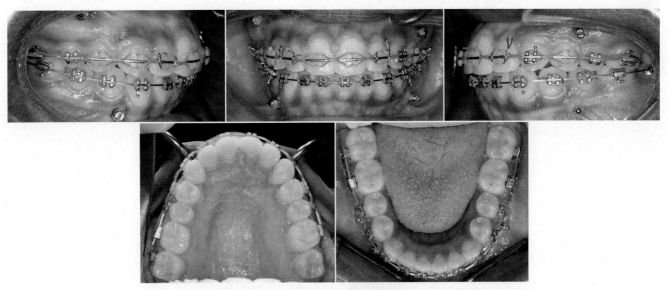

Figure 17-1-6   Finishing and settling of occlusion.

■ FINAL RESULTS

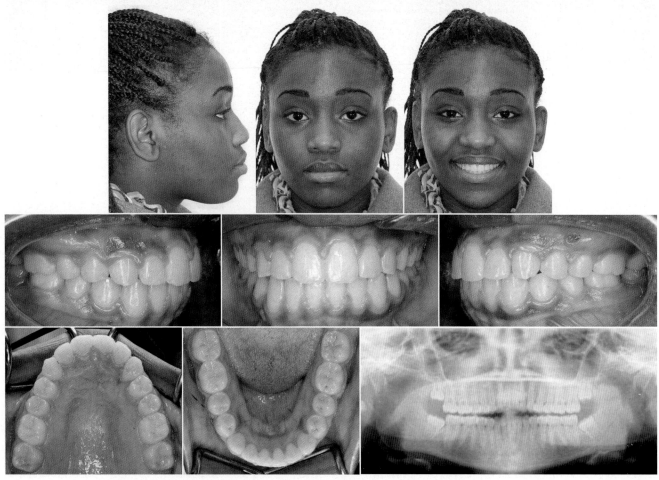

Figure 17-1-7   Posttreatment extraoral/intraoral photographs and panoramic radiograph.

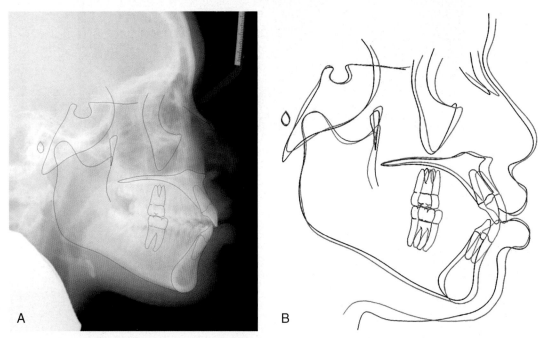

Figure 17-1-8   **A,** Posttreatment lateral cephalogram. **B,** Superimposition. *Black,* pretreatment; *red,* posttreatment.

Why were miniscrews placed for this treatment?
When the occlusion in the buccal segment is ideal, a targeted approach addressing the main problems (impacted canines and maxillary diastema) while minimizing the side effects on the anchor teeth is achieved through indirect anchorage drawn from interdental miniscrews. Tight control of the anchorage units increases treatment efficiency.

Section 7

Adjunctive Orthodontic Treatment

CASE 18-1

Vertical Ridge Development in Severe Attachment Loss of a Maxillary Central Incisor*

A 30-year-old female patient was referred by her periodontist regarding an anterior deep bite and excessive attachment loss on the maxillary left central incisor. Medical and dental histories were noncontributory, and findings from a temporomandibular joint (TMJ) examination were normal with adequate range of jaw movements.

■ PRETREATMENT

Extraoral Analysis (Fig. 18-1-1)

Facial Form	Euryprosopic
Facial Symmetry	No gross asymmetries noticed
Chin Point	Coincidental with facial midline
Occlusal Plane	Normal
Facial Profile	Normal for ethnicity
Facial Height	Upper Facial Height/Lower Facial Height: Normal
	Lower Facial Height/Throat Depth: Reduced
Lips	Competent, Upper: Slightly Protrusive, Lower: Protrusive
Nasolabial Angle	Acute
Mentolabial Sulcus	Normal

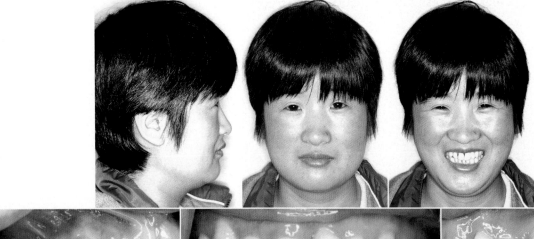
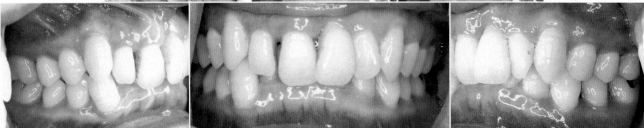

Figure 18-1-1 Pretreatment extraoral/intraoral photographs.

*Portions of Case 18-1 from Uribe F, Taylor T, Shafer D, Nanda R. A novel approach for implant site development through root tipping. *Am J Orthod Dentofacial Orthop*. 2010;138:649-655.

Smile Analysis (Fig. 18-1-2)

Smile Arc	Flat
Incisor Display	Rest: 2 mm
	Smile: 10 mm (100%)
Lateral Tooth Display	Second premolar to second premolar
Buccal Corridor	Narrow
Gingival Tissue	Margins: Gingival recession of maxillary left central incisor due to attachment loss; margin of right canine more gingival due to vertical positional height discrepancy
	Papilla: Absent between maxillary central incisors and between right maxillary central and lateral incisors due to periodontal bone loss
	Severe localized attachment loss of maxillary left central incisor with alveolar bone crest in the apical third of the root
Dentition	Tooth size and proportion: Normal
	Tooth shape: Normal
	Axial inclination: Maxillary and mandibular incisors are retroclined
	Connector space and contact area: No contact between maxillary right central and right lateral incisors
Incisal Embrasure	Normal
Midlines	Mandibular dental midline 1 mm to the right of the facial midline

Intraoral Analysis (see Fig. 18-1-2)

Teeth Present	7654321/1234567
	7654321/1234567
Molar Relation	Class I on left side and Class II end on right side
Canine Relation	Class I on left side and Class II end on right side
Overjet	2 mm
Overbite	8 mm (100%)
Maxillary Arch	U shaped, symmetric with 4 mm of crowding
Mandibular Arch	U shaped with 2 mm of crowding, deep curve of Spee
Oral Hygiene	Fair

Functional Analysis

Swallowing	Normal adult pattern
Temporomandibular joint	Normal with adequate range of jaw movements

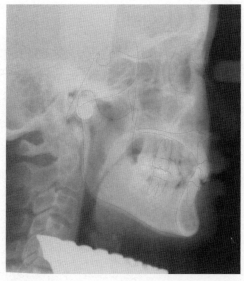

Parameter	Norm	Value
SNA (°)	82	86
SNB (°)	80	82
ANB (°)	2	4
FMA (°)	24	24
MP-SN (°)	32	30
U1-NA (mm/°)	4/22	6/10
L1-NA (mm/°)	4/25	1/11
IMPA (°)	95	79
U1-L1 (°)	130	157
OP-SN (°)	14	10
Upper Lip – E Plane (mm)	−4	−2
Lower Lip – E Plane (mm)	−2	−1
Nasolabial Angle (°)	103	105

Figure 18-1-2 Pretreatment lateral cephalogram with tracing and cephalometric analysis.

Diagnosis and Case Summary

A 30-year-old female patient had orthognathic soft and hard tissue profiles with short lower facial height and flat mandibular plane angle. She had a Class II subdivision left malocclusion with significant attachment loss on the maxillary left central incisor, mild angular bone defects related to the mandibular first molars, and a deep overbite with supraerupted mandibular incisors.

PROBLEM LIST			
Pathology/Others	Gingival recession on maxillary left central incisor due to severe localized attachment loss extending to the apical third of the root Angular bone defects on mandibular first molars		
Alignment	Maxillary arch crowding: 4 mm Mandibular arch crowding: 2 mm		
Dimension	**Skeletal**	**Dental**	**Soft Tissue**
Anteroposterior		Class II end on molar and canine relationship on the right side Retroclined maxillary and mandibular incisors	Slightly protrusive lips
Transverse		Lower midline 1 mm to the right of the facial midline	
Vertical	Decreased mandibular plane angle	OB: 8 mm (100%) Deep curve of Spee in mandibular arch due to supraerupted mandibular incisors	

OB, overbite.

TREATMENT OBJECTIVES			
Pathology/Others	Extrude maxillary left central incisor to obtain alveolar bone height for prosthetic implant placement Debridement and maintenance of angular bone defects with respect to mandibular first molars Close monitoring of the periodontium and referrals for maintenance visits every 3 months		
Alignment	Flare maxillary and mandibular anterior teeth for correction of crowding in maxillary and mandibular arch		
Dimension	**Skeletal**	**Dental**	**Soft Tissue**
Anteroposterior		Correct Class II end on relation on the right side by extraction of the right first premolar Flare maxillary and mandibular anterior teeth to improve inclination	
Transverse		Improve mandibular midline to match facial midline	
Vertical		Segmentally intrude mandibular incisors and left canine to level the curve of Spee and improve anterior deep bite	

Treatment Options

The treatment alternatives for the localized periodontal problem were the following:

The first option included extraction of the maxillary left central incisor, guided bone regeneration, and prosthetic implant placement to replace the maxillary left central incisor.

The second option included extraction of the maxillary left central incisor, guided bone regeneration, and orthodontic substitution of the maxillary left lateral incisor into the place of the left central incisor and prosthetic implant to replace maxillary left lateral incisor.

The third option included orthodontic extrusion of the maxillary left central incisor (after debridement of the anterior region in conjunction with periodontal maintenance visits every 3 months) to develop the alveolar bone because the maxillary central incisor is erupted incisally. The advantage could be that a greater amount of bone might be obtained in both height and width for an ideal implant site. Aesthetically, the gingival tissue would follow coronally, thereby matching the contralateral tooth and achieving optimal soft tissue contours. Moreover, as the maxillary central incisor is erupting, the root of the incisor can be tipped mesially so that greater mesiodistal width of bone develops. This option was chosen by the interdisciplinary team and patient.

TREATMENT SEQUENCE AND BIOMECHANICAL PLAN

Maxilla	Mandible
Refer the patient to the periodontist for full-mouth scaling and root planning and attain disease-free state.	Refer the patient to the periodontist for full-mouth scaling and root planning and attain disease-free state.
Bond first molars and left central incisor. Extrusion arch with .018 inch CNA, place 10 g of extrusive force on the maxillary left central incisor. Sequentially reduce incisal edge as incisor is extruded (perform elective endodontic treatment with calcium hydroxide fill).	Bond first molars and first and second premolars, segmentally align until a .017 × .025 inch SS wire. Bond .018 inch SS wire on the labial aspect of incisors and left canine. .018 inch CNA intrusion arch from the first molars extended anteriorly to be tied onto the wire bonded on the incisors. Place 40 g of intrusive force.
Bond rest of the arch, reposition the bracket on the maxillary left central incisor to sequentially tip the root mesially. Sequentially align with .016, .018 and .016 × .022 inch NiTi arch wires.	Continue leveling with .016 × .022 inch CNA after intrusion of the anterior segment.
Continue leveling with .019 × .025 inch CNA.	Continue leveling with .017 × .025 inch SS arch wire.
Extract maxillary right first premolar and close the space by distalizing the right canine into Class I and mesialize the right first molar into Class II.	Continue leveling with .019 × .025 inch SS arch wire.
Finish the occlusion with .016 × .022 inch CNA.	Finish the occlusion with .016 × .022 inch CNA.
Debond and deliver wrap around retainer.	Debond and deliver Hawley retainer.
Extract maxillary left central incisor, place prosthetic implant to restore it.	
6-month recall appointment for retention check.	6-month recall appointment for retention check.

CNA, Connecticut new arch wire; *NiTi,* nickel titanium; *SS,* stainless steel.

TREATMENT SEQUENCE

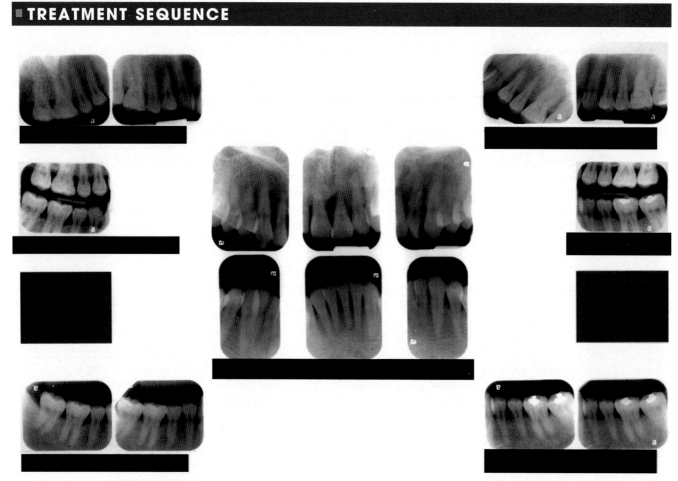

Figure 18-1-3 Full-mouth periapical radiographs depicting the areas of localized angular bone loss.

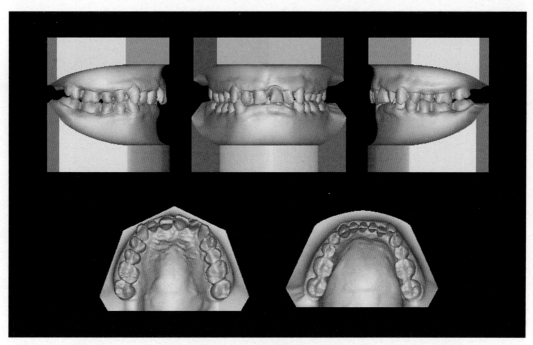

Figure 18-1-4   Pretreatment digital models.

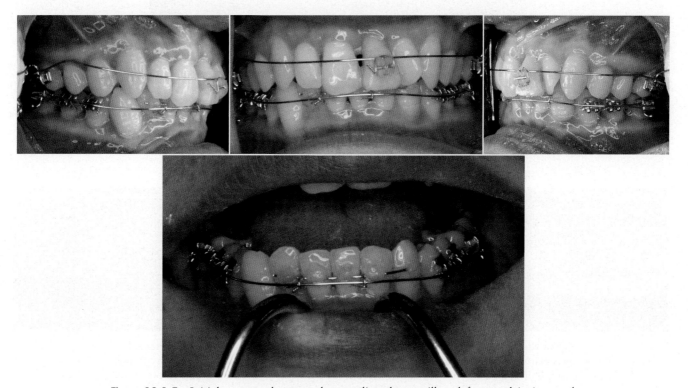

Figure 18-1-5   Initial segmental approach extruding the maxillary left central incisor and intruding the mandibular anterior segment.

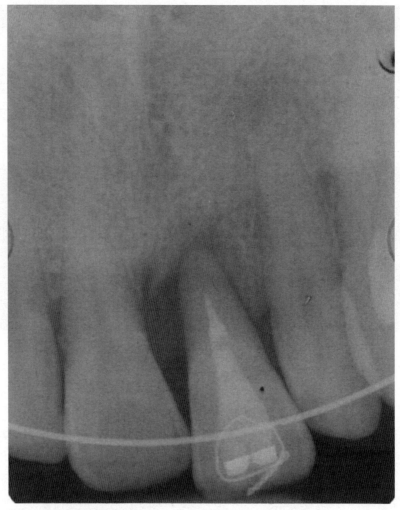

Figure 18-1-6 Elective endodontic treatment of the maxillary incisor was necessary as the forced eruption progressed.

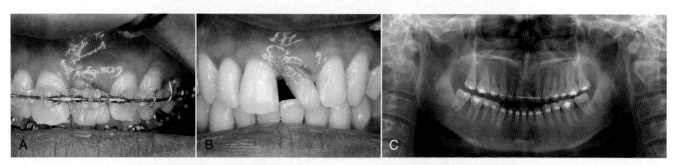

Figure 18-1-7 **A,** The maxillary central incisor was tipped mesially, and a composite buildup was placed in the mesial aspect for cosmetic reasons. Note the interproximal papilla compression. **B,** The maxillary incisor tipped without the aesthetic composite buildup before extraction. Note the gingival height gain. **C,** The panoramic radiograph shows the amount of incisor tipping achieved.

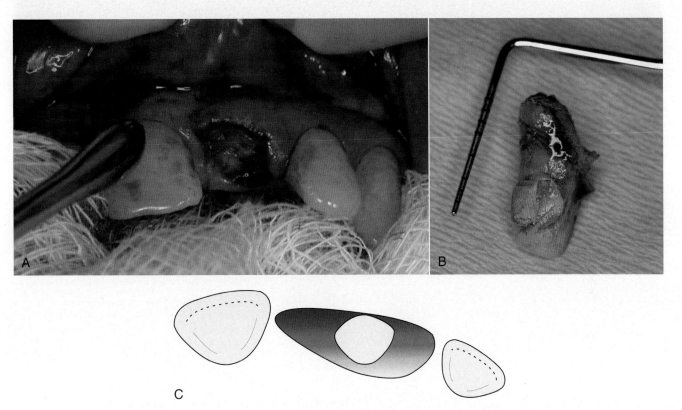

Figure 18-1-8 Flapless approach to implant placement. **A,** Note the papillary preservation and the bone volume achieved buccolingually and mesiodistally. **B,** The extracted tooth and root. **C,** Occlusal view showing the difference in cross-sections of the root when tipped (*orange–shaded area*) versus vertically extruded (*light yellow-shaded area*).

■ **FINAL RESULTS**

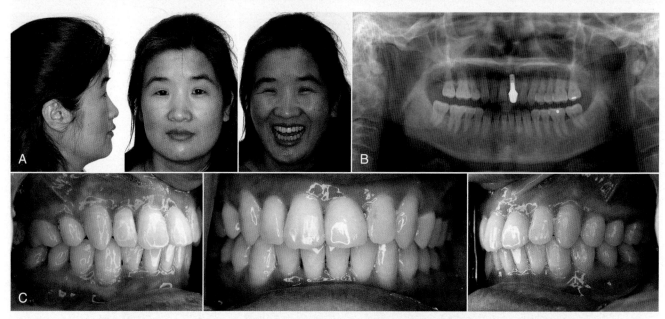

Figure 18-1-9 **A,** Extraoral photographs with the final implant restoration. *Note:* After the endosseous implant fixture placement, an abutment and acrylic crown were immediately placed. Permanent crown was delivered 2 months later. **B,** Posttreatment panoramic radiograph. **C,** Posttreatment intraoral photographs with the final restoration on the left maxillary central incisor implant.

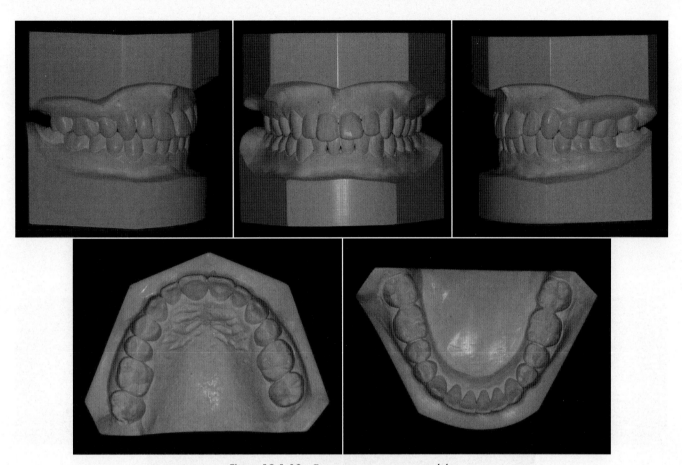

Figure 18-1-10   Posttreatment stone models.

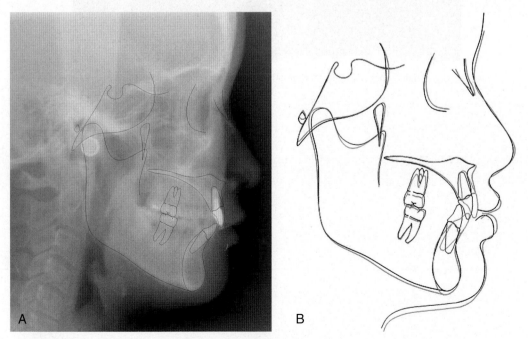

Figure 18-1-11   **A,** Posttreatment lateral cephalogram with tracing. **B,** Cephalometric superimposition. *Black,* pretreatment; *green,* posttreatment.

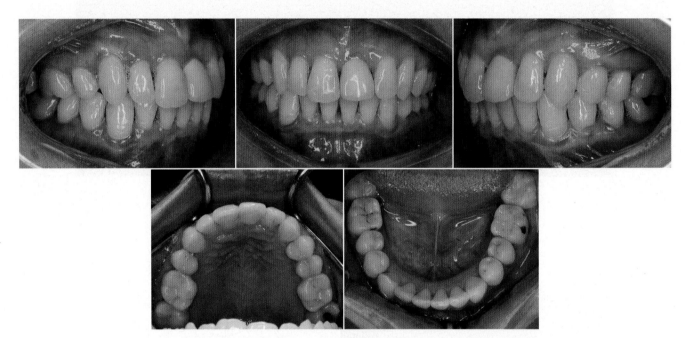

Figure 18-1-12 Six-year postretention intraoral photographs.

Why was the forced eruption performed at a slow rate and with a low-force magnitude?

The amount of attachment loss was excessive as evident from the initial periapical radiographs. Mobility of the left central incisor was also significant. A high-force, fast approach would have likely extracted the tooth without the possibility of developing the alveolar bone. It can also be noticed that there was a significant vertical soft tissue migration of the gingival margin of the central incisor with this slow low-force approach, which was maintained in the long term after the implant placement.

Why was the intrusion of the anterior segment initiated without brackets?

As a result of the deep bite, interocclusal space for bracket bonding was absent. Because these mandibular anterior teeth were bonded with a wire, there was no occlusal interference that could traumatize the maxillary anterior teeth during the intrusion process. The mandibular anterior teeth acted as a single unit that received the intrusion arch through which the required intrusion was achieved to correct the overbite. This intrusion allowed for extruding the left maxillary incisor for alveolar ridge development.

CASE 19-1

Autotransplantation of Second Premolars into the Site of Extracted Maxillary Central Incisors Due to Trauma

A 12-year-old prepubertal male patient's chief complaint was crowding in the upper front region of the jaw. Medical history was noncontributory. Dental history revealed an incident of dental trauma 2 years prior (avulsion with reimplantation), resulting in loss of vitality and ankyloses of maxillary incisors. Findings from a temporomandibular joint (TMJ) examination were normal with adequate range of jaw movements.

■ PRETREATMENT

Extraoral Analysis (Fig. 19-1-1)

Facial Form	Mesoprosopic
Facial Symmetry	No gross asymmetries noticed
Chin Point	Coincidental with facial midline
Occlusal Plane	Normal
Facial Profile	Straight
Facial Height	Upper Facial Height/Lower Facial Height: Normal
	Lower Facial Height/Throat Depth: Normal
Lips	Slight incompetence due to left maxillary incisor proclination, Upper: Normal; Lower: Protrusive
Nasolabial Angle	Normal
Mentolabial Sulcus	Normal

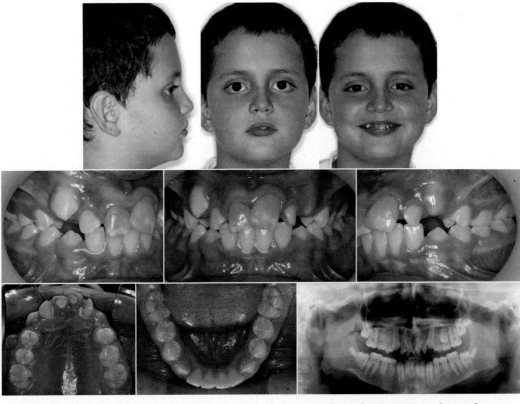

Figure 19-1-1   Pretreatment extraoral/intraoral photographs and panoramic radiograph.

Smile Analysis (Fig. 19-1-2)

Smile Arc	Consonant, maxillary incisors impinging on the lower lip
Incisor Display	Rest: 1 mm
	Smile: 8 mm of maxillary incisor display
Lateral Tooth Display	First premolar to first premolar
Buccal Corridor	Narrow
Gingival Tissue	Margins: Irregular with maxillary central incisors more gingival, especially left incisor
	Papilla: Present between centrals, not present between central and lateral incisors due to diastemas; thin biotype and width of attached gingiva on the labial aspect of the mandibular central incisors
Dentition	Tooth size and proportion: Normal
	Maxillary central incisors are nonvital, ankylosed, and discolored due to previous dentoalveolar trauma
	Maxillary lateral incisors are small in mesiodistal dimension
	Tooth shape: Rounded morphology of the incisal edges of the maxillary lateral incisor
	Axial inclination: Maxillary teeth inclined labially
	Connector space: Present between centrals, not present between central and lateral incisors due to diastemas
Incisal Embrasure	Not defined between maxillary central incisors as these overlap; not present between central and lateral incisors and lateral incisors and canines
Midlines	Maxillary and mandibular dental midlines are coincidental with facial midline

Intraoral Analysis (see Fig. 19-1-2)

Teeth Present	654321/1234E6 (Unerupted 7s, 8s, and maxillary left 5)
	654321/123456
Molar Relation	Class I bilaterally
Canine Relation	Class II end on bilaterally
Overjet	6 mm
Overbite	3 mm
Maxillary Arch	U shaped and symmetric with 4 mm of spacing
Mandibular Arch	U shaped with spacing of 2 mm and normal curve of Spee
Oral Hygiene	Fair

Functional Analysis

Swallowing	Normal adult pattern
Temporomandibular joint	Normal with adequate range of jaw movements

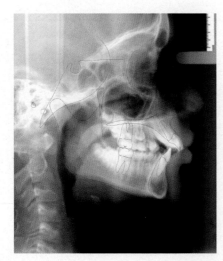

Parameter	Norm	Value
SNA (°)	82	80
SNB (°)	80	77
ANB (°)	2	3
FMA (°)	24	22
MP-SN (°)	32	30
U1-NA (mm/°)	4/22	6.5/33
L1-NA (mm/°)	4/25	3.5/26
IMPA (°)	95	98
U1-L1 (°)	130	117
OP-SN (°)	14	12
Upper Lip – E Plane (mm)	−4	−1
Lower Lip – E Plane (mm)	−2	2
Nasolabial Angle (°)	103	116

Figure 19-1-2 Pretreatment lateral cephalogram with tracing and cephalometric analysis.

Diagnosis and Case Summary

A 12-year-old prepubertal male patient had straight soft and hard tissue profiles. He had a Class I malocclusion with flared maxillary incisors, an acute interincisal angle, a protrusive lower lip, and ankylosed maxillary central incisors secondary to dental trauma.

PROBLEM LIST			
Pathology/Others	Maxillary central incisors are nonvital and ankylosed and discolored secondary to dental trauma Reduced maxillary lateral incisors' mesiodistal width Rounded incisal edges of maxillary lateral incisors Thin biotype of mandibular central incisors		
Alignment	4 mm of spacing present in maxillary arch 2 mm of spacing present in mandibular arch		
Dimension	**Skeletal**	**Dental**	**Soft Tissue**
Anteroposterior		OJ: 6 mm Acute interincisal angle Flared maxillary incisors Class II canines	Obtuse nasolabial angle Protrusive lower lip
Vertical		Highly placed maxillary canines	
Transverse			

OJ, overjet.

TREATMENT OBJECTIVES			
Pathology/Others	Extract ankylosed central incisors and auto transplant with maxillary second premolars Contour lingual aspect of autotransplants for proper interocclusal space; place composite veneers to obtain proper central incisor crown morphology Restore mesiodistal width of the maxillary lateral incisors with composite veneers		
Alignment	Close maxillary and mandibular spacing by retracting the anterior teeth		
Dimension	**Skeletal**	**Dental**	**Soft Tissue**
Anteroposterior		Retract maxillary anterior teeth to improve overjet, flared maxillary incisors, and interincisal angle	
Vertical		Erupt maxillary canine into the arch	Periodontal aesthetic recontouring of maxillary anterior teeth prior to composite restorations
Transverse			

Treatment Options

Three treatment options were presented to the patient.

Option 1 involved the extraction of the ankylosed maxillary central incisors and replacement with prosthetic implants. The disadvantage of this option is that because the patient is still growing, placement of endosseous implants needs to be delayed until adulthood.

Option 2 required extraction of ankylosed maxillary incisors and protraction of the maxillary arch to substitute maxillary lateral incisors in place of the maxillary central incisors and maxillary canines in place of the maxillary lateral incisors, as well as to substitute the maxillary first premolars in place of the maxillary canines. The disadvantage of this option is the prolonged treatment time involved with the protraction of the entire maxillary arch. An alternative similar option would require the extraction of mandibular first or second premolars to finish in a Class I molar occlusion. This plan is easier to deliver from a biomechanical perspective as it requires a simple space closure approach. However, this plan has the risk of significantly retracting the incisors which may impact the profile.

Option 3 entailed the extraction of the ankylosed maxillary incisors, replacing these with the autotransplantation of the maxillary second premolars. These teeth are recontoured during treatment and restored at the end of orthodontic treatment to mimic the size and shape of the central incisors.

The patient chose the third option.

TREATMENT SEQUENCE AND BIOMECHANICAL PLAN

Maxilla	Mandible
Extract maxillary central incisors atraumatically, autotransplant maxillary second premolars in place of maxillary incisors, and secure them with sutures. Wait for 3 months for optimal healing and monitor for the continuation of root formation.	
Band molars, bond maxillary arch, and initiate leveling using .016, .018, and .016 × .022 inch NiTi arch wires. Sequentially reshape autotransplanted premolars by reducing the palatal surface.	Band molars, bond maxillary arch, and initiate leveling with .016, .018, .016 × .022 inch NiTi arch wires.
Level with .017 × .025 and .019 × .025 inch NiTi arch wire. Prescribe Class III elastics to protract maxillary molar mesially into Class II.	Continue leveling with .017 × .025 and .019 × .025 inch NiTi arch wire.
.016 × .025 inch CNA with finishing bends.	.016 × .025 inch CNA with finishing bends.
Debond and deliver wrap around retainer.	Debond and deliver Hawley retainer.
Refer for periodontal aesthetic contouring of the gingival tissue in the maxillary anterior segment and composite veneers.	
6-month recall appointment for retention check.	6-month recall appointment for retention check.

CNA, Connecticut new arch wire; *NiTi,* nickel titanium.

■TREATMENT SEQUENCE

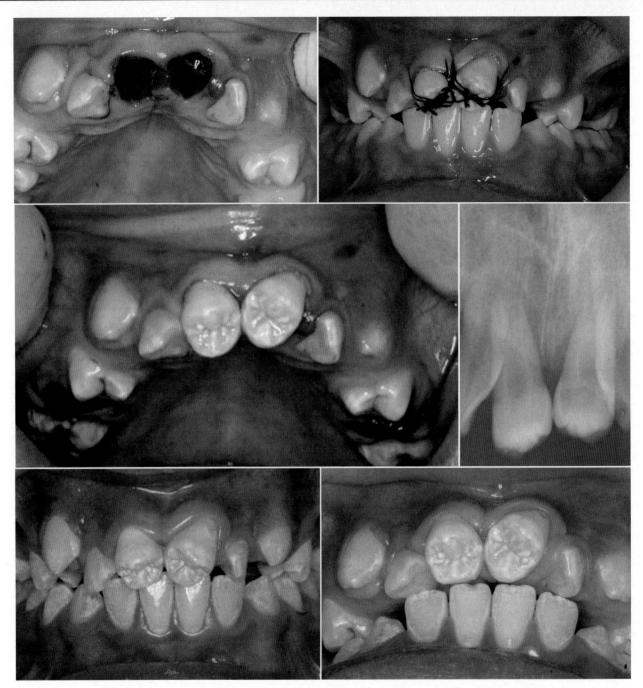

Figure 19-1-3 Extraction of ankylosed maxillary central incisor and autotransplantation with maxillary second premolars.

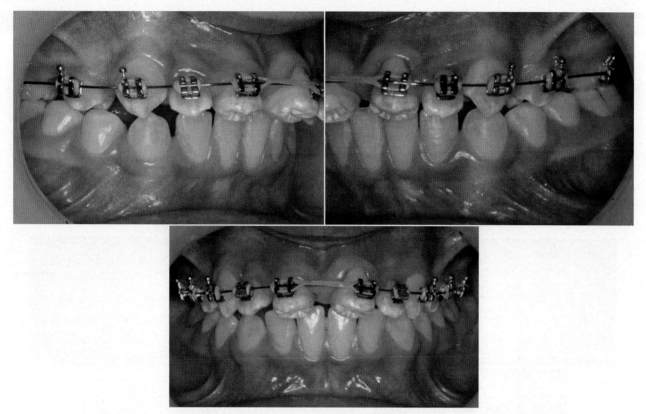

Figure 19-1-4   Initial leveling of maxillary arch.

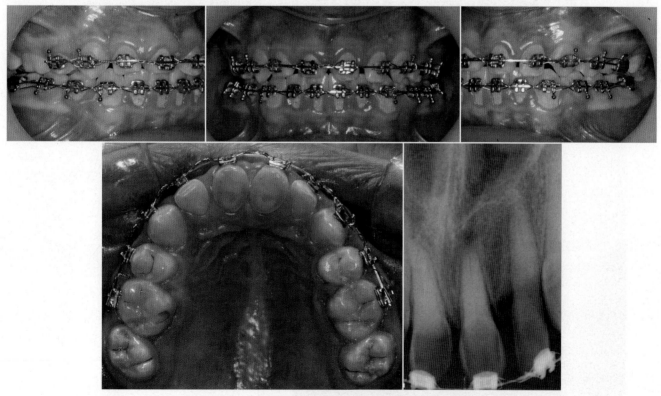

Figure 19-1-5   Finishing stage. Reshaped maxillary premolars (in the place of maxillary incisors). Periapical radiographs showing normal periapical architecture. Maxillary anterior teeth will be restored with composite veneers.

■FINAL RESULTS

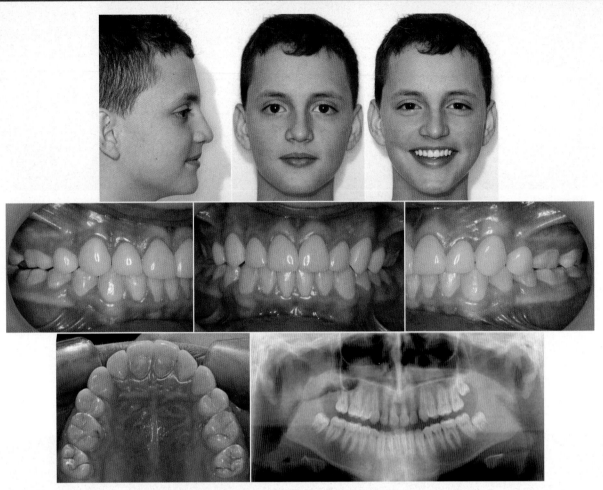

Figure 19-1-6   Posttreatment extraoral/intraoral photographs and panoramic radiograph. Mesiodistal dimension of the maxillary incisors restored with composite veneers.

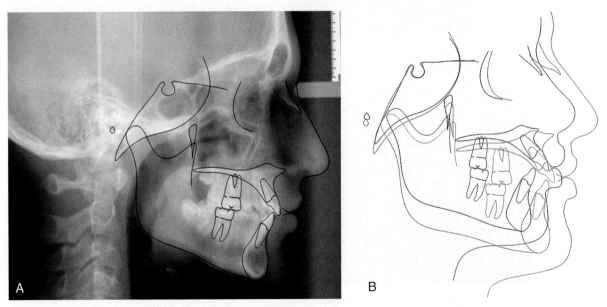

Figure 19-1-7   **A,** Posttreatment lateral cephalogram. **B,** Superimposition. *Black,* pretreatment; *green,* posttreatment.

What is the ideal age for autotransplantation of premolars?

The ideal age for autotransplantation is around 10. More important, however, is the assessment of the root development. The long-term prognosis of the tooth is best when two thirds to three quarters of the root are formed, which on average coincides with the chronologic age mentioned earlier. In this patient, root formation was more developed, but the apex was still open, which is favorable for preservation of tooth vitality.

It is also important to mention that the root formation continues in the new transplanted site.

Is root canal therapy necessary for autotransplanted teeth?

Root canal therapy is not necessary. Because the tooth has an open apex, the viability of the tooth is often preserved. It is important, though, to note that obliteration of the root is observed with time. Nonetheless, vitality of the tooth is still present.

Section 8

Aesthetics

CASE 20-1
Orthognathic Surgery and Reduction of the Open Gingival Embrasures "Black Triangles" to Maximize Facial and Smile Aesthetics

An adult female patient was interested in improving her facial aesthetics and smile. She had a convex soft and hard tissue profile with missing teeth distal to the first premolar in the mandibular right buccal segment. Dentally, the patient presented with a Class II malocclusion subdivision right. Orthognathic surgery with mandibular advancement was planned. Implants to restore the missing second premolar and first molar were to be placed after orthodontic treatment. During the presurgical orthodontic phase the extraction of the left first premolar was planned to maximize the mandibular advancement. Also, for an increase in the lower facial height, the lower occlusal plane was leveled after surgery. Finally, interproximal reduction was performed so that the open gingival embrasures observed after aligning the maxillary teeth could be addressed. This procedure was able to fill the open gingival embrasure by displacing the interproximal contact apically and the papilla incisally through tissue compression.

▪ PRETREATMENT

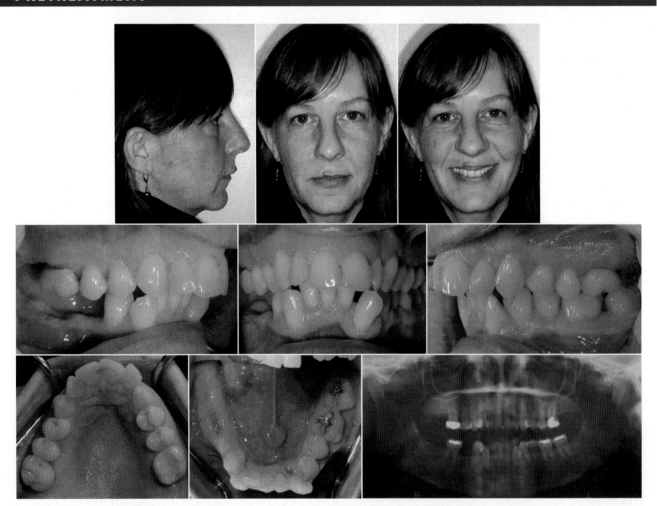

Figure 20-1-1 Pretreatment extraoral/intraoral photographs and panoramic radiograph.
Note: Panoramic radiograph before extraction of mandibular right first molar.

■ TREATMENT SEQUENCE

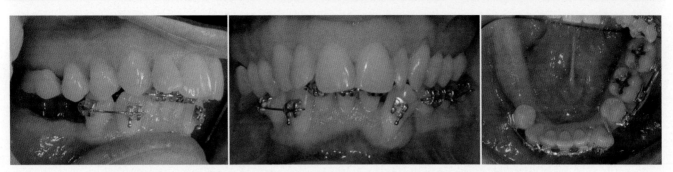

Figure 20-1-2 Presurgical photos depicting the two occlusal planes in the mandible to be leveled after surgery by extrusion of the posterior segment to increase the lower facial height.

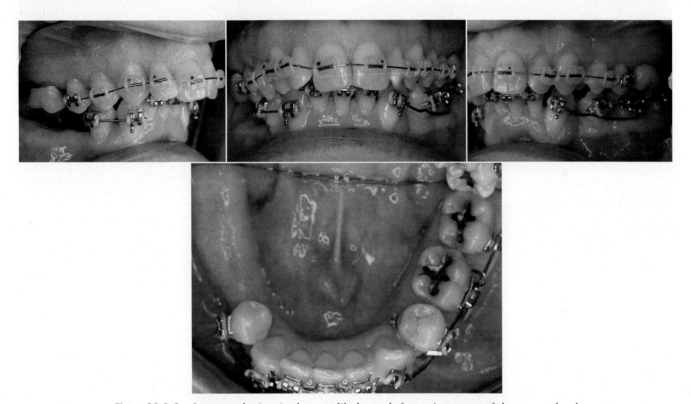

Figure 20-1-3 Segmented wires in the mandibular arch for maintenance of the two occlusal planes before surgery. Retraction of mandibular left canine with uprighting spring.

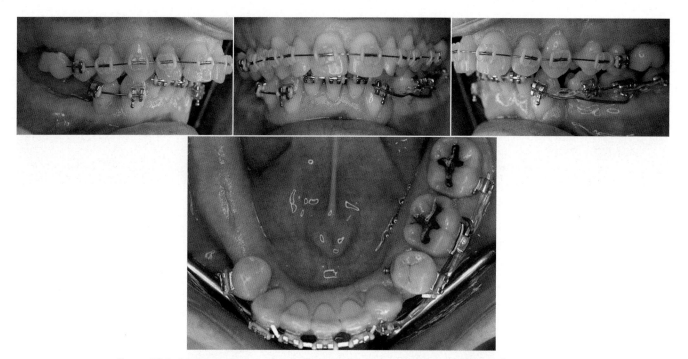

Figure 20-1-4   Continuation of mandibular left canine retraction with uprighting spring.

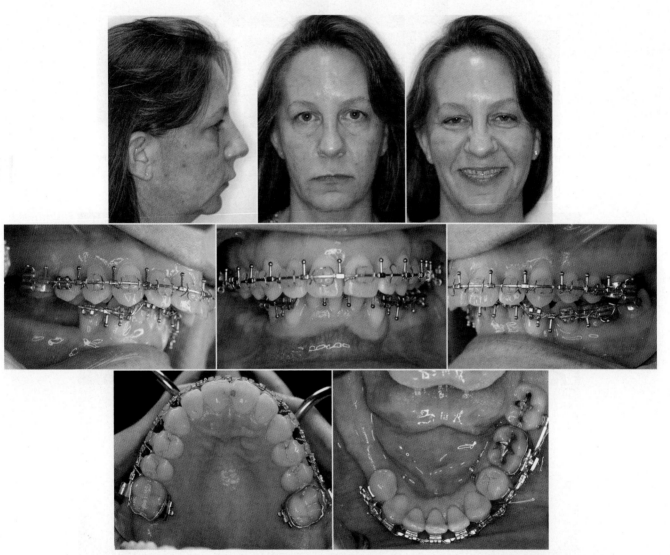

Figure 20-1-5 Presurgical extraoral and intraoral photographs. Note the significant facial convexity and reduced lower facial height and deep mentolabial fold. Mandibular surgical continuous wire with two planes of occlusion. Mandibular arch to be leveled after surgery with extrusion of posterior teeth.

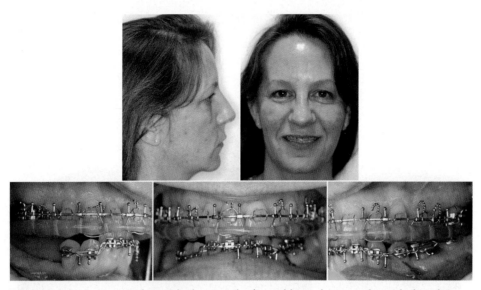

Figure 20-1-6 Postsurgical records showing the favorable aesthetic results with the advancement and increased lower facial height. Surgical splint to be removed distal of the maxillary lateral incisors to erupt the posterior teeth into occlusion in the orthodontic postsurgical phase.

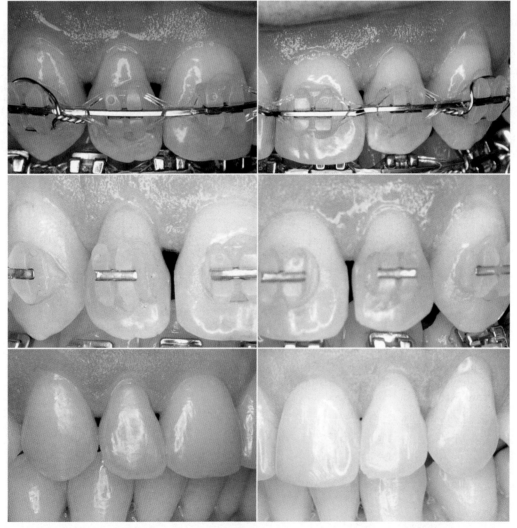

Figure 20-1-7 Reduction of the open gingival embrasures in the maxilla with interproximal reduction. The result is a larger connector space, displacement to the contact apically, and compression of the papilla.

■ FINAL RESULTS

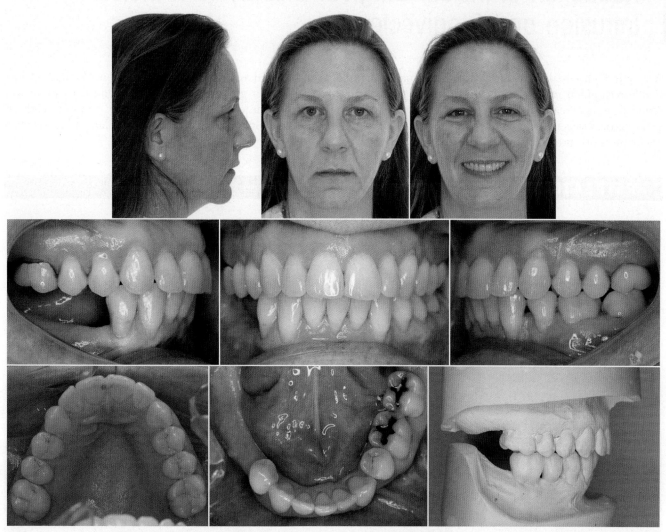

Figure 20-1-8   Posttreatment records depicting the favorable skeletal, smile, and occlusal changes. The patient required implant placement on the right buccal segment. The wax-up shows the occlusal relationship planned for implant placement.

CASE 20-2
Reduction of Incisal Gingival Display with Incisor Intrusion and Gingivectomy

A young adult female presented with supraerupted maxillary incisors and an altered passive eruption. She had a Class II subdivision left malocclusion. An intrusion arch was used to reduce her gingival display. Although the overbite was reduced, a significant amount of gingival tissue was present around the crowns of the maxillary anterior teeth. A gingivectomy was performed to complement the intrusion of the incisors to reduce the gingival display and reestablish adequate tooth proportions on the maxillary incisors.

▪ PRETREATMENT

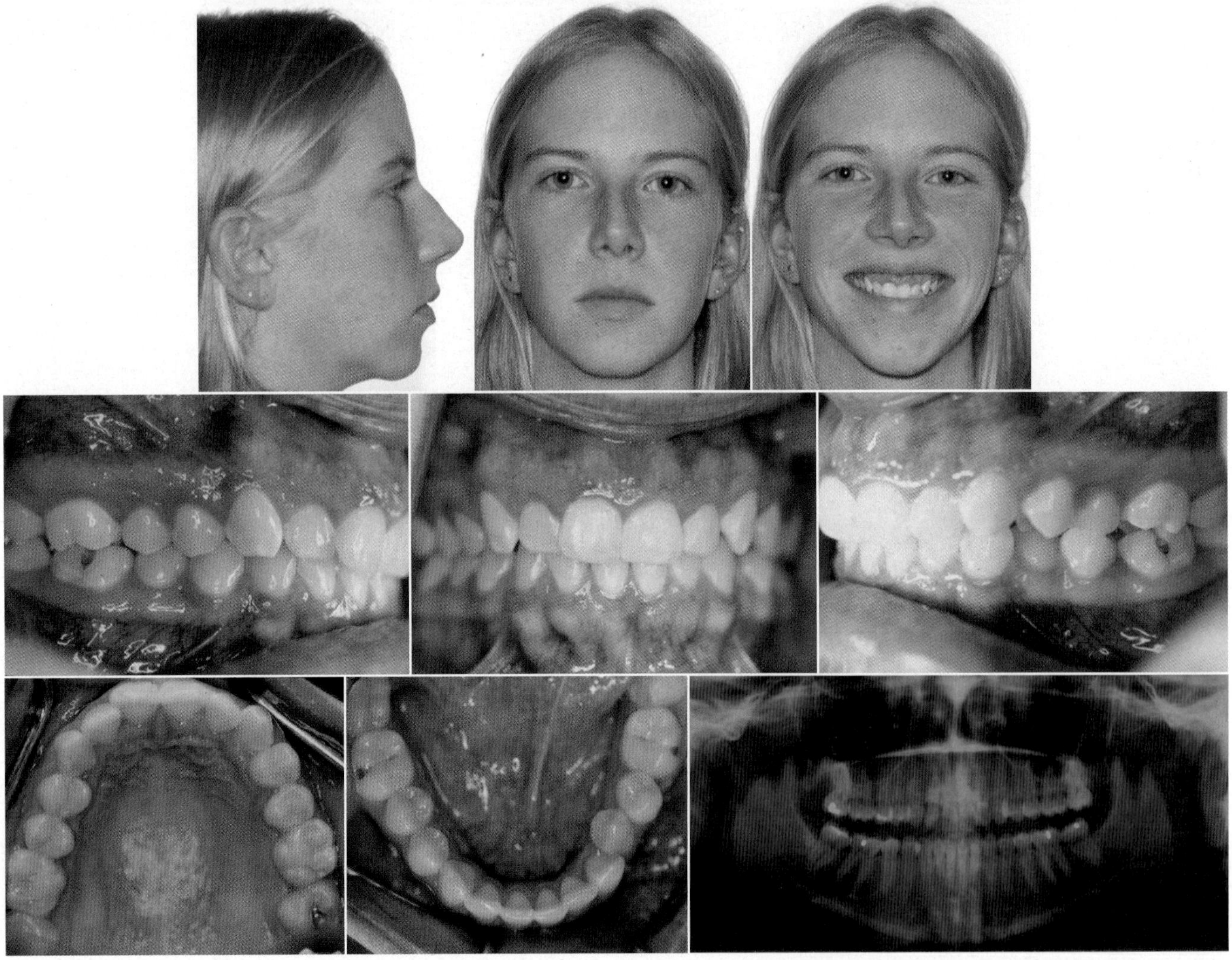

Figure 20-2-1   Pretreatment intraoral/extraoral photographs and panoramic radiograph.

■ FINAL RESULTS

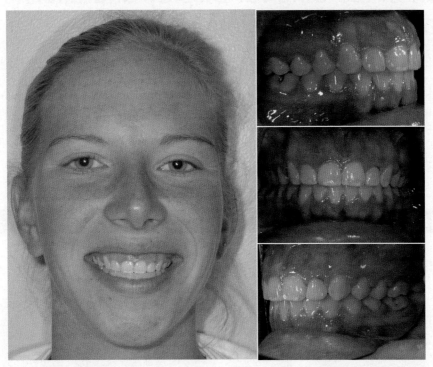

Figure 20-2-2 Postorthodontic intraoral/extraoral photographs showing improvement in gingival display after intrusion of the maxillary anterior segment.

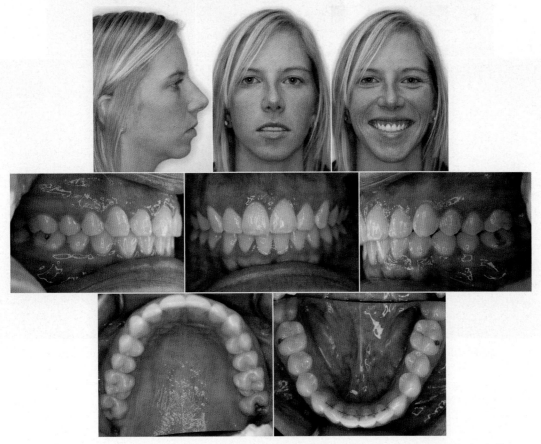

Figure 20-2-3 Postgingivectomy intraoral/extraoral photographs showing reduced gingival display.

CASE 20-3
Reduction of the Gingival Display and Midline Correction with an Intrusion Arch

A postpubertal female patient had an increased gingival display and Class II subdivision right malocclusion. The objective for her was to intrude the maxillary incisors to normalize the incisor display and at the same time correct the Class II malocclusion with molar tip back on the right side.

An intrusion arch was used for the intrusion of the maxillary incisors while simultaneously tipping back the right buccal segment to achieve a Class I molar occlusion and reduce the gingival display.

■ PRETREATMENT

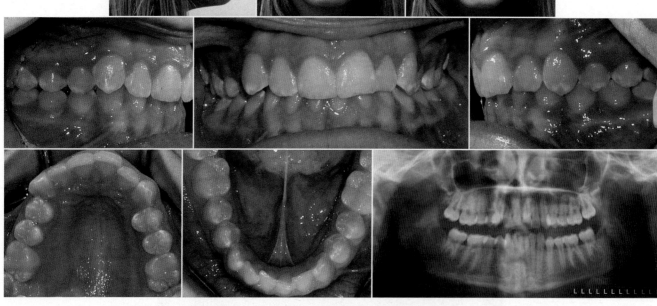

Figure 20-3-1   Pretreatment intraoral/extraoral photographs and panoramic radiograph.

■ TREATMENT SEQUENCE

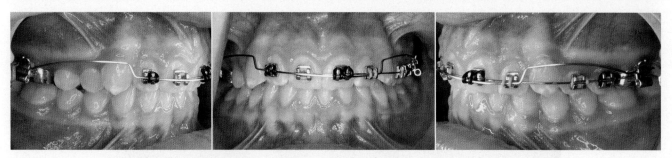

Figure 20-3-2   Intrusion arch resulting in maxillary incisor intrusion and tip back of right first molar.

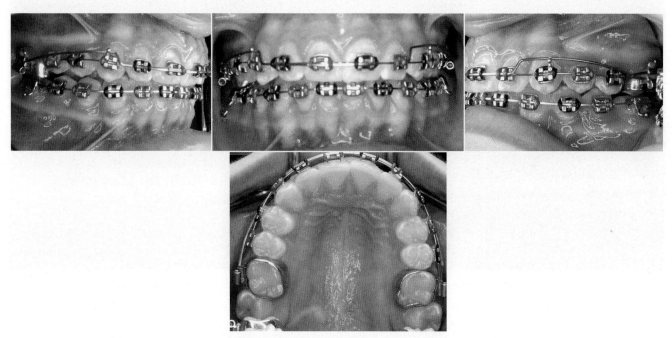

Figure 20-3-3   Continued tip back of the maxillary right first molar for the correction of Class II molar on the right side.

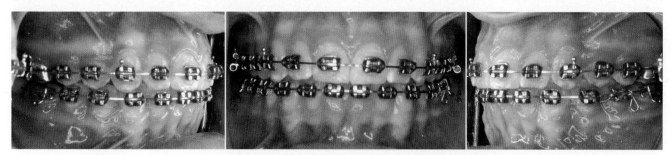

Figure 20-3-4   Finishing of the occlusion.

FINAL RESULTS

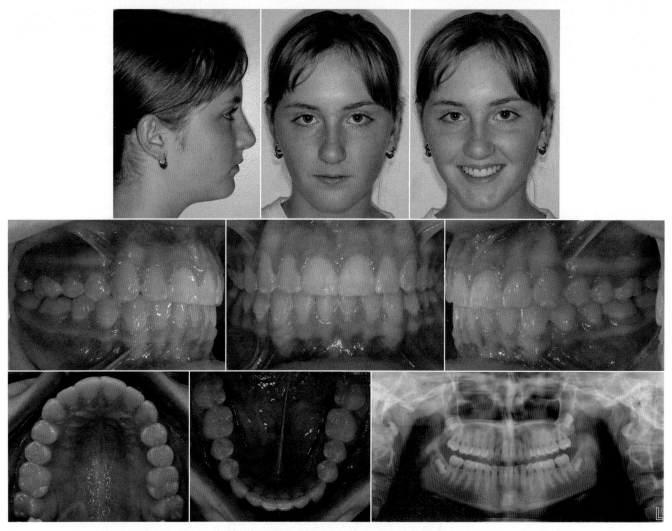

Figure 20-3-5   Postorthodontic intraoral/extraoral photographs and panoramic radiograph.

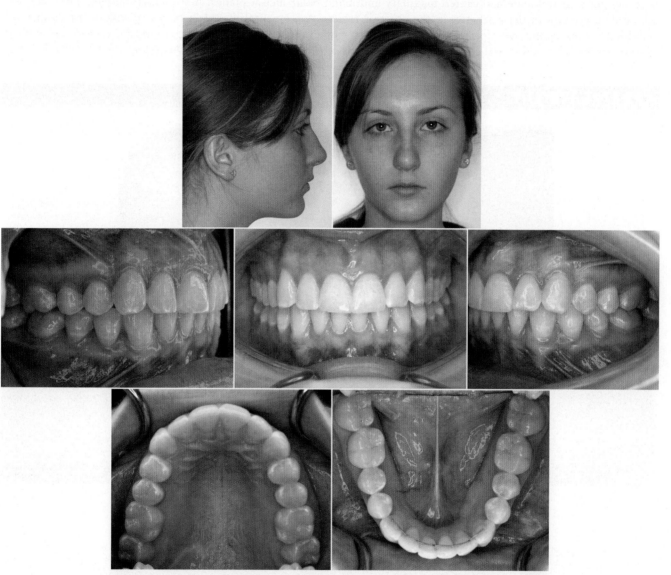

Figure 20-3-6 Postretention intraoral/extraoral photographs and panoramic radiograph 5 years after the end of orthodontic treatment.

Incisal Cant Correction and Composite Restoration in Maxillary Anterior Teeth

A young postpubertal male had canted maxillary and mandibular incisal planes. A sequential targeted approach was followed to reestablish the aesthetics in the anterior region. A segmental intrusion of the maxillary left canine and mandibular right canine were performed to level both canted incisal planes. Finally, composite veneers are used to reconstruct the fractured incisal edge of the maxillary left central incisor and the distal aspect of the left lateral incisor.

■ PRETREATMENT

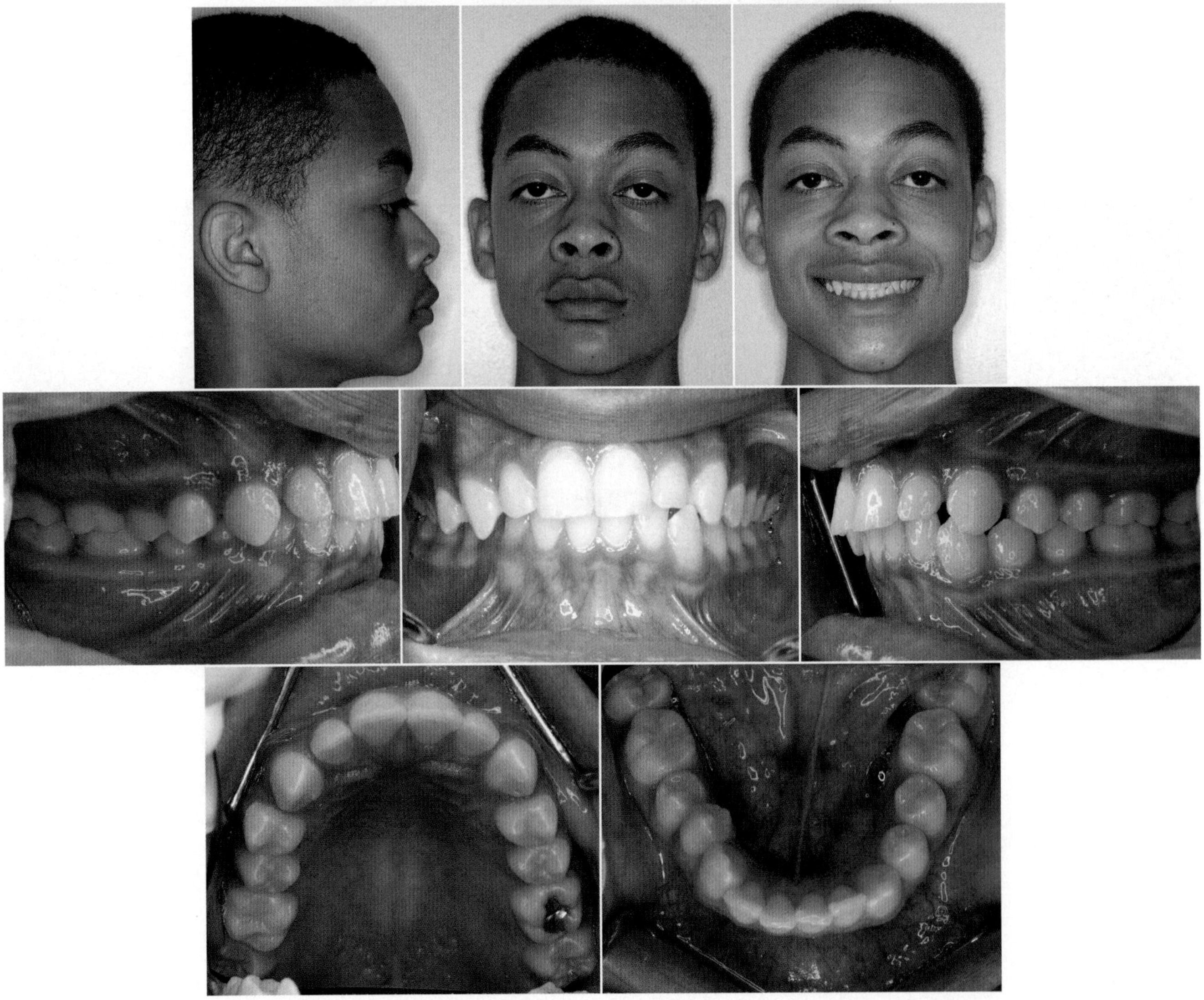

Figure 20-4-1 Pretreatment intraoral/extraoral photographs.

◾ TREATMENT SEQUENCE

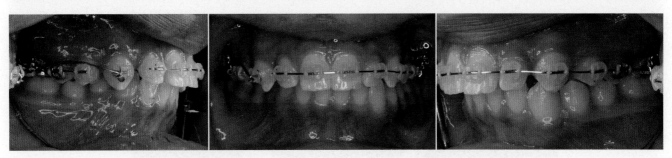

Figure 20-4-2   Maxillary right canine intrusion with help of a cantilever.

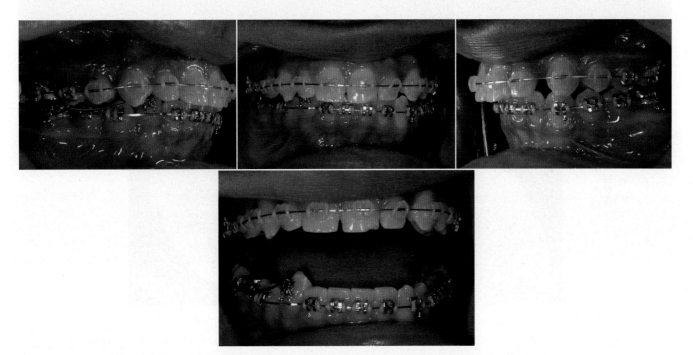

Figure 20-4-3   Mandibular right canine intrusion with help of a cantilever.

FINAL RESULTS

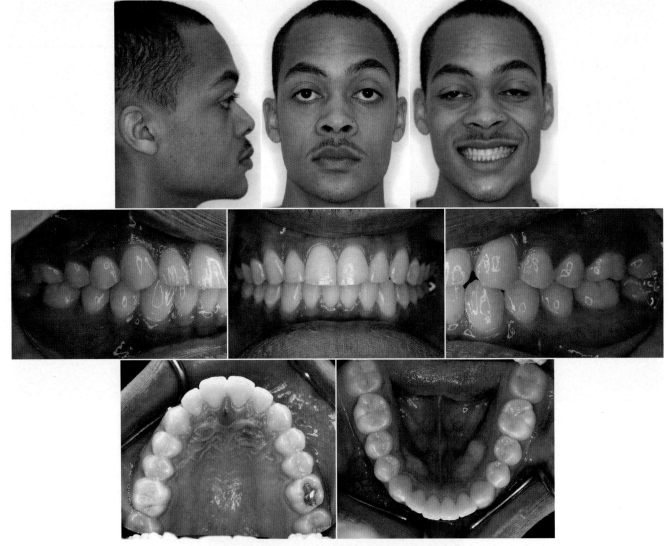

Figure 20-4-4   Postorthodontic intraoral/extraoral photographs.

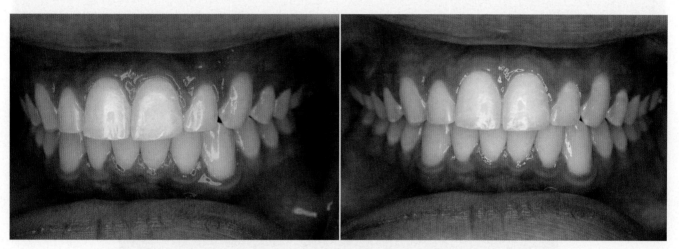

Figure 20-4-5 Final intraoral/extraoral photographs after composite restoration of the distal aspect of the left lateral incisor and incisal edge of left central incisor.

CASE 20-5
Orthodontic Extrusion to Match Gingival Margins and Composite Veneers on Maxillary Anterior Teeth

An adult female patient was interested in enhancing the aesthetics of her anterior teeth. The mesiodistal width of the maxillary incisors was reduced, and the gingival height of the maxillary right lateral incisor was more apical than the contralateral and at the same level of the central incisors and canines. The treatment plan to maximize the smile aesthetics required extrusion of the right maxillary lateral incisor and space appropriation for composite buildups of the four incisors.

■ PRETREATMENT

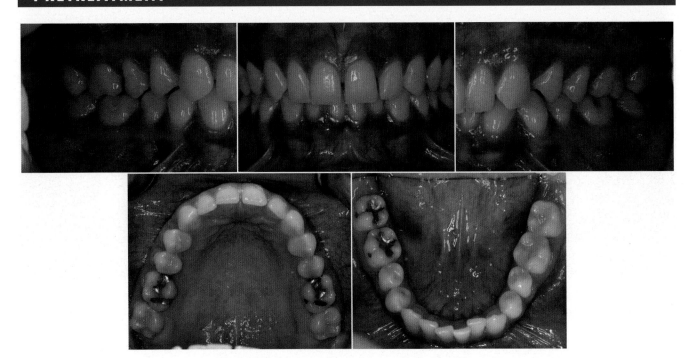

Figure 20-5-1   Pretreatment intraoral photographs.

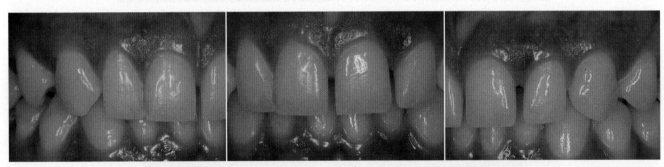

Figure 20-5-2   Pretreatment intraoral photographs showing gingival discrepancy in maxillary anterior region.

■ TREATMENT SEQUENCE

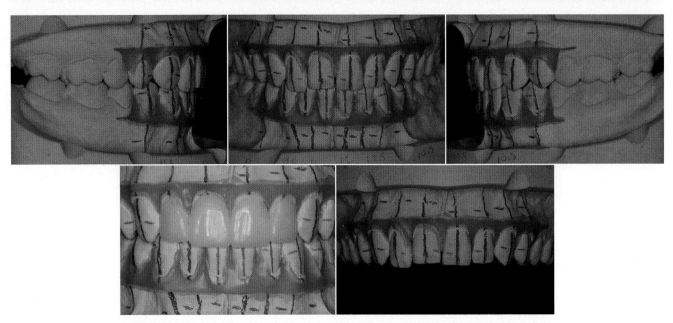

Figure 20-5-3 Diagnostic wax-up. Note the extrusion of the right lateral incisor to match the gingival height of the contralateral tooth.

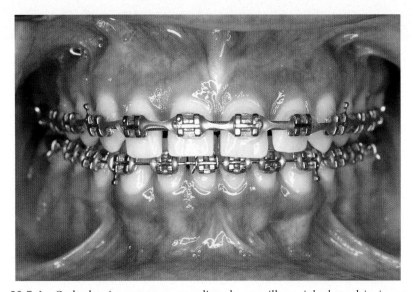

Figure 20-5-4 Orthodontic treatment extruding the maxillary right lateral incisor to level the gingival margins and obtain proper space appropriation for composite buildups in the maxillary incisors with enameloplasty of the incisal edge of the right maxillary lateral incisor.

■ FINAL RESULTS

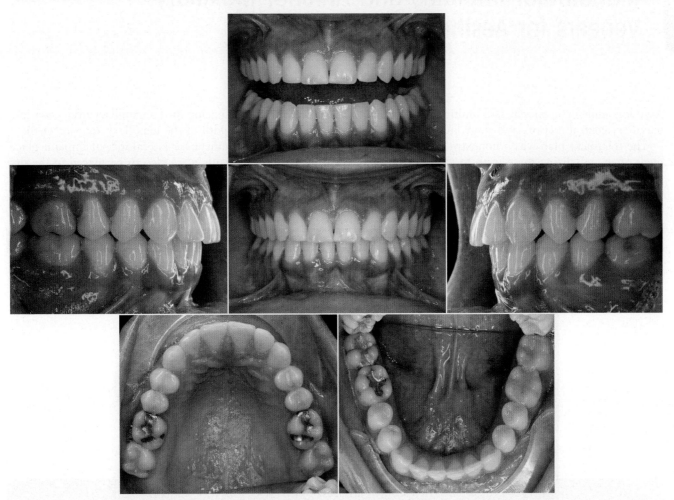

Figure 20-5-5 Postprosthetic final intraoral photographs. Anterior spacing restored with composite veneers after matching the gingival margins.

CASE 20-6
Mandibular Implants and Anterior Maxillary Veneers for Aesthetics

A young adult male patient had multiple congenitally missing teeth. He had spacing in the maxillary arch with long maxillary central incisors and short lateral incisors and reduced mesiodistal width of the maxillary anterior teeth.

The treatment plan was a nonextraction approach and implant site development for lateral incisor implant placement after mesializing these teeth to the position of the central incisors. Implants were also to be placed in the first premolar sites where space was to be developed. The maxillary anterior space was to be distributed appropriately for veneers to be placed from first premolar to contralateral first premolar.

■ PRETREATMENT

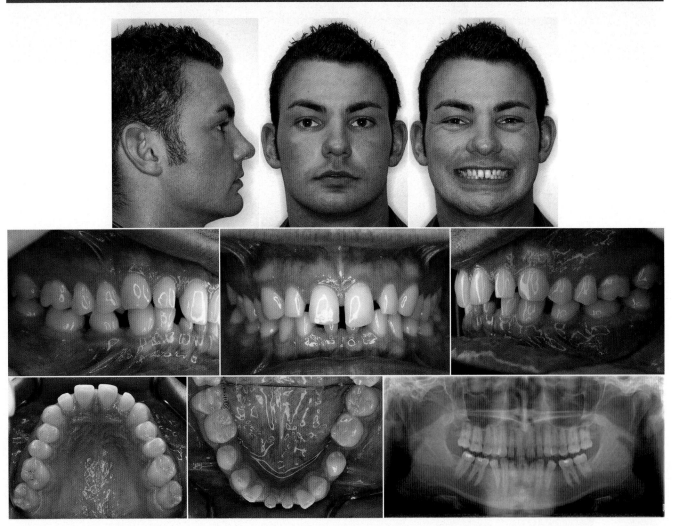

Figure 20-6-1   Pretreatment extraoral/intraoral photographs and panoramic radiograph.

■TREATMENT SEQUENCE

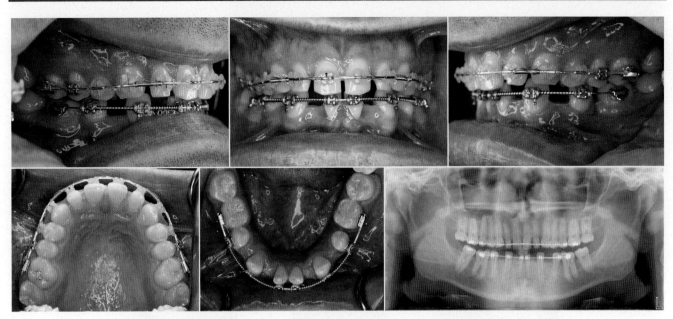

Figure 20-6-2   Maintaining space in the maxillary arch with the help of passive coil springs. In the lower arch, open coil springs between canine and lateral incisors to mesialize the lateral incisors in place of the central incisors and to create bone width for prosthetic implant placement in place of the lateral incisors.

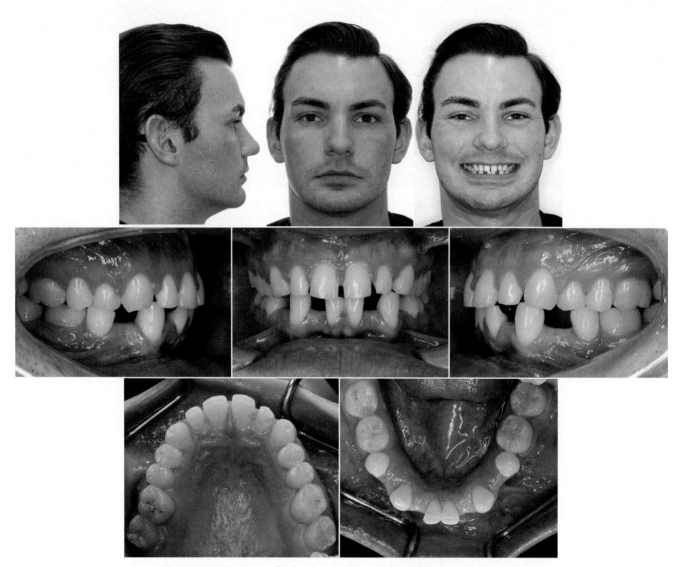

Figure 20-6-3   Postorthodontic treatment intraoral/extraoral pictures.

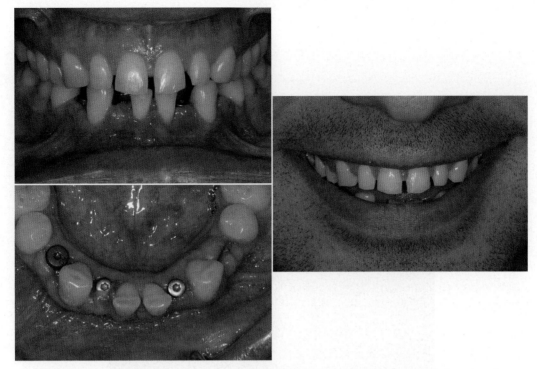

Figure 20-6-4   Preprosthetic assessment of smile and spaces. Implants placed in lower arch.

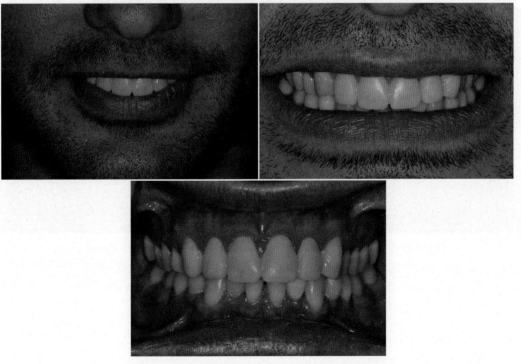

Figure 20-6-5   Smile and intraoral frontal pictures showing the temporary restorations in place.

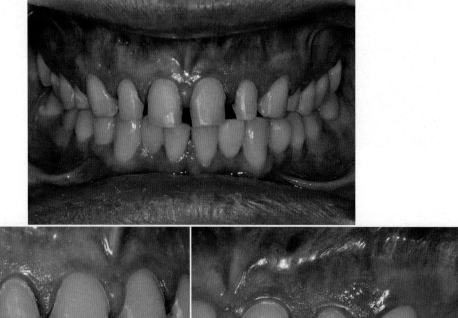

Figure 20-6-6   Tooth preparation in maxillary anterior region for veneers.

FINAL RESULTS

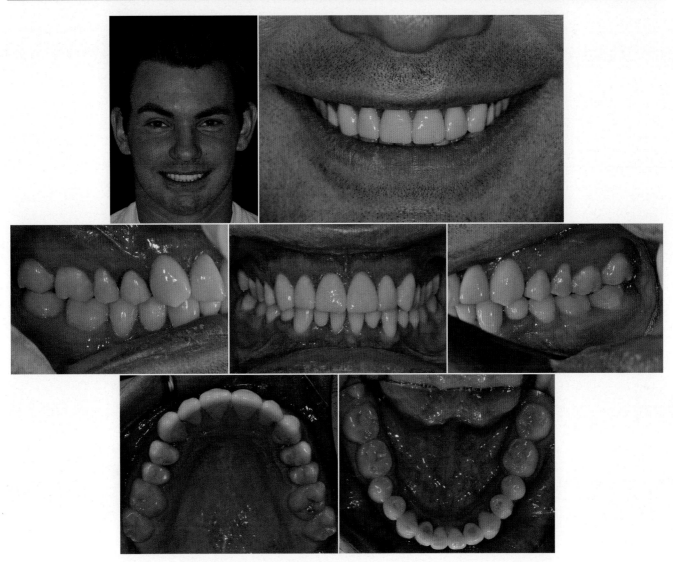

Figure 20-6-7 Postprosthetic final intraoral/extraoral pictures.

Pages followed by *f* indicate figures; *t*, tables.